ALTERNATE EDITION

Fit & Well

Core Concepts and Labs in Physical Fitness and Wellness

THIRD EDITION

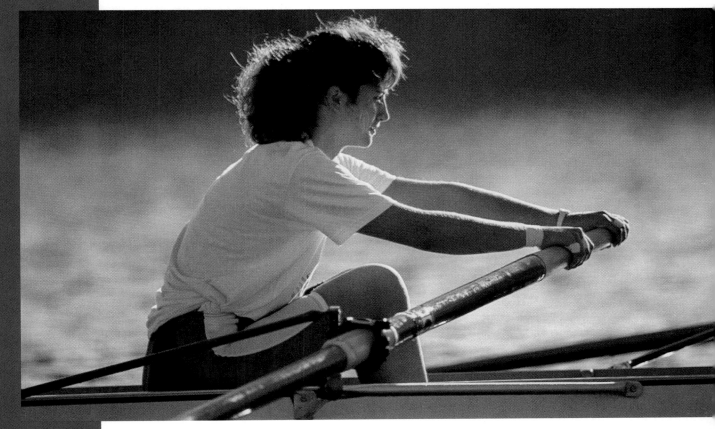

Thomas D. Fahey
California State University, Chico

Paul M. Insel
Stanford University

Walton T. Roth
Stanford University

Mayfield Publishing Company
Mountain View, California
London • Toronto

Library of Congress Cataloging-in-Publication Data
Fahey, Thomas D. (Thomas Davin)
    Fit and well : core concepts and labs in physical fitness and wellness / Thomas D. Fahey, Paul M. Insel, Walton T. Roth.—3rd ed.
       p.   cm.
    Includes bibliographical references and index.
    ISBN 0-7674-0535-8
    1. Physical fitness.   2. Health.   I. Insel, Paul M.   II. Roth, Walton T.   III. Title.
GV481.F26   1998
613.7'043—DC21

                                  98-21016
                                       CIP

Alternate edition (Chapters 1–11) ISBN: 0-7674-0537-4

Manufactured in the United States of America
10 9 8 7 6 5 4

Mayfield Publishing Company
1280 Villa Street
Mountain View, CA 94041

Sponsoring editor, Michele Sordi; *developmental editors,* Kirstan Price, Susan Shook, Megan Rundel, and Kathleen Engelberg; *production editor,* Julianna Scott Fein; *manuscript editor,* Margaret Moore; *art director, text designer,* Jeanne M. Schreiber; *cover designer,* Laurie Anderson; *cover photo,* © Philip and Karen Smith/Tony Stone Images; *art manager,* Robin Mouat; *illustrators,* Joan Carol, Kristin Mount, Judy and John Waller, and Susan Seed; *photo researcher,* Brian Pecko; *manufacturing manager,* Randy Hurst. The text was set in 10.5/12 Berkeley Book by GTS Graphics, Inc., and printed on acid-free 45# Chromatone by Banta Book Group.

The Internet addresses listed in the text were accurate at the time of publication. The inclusion of a Web site does not indicate an endorsement by the authors or Mayfield Publishing Company, and Mayfield does not guarantee the accuracy of the information presented at these sites.

Sources for Appendix C Arbys, http://www.arbysrestaurant.com, Burger King, http://www.burgerking.com, Domino's Pizza, http://www.dominos.com, Jack in the Box, 1998, *Jack'sNutrition Facts,* http://www.jackinthebox.com, KFC, http://www.kfc.com, McDonald's, March, 1998 *Nutrition Facts,* http://www.mcdonalds.com, Taco Bell, 1997, *Nutritional Guide,* http://www.tacobell.com, Wendy's, 1998, *Nutrition/Ingredient Guide,* http://www.wendys.com

Photo Credits

Title Page © David Madison

Chapter 1 p. 1, © J. Nordell/The Image Works; p. 3, © Myrleen Ferguson Cate/PhotoEdit; p. 12, © Mary Kate Denny/PhotoEdit

Chapter 2 p. 19, © Charles Gupton/Stock Boston; p. 22, © Steven Ferry/P & F Communications; p. 24, © Michael Newman/PhotoEdit; p. 30, © Michael Newman/PhotoEdit

Chapter 3 p. 39, © Michael Newman/PhotoEdit; p. 45, © Alán Gallegos/AG Photograph; p. 50, Courtesy Shirlee Stevens; p. 56, © Bob Daemmrich/The Image Works; p. 64, Courtesy Shirlee Stevens

Chapter 4 p. 69, © David Madison; p. 73, 74, 79, Courtesy Neil A. Tanner; p. 84, 85T, Courtesy Shirlee Stevens; p. 85B, Courtesy Neil A. Tanner; p. 86T, Courtesy Shirlee Stevens; p. 86B, 87, 88, 89T, Courtesy Neil A. Tanner; p. 89B, Courtesy Shirlee Stevens; p. 90T, Courtesy Neil A. Tanner; p. 90B, 91, 92T, Courtesy Shirlee Stevens; p. 92B, Courtesy Neil A. Tanner; p. 93, Courtesy Shirlee Stevens; p. 94T, Courtesy Neil A. Tanner; p. 94B, Courtesy Shirlee Stevens; p. 99, 100, Photos furnished by Universal Gym Equipment, Inc., Cedar Rapids, Iowa; p. 101, 103, 104, 106, Courtesy Neil A. Tanner

Chapter 5 p. 109, © J. Sohm/The Image Works; p. 114, 115, 116T, 116M, Courtesy Shirlee Stevens; p. 116B, 117T, Courtesy Neil A. Tanner; p. 117M, 117B, 118, Courtesy Shirlee Stevens; p. 119, 123T, Courtesy Neil A. Tanner; p. 123B, 124, 125T, 125M, Courtesy Shirlee Stevens; p. 125B, Courtesy Neil A. Tanner; p. 129, Courtesy Shirlee Stevens; p. 130, Courtesy Neil A. Tanner

Chapter 6 p. 137, © Mark Richards/PhotoEdit; p. 144, Courtesy Shirlee Stevens; p. 145, © Frank Siteman/Stock Boston; p. 150, Courtesy Shirlee Stevens

Chapter 7 p. 157, © Alán Gallegos/AG Photograph; p. 158, © Bonnie Kamin; p. 167, © Melanie Carr/Zephyr Images

Chapter 8 p. 183, © Alán Gallegos/AG Photograph; p. 191, © Bonnie Kamin; p. 209, © David Young-Wolff/PhotoEdit

Chapter 9 p. 227, © Bob Daemmrich/Stock Boston; p. 232, © Lawrence Migdale/Stock Boston; p. 234, © Ben Barnhart/Offshoot Stock; p. 238, © Bill Davila/Retna, Ltd.

Chapter 10 p. 253, © Bob Daemmrich/The Image Works; p. 257, © Michael Grecco/Stock Boston; p. 260, © John Nordell/The Image Works; p. 262, © Dorothy Littell Grecco/The Image Works

Chapter 11 p. 273, © NIH/Custom Medical Stock Photo; p. 277, © Joel Gordon; p. 281, © Christopher Brown/Stock Boston; p. 284, © Lawrence Migdale/Stock Boston

Chapter 12 p. 291, © AMC/Custom Medical Stock Photo; p. 293, © Matthew Neal McVay/Stock Boston; p. 297, © Joel Gordon; p. 303, © Richard Lord/The Image Works

Chapter 13 p. 311, © Alán Gallegos/AG Photograph; p. 313, © Amanda Merullo/Stock Boston; p. 318, © David Young-Wolff/PhotoEdit; p. 326, © Michael Newman/PhotoEdit

Chapter 14 p. 337, © Mark C. Burnett/Stock Boston; p. 340, © Mark Richards/PhotoEdit; p. 347, © Mary Kate Denny/PhotoEdit; p. 350, © Joel Gordon

Chapter 15 p. 357, © John Cleare/Offshoot Stock; p. 360, © Jennifer Bishop/Actuality, Inc.; p. 364, © Charles Harbutt/Actuality, Inc.; p. 369, © Susan Van Etten/PhotoEdit

Preface

For today's fitness-conscious student, *Fit and Well: Alternate Edition* combines the best of two worlds. In the area of physical fitness, *Fit and Well* offers expert knowledge based on the latest findings in exercise physiology and sports medicine, along with tools for self-assessment and guidelines for becoming fit. In the area of wellness, it offers accurate, current information on today's most important health-related topics and issues, again with self-tests and guidelines for achieving wellness. To create this book, we have drawn on our combined expertise and experience in exercise physiology, athletic training, personal health, scientific research, and teaching. This special Alternate Edition contains the first 11 of the 15 chapters that appear in the full version of *Fit and Well*.

OUR AIMS

Our aims in writing this book can be stated simply:

- To show students that becoming fit and well greatly improves the quality of their lives
- To show students how they can become fit and well
- To motivate students to make healthy choices and to provide them with tools for change

The first of these aims means helping students see how their lives can be enhanced by a fit and well lifestyle. This book offers convincing evidence of a simple truth: To look and feel our best, to protect ourselves from degenerative diseases, and to enjoy the highest quality of life, we need to place fitness and wellness among our top priorities. *Fit and Well* makes clear both the imprudence of our modern, sedentary lifestyle and the benefits of a wellness lifestyle.

Our second aim is to give students the tools and information they need to become fit and well. This book provides students with everything they need to create their own personal fitness programs, including instructions for fitness tests, explanations of the components of fitness and guidelines for developing them, descriptions and illustrations of exercises, sample programs, and more. In addition, *Fit and Well* provides accurate, up-to-date, scientifically based information about other key topics in wellness, including nutrition, weight management, stress, and cardiovascular health.

In providing this material, we have pooled our efforts. Thomas Fahey has contributed his knowledge as an exercise physiologist, teacher, and author of numerous exercise science textbooks. Paul M. Insel and Walton T. Roth have contributed their knowledge of current topics in health as the authors of the leading personal health textbook, *Core Concepts in Health*.

Because we know this expert knowledge can be overwhelming, we have balanced the coverage of complex topics with student-friendly features designed to make the book accessible. Written in a straightforward, easy-to-read style and presented in a colorful, open format, *Fit and Well* invites the student to read, learn, and remember. Boxes, labs, tables, figures, artwork, photographs, and other features add interest to the text and highlight areas of special importance.

Our third aim is to involve students in taking responsibility for their health. *Fit and Well* makes use of interactive features to get students thinking about their own levels of physical fitness and wellness. We offer students assessment tools and laboratory activities to evaluate themselves in terms of each component of physical fitness and each major wellness area, ranging from cardiorespiratory endurance and muscular strength to stress and heart disease.

We also show students how they can make difficult lifestyle changes by using the principles of behavior change. Chapter 1 contains a step-by-step description of this simple but powerful tool for change. The chapter not only explains the five-step process but also offers a wealth of tips for ensuring success. Behavior management aids, including personal contracts, behavior checklists, and self-tests, appear throughout the book. *Fit and Well*'s combined emphasis on self-assessment, self-development in each area of wellness, and behavior change ensures that students not only are inspired to become fit and well but also have the tools to do so.

When students use these tools to make significant lifestyle changes, they begin to realize that they are in charge of their health—and their lives. From this realization comes a sense of competence and personal power. Perhaps our overriding aim in writing *Fit and Well* is to convey the fact that virtually everyone has the ability to understand, monitor, and make changes in his or her own level of fitness and wellness. By making healthy choices from an early age, individuals can minimize the amount of professional medical care they will ever require. Our hope is that *Fit and Well* will help people make this exciting discovery—that they have the power to shape their own futures.

CONTENT AND ORGANIZATION OF THE THIRD EDITION

The basic content of *Fit and Well* remains unchanged in the third edition. Chapter 1 provides an introduction to fitness and wellness and explains the principles of behavior change. Chapters 2–7 focus on the various areas of physical fitness. Chapter 2 provides an overview, discussing the five components of fitness, the principles of physical training, and the factors involved in designing a well-rounded, personalized exercise program. Chapter 3 provides basic information on how the cardiorespiratory system functions, how the body produces energy for exercise, and how to create a successful cardiorespiratory fitness program. Chapters 4, 5, and 6 look at muscular strength and endurance, flexibility, and body composition, respectively. Chapter 7 "puts it all together," describing the nature of a complete fitness program that develops all the components of fitness. This chapter also includes several sample exercise programs for developing overall fitness.

Chapters 8, 9, and 10 treat three important areas of wellness promotion: nutrition, weight management, and stress management, respectively. It is in these areas that individuals have some of the greatest opportunities for positive change. Chapter 11 focuses on one of the most important reasons for making lifestyle changes: cardiovascular disease, the leading cause of death among Americans. Students learn the basic risk factors for cardiovascular disease and how they can make lifestyle changes to reduce their risk.

For the third edition, each chapter was carefully reviewed, revised, and updated. The latest information from scientific and wellness-related research is incorporated in the text, and newly emerging topics are discussed. The following list gives a sample of some of the new and updated material included in the third edition of *Fit and Well:*

- The Surgeon General's report on physical activity and health
- Exercise recommendations from the American College of Sports Medicine
- The 1998 Dietary Reference Intakes for vitamins and minerals, including recommendations for supplements
- Energy (ATP) production for exercise
- Stress-management techniques

- Exercise and dietary recommendations for special population groups and people with special health concerns
- Prescription drugs for weight loss
- Dietary fats and health
- Eating disorders
- Safe use of air bags

Research in the areas of health and wellness is ongoing, with new discoveries, advances, trends, and theories reported nearly every week. For this reason, no wellness book can claim to have the final word on every topic. Yet within these limits, *Fit and Well* does present the latest available information and scientific thinking on important wellness topics. Taken together, the chapters of the book provide students with a complete, up-to-date guide to maximizing their well-being, now and through their entire lives.

FEATURES OF THE THIRD EDITION

This edition of *Fit and Well* builds on the features that attracted and held our readers' interest in previous editions. These features are designed to help students increase their understanding of the key concepts of wellness and to make better use of the book.

Laboratory Activities

To help students apply the principles of fitness and wellness to their own lives, *Fit and Well* includes **laboratory activities** for classroom use. These hands-on activities give students the opportunity to assess their current level of fitness and wellness, to create plans for changing their lifestyle to reach wellness, and to monitor their progress. They can assess their level of cardiorespiratory endurance, for example, or their daily energy balance; they can design a program to improve muscular strength or meet weight-loss goals; and they can explore their risk of developing cardiovascular disease. Labs are found at the end of each chapter; they are perforated for easy use.

 Many of the laboratory activities in the text can also be found on the Lab Activities and Fitness Log Software, a student supplement described later in the preface. Labs that appear in the software are indicated with a disk icon. For a complete list of laboratory activities, see p. xvi in the table of contents.

Illustrated Exercise Sections

To ensure that students understand how to perform important exercises and stretches, *Fit and Well* includes three separate **illustrated exercise sections,** one in Chapter 4 and two in Chapter 5. The section in Chapter 4 covers a total of 22 exercises for developing muscular strength and endurance, as performed both with free weights and on Nautilus equipment. One section in Chapter 5 presents 12 stretches for flexibility, and the other presents 11 exercises to stretch and strengthen the lower back. Each exercise is illustrated with one or more full-color photographs showing proper technique.

Sample Programs

To help students get started, Chapter 7 offers seven complete **sample programs** designed to develop overall fitness. The programs are built around four popular cardiorespiratory endurance activities: walking/jogging/running, bicycling, swimming, and—new to the third edition—in-line skating. They also include weight training and stretching exercises. Each one includes detailed information and guidelines on equipment and technique; target intensity, duration, and frequency; calorie cost of the activity; record keeping; and adjustments to make as fitness improves. The chapter also includes general guidelines for putting together a personal fitness program—setting goals; selecting activities; setting targets for intensity, duration, and frequency; making and maintaining a commitment; and recording and assessing progress.

Boxes

Boxes are used in *Fit and Well* to explore a wide range of current topics in greater detail than is possible in the text itself. Boxes fall into five different categories, each marked with a special icon and label.

Tactics and Tips boxes distill from the text the practical advice students need to apply information to their own lives. By referring to these boxes, students can easily find information about such topics as becoming more active, rehabilitating athletic injuries, exercising in hot weather, proper weight training technique, reducing fat in the diet, helping a friend who has an eating disorder, breathing techniques for stress reduction, and many others.

Critical Consumer boxes are designed to help students develop and apply critical thinking skills, thereby enabling them to make sound choices related to health and well-being. Critical Consumer boxes provide specific guidelines for choosing fitness centers and exercise footwear and equipment; for evaluating health news and commercial weight-loss programs; and for using food labels to make informed dietary choices.

A Closer Look boxes highlight current topics and issues of particular interest to students. These boxes focus on such topics as benefits of physical activity, exercise ma-

chines versus free weights, diabetes, risk factors for low-back pain, health implications of obesity, osteoporosis, and many others.

Dimensions of Diversity boxes focus on the important theme of diversity. Most wellness issues are universal; we all need to exercise and eat well, for example. However, certain differences among people—based on gender, socioeconomic status, ethnicity, age, and other factors—do have important implications for wellness. Dimensions of Diversity boxes give students the opportunity to identify special wellness concerns that affect them because of who they are, as individuals or as members of a group. Topics of Dimensions of Diversity boxes include fitness for people with disabilities, gender differences in cardiorespiratory endurance, and ethnic foods.

Wellness Connection boxes highlight important links among the different dimensions of wellness—physical, emotional, social/interpersonal, intellectual, spiritual, and environmental—and emphasize that all the dimensions must be developed in order for an individual to achieve optimal health and well-being. Included in Wellness Connection boxes are topics such as how exercise improves mood and mental functioning and how social support affects overall health.

Vital Statistics

Vital Statistics tables and figures highlight important facts and figures in an accessible format. From tables and figures marked with the Vital Statistics label, students learn about such matters as the leading causes of death for Americans and the factors that play a part in each one; the relationship between level of physical fitness and mortality; the most popular fitness activities; populations of special concern for obesity; and a wealth of other information. For students who learn best when material is displayed graphically or numerically, Vital Statistics tables and figures offer a way to grasp information quickly and directly.

Common Questions Answered

Sections called **Common Questions Answered** appear at the ends of Chapters 2–11. In these student-friendly sections, the answers to the most-often-asked questions are presented in easy-to-understand terms. Included are such questions as, Are there any stretching exercises I shouldn't do? Do I need more protein in my diet when I train with weights? If I stop weight training, will my muscles turn to fat? and, How can I safely gain weight?

Quick-Reference Appendixes

Included at the end of the book are four appendixes containing vital information in an easy-to-use format.

Appendix A, Injury Prevention and Personal Safety, is a reference guide to preventing and treating common injuries, whether at home, at work, at play, or on the road. It includes such information as how to treat poisoning, choking, and burns; how to prevent injuries from falls, fires, and motor vehicle crashes; how to be safe when walking, jogging, and biking; and how to protect oneself from assault and rape, including acquaintance rape. It also provides information on giving emergency care when someone else's life is in danger. A chart shows proper technique for administering the Heimlich maneuver and performing rescue breathing.

Appendix B, Nutritional Content of Common Foods, allows students to assess their daily diet in terms of 11 nutrient categories, including protein, fat, saturated fat, fiber, added sugar, cholesterol, and sodium. Keyed to the software available with the text, this guide puts vital nutritional information at students' fingertips.

Appendix C, Nutritional Content of Popular Items from Fast-Food Restaurants, provides a breakdown of the nutritional content of the most commonly ordered menu items at eight popular fast-food restaurants. Especially useful are the facts about fat and sodium in different items and about the proportion of fat calories to total calories.

Appendix D, Monitoring Your Progress, is a log that enables students to record and summarize the results of the assessment tests they complete as part of the laboratory activities. With space for preprogram and postprogram assessment results, the log provides an easy way to track the progress of a behavior change program.

Built-In Behavior Change Workbook

The new built-in Behavior Change Workbook complements the lifestyle management model presented in Chapter 1. Based on the behavior change activities that appeared in the second edition, the workbook contains 15 separate activities. It guides students in developing a successful program by walking them through each of the steps of behavior change—from choosing a target behavior to completing and signing a contract. It also includes activities to help students overcome common obstacles to behavior change.

LEARNING AIDS

Several specific learning aids have been incorporated in *Fit and Well*. At the beginning of each chapter, under the heading **Looking Ahead,** five or six questions preview the main points of the chapter for the student and serve as learning objectives. Within each chapter, important terms appear in boldface type and are defined on the same page of text in a **running glossary,** helping students handle new vocabulary.

Chapter summaries offer students a concise review and a way to make sure they have grasped the most important concepts in the chapter. Also found at the end of chapters are **selected bibliographies** and sections called **For More Information.** These sections list books, journal articles, newsletters, organizations, hotlines, and Web sites that may be of interest to students, as well as further resources that can often be found on campus or in the community.

TEACHING TOOLS

Available with the third edition of *Fit and Well* is a comprehensive package of supplementary materials designed to enhance teaching and learning. Included in the package are the following items:

- Instructor's Resource Binder
- Transparency acetates
- Image Bank and PowerPoint® Presentation CD-ROM
- Students on Health and Wellness: Custom Video to Accompany *Fit and Well*
- Computerized test bank
- Nutritional analysis software
- Mayfield *Fit and Well* Web site
- Nutrition and Weight Management Journal
- Daily Fitness Log
- Lab Activities and Fitness Log Software
- Internet guide

The **Instructor's Resource Binder** contains a variety of helpful teaching materials in an easy-to-use form:

- The **Instructor's Resource Guide,** prepared for the third edition by Meredith Busby at the University of North Carolina, Chapel Hill, includes learning objectives; extended chapter outlines; lists of additional resources, including books and articles, videos, software, Internet sites, and other multimedia tools; and descriptions of the labs and transparencies.

- The new **Internet Handbook** includes a brief introduction to the Internet, a complete directory of all the sites listed in the text and Instructor's Resource Guide, guidelines for evaluating information from the Internet, and student Internet activities.

- The **Examination Questions,** completely revised and updated for the third edition by John D. Emmett, Eastern Illinois University, include over 1000 true/false, multiple choice, and essay questions.

- Over 70 **Additional Laboratory Activities,** formatted for easy duplication and distribution, supplement the labs that are included in the text.

- Over 100 **Transparency Masters and Handouts** are provided as additional lecture resources.

The set of **transparency acetates** includes 50 acetates, half of which are in color. The transparencies provide material suitable for lecture and demonstration purposes and complement the transparency masters in the Instructor's Resource Binder.

New to the third edition, the **Image Bank and Power-Point® Presentation CD-ROM** includes an image bank of over 80 images from the third edition that can be displayed, printed, or imported into presentation software. The PowerPoint slides, prepared by Christopher M. Janelle at the University of Florida, can be customized to fit any lecture. The CD-ROM also includes material from the Instructor's Resource Guide in editable format as well as versions of selected transparency acetates and masters suitable for use with presentation software. It is compatible with both IBM and Macintosh computers.

Also new to the third edition is **Students on Health and Wellness: Custom Video to Accompany** *Fit and Well.* Filmed with students at college campuses across the country, this unique video is designed to stimulate critical thinking and class discussion. The 8- to 10-minute segments focus on key wellness concerns—fitness, nutrition, stress, intimate relationships, alcohol, tobacco, STDs, and personal safety. The accompanying Instructor's Video Guide provides summaries of each segment and discussion questions.

The **computerized test bank** (Microtest III from Chariot Software Group) allows instructors to design tests using the questions from the test item file and/or their own questions. It is available for Macintosh and Windows. **DINE Healthy software** provides an easy way for students to evaluate the nutritional value of their current diet; it also includes an exercise section that allows students to track their energy expenditures. **Other videos, software, and multimedia,** on topics such as weight training, body composition, healthy diets, and heart disease prevention, are also available.

Also new to the third edition is the **Mayfield** *Fit and Well* **Web site** (http://www.mayfieldpub.com/fahey). The site includes up-to-date links to useful Internet resources, student study questions that provide immediate feedback, a customized syllabus builder for instructors, and more.

Several practical items for students can be shrink-wrapped with the textbook:

- The **Nutrition and Weight Management Journal,** new to the third edition of *Fit and Well,* guides students in assessing their current diet and making appropriate changes.
- The **Daily Fitness Log** is a 48-page booklet that contains logs for students to plan and track the progress of their general fitness and weight training programs for up to 40 weeks.

- The **Lab Activities and Fitness Log Software** presents lab activities and fitness logs in an electronic format (Macintosh or Windows). The software calculates and prints out the results of selected self-assessments and fitness tests; it also includes information about behavior change and a behavior change contract. Students can print out their logs and graph the progress of their fitness program. A disk icon indicates which lab activities from the text are also found on the software; see p. xvi in the table of contents for a complete list.
- Also new to the third edition is *Mayfield's Quick View Guide to the Internet for Students of Health and Physical Education,* by Jennifer Campbell and Michael Keene at the University of Tennessee, Knoxville. It provides step-by-step instructions on how to access the Internet; how to find, evaluate, and use information about wellness; how to communicate via e-mail and chat rooms; how to use listservs and newsgroups; and many other topics. If you have any questions concerning the book or teaching package, please call your local Mayfield sales representative or the Marketing and Sales Department at 800-433-1279. You may also e-mail Mayfield at calpoppy@mayfieldpub.com.

A NOTE OF THANKS

Many people have contributed to the production of *Fit and Well.* The book has benefited from their thoughtful commentaries, expert knowledge, and helpful suggestions. We are deeply grateful for their participation in the project.

Academic reviewers of the first edition:

Liz Applegate, University of California, Davis
E. Harold Blackwell, Lamar University
Laura L. Borsdorf, Ursinus College
Vicki Boye, Concordia College
William J. Considine, Springfield College
Arlene Crosman, Linn-Benton Community College
Robert Cross, Salisbury State University
Jean F. Dudney, San Antonio College
Eunice Goldgrabe, Concordia College
Susan J. Hibbs, Bloomsburg University of Pennsylvania
William Hottinger, Wake Forest University
Kenneth W. Kambis, College of William and Mary
Russell R. Pate, University of South Carolina
Charles J. Pelitera, Canisius College
Margaret A. Peterson, Central Oregon Community College
Jacalyn J. Robert, Texas Tech University
Rob Schurrer, Black Hills State University
Eugenia S. Scott, Butler University
Charles R. Seager, Miami-Dade Community College

J. L. Sexton, Fort Hays State University
Jack Stovall, Salisbury State University
Karen Teresa Sullivan, Marymount University
Glenn R. West, Transylvania University
Anthony Zaloga, Frostburg State University

Academic reviewers of the second edition:

Viviane L. Avant, University of North Carolina-Charlotte
Elaine H. Blair, Indiana University of Pennsylvania
Susan Brown, Johnson County Community College
Arlene Crosman, Linn-Benton Community College
Todd Crowder, U.S. Military Academy
Michael A. Dupper, University of Mississippi
Richard J. Fopeano, Rowan College of New Jersey
Mike Johnson, Berea College
Patricia A. Miller, Anderson University
Roland J. Schick, Tyler Junior College
Rob Schurrer, Black Hills State University
Mark G. Urtel, Indiana University-Purdue University-
  Indianapolis
Ann Ward, University of Wisconsin-Madison
Christopher J. Womack, Longwood College

Academic reviewers of the third edition text:

Phil Bogle, Eastern Michigan University
Anita D'Angelo, Florida Atlantic University
Carol A. Giroud, Monmouth University
Joyce Huner, Macomb Community College
Shahla Kahn, Kennesaw State University
Jeanne M. Mathias, Binghamton University
Steve Sansone, Chemeketa Community College
Susan T. Saylor, Shelton State Community College

Academic reviewers of the third edition teaching tools:

Mary Jo Adams, Illinois State University
Barbara Coleman, Northern Michigan University
Robert Femat, El Paso Community College

Dorothy P. Haugen, Bethel College
Elizabeth Fell Kelly, Monroe Community College
Christine M. Miskec, Mankato State University
Rob Schurrer, Black Hills State University
Lois M. Smith, University of Maryland, Eastern Shore

Special fitness consultants:

Warren D. Franke, Iowa State University
David C. Nieman, Appalachian State University
Michael Pollock, University of Florida

Technology focus group participants:

Ken Allen, University of Wisconsin, Oshkosh
Lisa Farley, Butler University
Barbara Greenburg, Butler University
Bill Johnson, Stephen F. Austin State University
Rita Nugent, University of Evansville
Patricia Dotson Pettit, Nebraska Wesleyan University
Carol Plugge, Lamar University
Steve Sedbrook, Fort Hays State University
Marilyn Strawbridge, Butler University

We are also grateful to the staff of Mayfield Publishing Company and the *Fit and Well* book team, without whose efforts the book could not have been published. Special thanks to Michele Sordi, sponsoring editor; Kirstan Price, Susan Shook, Megan Rundel, and Kate Engelberg, developmental editors; Julianna Scott Fein, production editor; Jeanne M. Schreiber, art director; Robin Mouat, art manager; Marty Granahan, permissions editor; Brian Pecko, photo researcher; Randy Hurst, manufacturing manager; Heather Collins, production assistant; Michelle Rodgerson, marketing manager; and Jay Bauer, product manager.

Thomas D. Fahey
Paul M. Insel
Walton T. Roth

CHAPTER 7

Putting Together a Complete Fitness Program   157

CHAPTER 8

Nutrition   183

LABORATORY ACTIVITIES

Indicates a laboratory activity that is also found on the Lab Activities and Fitness Log Software.

Introduction to Wellness, Fitness, and Lifestyle Management

1

LOOKING AHEAD

After reading this chapter, you should be able to answer these questions about fitness, wellness, and behavior change:

- What is wellness?
- What are the major health problems in the United States today, and what are their principal causes?
- What behaviors are part of a fit and well lifestyle?
- What is physical fitness, and why is it important to wellness?
- What are the components of a behavior change program?

A first-year college student resolves to meet the challenge of making new friends. A long-sedentary senior starts riding her bike to school every day instead of taking the bus. A busy graduate student volunteers to plant trees in a blighted inner-city neighborhood. What do these people have in common? Each is striving for optimal health and well-being. Not satisfied to be merely free of major illness, these individuals want more. They want to live life actively, energetically, and fully, in a state of optimal personal, interpersonal, and environmental well-being. They have taken charge of their health and are on the path to wellness.

WELLNESS: THE NEW HEALTH GOAL

Wellness is an expanded idea of health. Many people think of health as being just the absence of physical disease. But wellness transcends this concept of health, as when individuals with serious illnesses or disabilities rise above their physical or mental limitations to live rich, meaningful, vital lives. Some aspects of health are determined by your genes, your age, and other factors that may be beyond your control. But true wellness is largely determined by the decisions you make about how to live your life. In this book, we will use the terms "health" and "wellness" interchangeably to mean the ability to live life fully—with vitality and meaning.

The Dimensions of Wellness

No matter what your age or health status, you can optimize your health in each of the following six interrelated dimensions. Wellness in any dimension is not a static goal but a dynamic process of change and growth (Figure 1-1).

Physical Wellness Optimal physical health requires eating well, exercising, avoiding harmful habits, making responsible decisions about sex, learning about and recognizing the symptoms of disease, getting regular medical and dental checkups, and taking steps to prevent injuries at home, on the road, and on the job. The habits you develop and the decisions you make today will largely determine not only how many years you will live, but the quality of your life during those years.

Emotional Wellness Optimism, trust, self-esteem, self-acceptance, self-confidence, self-control, satisfying relationships, and an ability to share feelings are just some of the qualities and aspects of emotional wellness. Maintaining emotional wellness requires monitoring and exploring your thoughts and feelings, identifying obstacles to emotional well-being, and finding solutions to emotional problems, with the help of a therapist if necessary.

Intellectual Wellness The hallmarks of intellectual health include an openness to new ideas, a capacity to question and think critically, and the motivation to master new skills, as well as a sense of humor, creativity, and curiosity. An active mind is essential to overall wellness; it detects problems, finds solutions, and directs behavior. People who enjoy intellectual wellness never stop learning. They seek out and relish new experiences and challenges.

Spiritual Wellness To enjoy spiritual health is to possess a set of guiding beliefs, principles, or values that give meaning and purpose to your life, especially during difficult times. Spiritual wellness involves the capacity for love, compassion, forgiveness, altruism, joy, and fulfillment. It is an antidote to cynicism, anger, fear, anxiety, self-absorption, and pessimism. Spirituality transcends the individual and can be a common bond among people. Organized religions help many people develop spiritual health. Many others find meaning and purpose in their lives on their own—through nature, art, meditation, political action, or good works.

Interpersonal and Social Wellness Satisfying relationships are basic to both physical and emotional health. We need to have mutually loving, supportive people in our lives. Developing interpersonal wellness means learning good communication skills, developing the capacity for intimacy, and cultivating a support network of caring friends and/or family members. Social wellness requires participating in and contributing to your community, country, and world.

Environmental, or Planetary, Wellness Increasingly, personal health depends on the health of the planet—from the safety of the food supply to the degree of violence in a society. Other examples of environmental threats to health are ultraviolet radiation in sunlight, air and water pollution, lead in old house paint, and second-hand tobacco smoke in indoor air. Wellness requires learning about and protecting yourself against such hazards—and doing what you can to reduce or eliminate them, either on your own or with others.

The six dimensions of wellness interact continuously, influencing and being influenced by one another. Making a change in one dimension often affects some or all of the others. For example, regular exercise (developing the

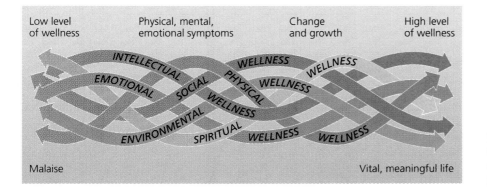

| Low level of wellness | Physical, mental, emotional symptoms | Change and growth | High level of wellness |

INTELLECTUAL WELLNESS
EMOTIONAL WELLNESS
SOCIAL WELLNESS
PHYSICAL WELLNESS
ENVIRONMENTAL WELLNESS
SPIRITUAL WELLNESS

Malaise

Vital, meaningful life

Figure 1-1 The wellness continuum.
Wellness is composed of six interrelated dimensions, all of which must be developed in order to achieve overall wellness.

physical dimension of wellness) can increase feelings of well-being and self-esteem (emotional wellness), which in turn can increase feelings of confidence in social interactions and achievements at work or school (interpersonal and social wellness). Maintaining good health is a dynamic process, and increasing your level of wellness in one area of life often influences many others. Some of the key links among different dimensions of wellness are highlighted in this text in boxes labeled Wellness Connection.

New Opportunities, New Responsibilities

Wellness is a relatively recent concept. A century ago, people considered themselves lucky just to survive to adulthood. A child born in 1890, for example, could expect to live only about 40 years. Many people died as a result of common **infectious diseases** and poor environmental conditions (unrefrigerated food, poor sanitation, air and water pollution). However, over the past 100 years, the average life expectancy has nearly doubled, thanks largely to the development of vaccines and antibiotics to prevent and fight infectious diseases and to public health campaigns to improve environmental conditions.

But a different set of diseases has emerged as our major health threat—**chronic diseases** such as cardiovascular disease (CVD), cancer, hypertension (high blood pressure), diabetes, osteoporosis, and cirrhosis of the liver. Of these diseases, the most widespread and devastating are heart disease, cancer, and stroke, the three leading causes of death for Americans today (Table 1-1). Treating these and other chronic, degenerative diseases is enormously expensive and extremely difficult. The best treatment for these diseases is prevention—people having a greater awareness about health and about taking care of their bodies.

The good news is that people do have some control over whether they develop CVD, cancer, and other chronic diseases. People make choices every day that either increase or decrease their risks for these diseases—choices involving things such as exercise, diet, and smoking and drinking habits. When researchers look at the actual behavioral and environmental causes of death in

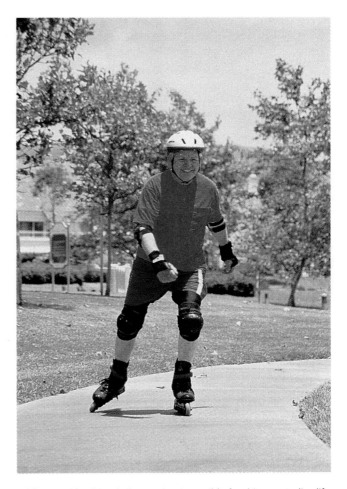

A lifetime of healthy choices makes it possible for this man to live life actively, energetically, and fully. To enjoy health and vigor later in life, people have to cultivate wellness while they are young.

the United States, it becomes clear that individuals can profoundly influence their own health risks (Table 1-2). This knowledge has led to the realization that wellness cannot be prescribed; physicians and other health care professionals can do little more than provide information, advice, and encouragement—the rest is up to each of us.

TABLE 1-1	*Leading Causes of Death in the United States*

Rank	Cause of Death	Number of Deaths	Percent of Total Deaths	Female/Male Ratio*	Lifestyle Factors
1	Heart disease	733,834	31.6	50/50	D I S A
2	Cancer	544,278	23.4	48/52	D I S A
3	Stroke	160,431	6.9	61/39	D I S
4	Chronic obstructive lung diseases	106,146	4.6	48/52	S
5	Unintentional injuries	93,874	4.0	34/66	S A
	Motor vehicle–related	(43,449)	(1.9)	(33/67)	
	All others	(50,425)	(2.2)	(35/65)	
6	Pneumonia and influenza	82,579	3.6	54/46	S
7	Diabetes mellitus	61,559	2.7	56/44	D I
8	HIV infection	32,655	1.4	7/93	
9	Suicide	30,862	1.3	19/81	A
10	Chronic liver disease and cirrhosis	25,135	1.1	34/66	A
	All causes	2,322,421			

Key: D Cause of death in which diet plays a part
 I Cause of death in which an inactive lifestyle plays a part
 S Cause of death in which smoking plays a part
 A Cause of death in which excessive alcohol consumption plays a part

*Ratio of females to males who died of each cause. For example, an equal number of women and men died of heart disease, but only about half as many women as men died of motor-vehicle-related injuries.

SOURCES: National Center for Health Statistics. 1997. Births and deaths: United States, 1996. *Monthly Vital Statistics Report* 46(1S2): 5. National Center for Health Statistics. 1997. Report of final mortality statistics, 1995. *Monthly Vital Statistics Report* 45(11): 23–25.

TABLE 1-2	*Actual Causes of Death in the United States*

Cause	Approximate Number of Deaths per Year
Tobacco	400,000
Diet and activity habits	300,000
Alcohol	100,000
Microbial agents	90,000
Toxic agents	60,000
Secondhand tobacco smoke	50,000
Motor vehicle crashes	40,000
Firearms	35,000
Sexual behavior	30,000
Illegal drug use	20,000

SOURCES: American Heart Association. National Center for Health Statistics. 1997. Births and deaths: United States, 1996. *Monthly Vital Statistics Report* 46(1S2): 5. McGinnis, J. M., and W. H. Foege. 1993. Actual causes of death in the United States. *Journal of the American Medical Association* 270(18): 2207–2212.

This chapter provides an overview of a lifestyle that promotes wellness and describes a method that can help you make lasting changes in your life to promote good health. The chapters that follow provide more detailed in-formation about fitness, nutrition, and other components of a wellness lifestyle. The book as a whole is designed to be used in a very real way, to help you take charge of your behavior and improve the quality of your life—to become fit and well.

Behaviors That Contribute to Wellness

A lifestyle based on good choices and healthy behaviors maximizes the quality of life. It helps people avoid dis-ease, remain strong and fit, and maintain their physical and mental health as long as they live (Figure 1-2). The most important behaviors and habits are described in the following sections.

Be Physically Active   Perhaps the single most impor-tant choice individuals can make to promote wellness is to be physically active. Unfortunately, a sedentary lifestyle is common among Americans today: More than 60% of Americans are not regularly physically active, and 25% are not active at all. The human body is designed to work best when it is active. It readily adapts to nearly any level of activity and exertion; in fact, **physical fitness** is de-fined as the ability of the body to adapt to the demands and stresses of physical effort. The more we ask of our bodies—our muscles, bones, heart, lungs—the stronger and more fit they become. However, the reverse is also

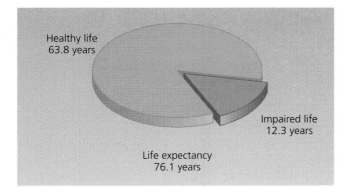

Healthy life
63.8 years

Impaired life
12.3 years

Life expectancy
76.1 years

VITAL STATISTICS

Figure 1-2   Quantity of life versus quality of life.   Due to improved medical and environmental practices, the average life expectancy of Americans increased greatly during the twentieth century. But quality of life is also an important consideration, and the typical American currently maintains good health for only about 85% of his or her life. Developing and maintaining a healthy lifestyle can both increase longevity and decrease the number of years of unhealthy life.
SOURCES: U.S. Department of Health and Human Services. 1997. *Healthy People 2000 Review, 1997*. Hyattsville, Md.: Public Health Service, DHHS Publication No. (PHS) 98-1256. National Center for Health Statistics. 1997. Births and deaths: United States, 1996. *Monthly Vital Statistics Report* 46(1S2): 31.

true: The less we ask of them, the less they can do. When our bodies are not kept active, they begin to deteriorate. Bones lose their density, joints stiffen, muscles become weak, and cellular energy systems begin to degenerate. To be truly well, human beings must be active.

The benefits of physical activity are both physical and mental, immediate and long term (see the box "Benefits of Regular Physical Activity"). In the short term, being physically fit makes it easier to do everyday tasks, such as lifting; it provides reserve strength for emergencies; and it helps people look and feel good. In the long term, being physically fit confers protection against chronic diseases and lowers the risk of dying prematurely (Figure 1-3). Physically active individuals are less likely to develop or die from heart disease, respiratory disease, high blood pressure, cancer, diabetes, and osteoporosis. Their cardiorespiratory systems tend to resemble those of people 10 or more years younger than themselves. As they get older, they may be able to avoid weight gain, muscle and bone loss, fatigue, and other problems associated with aging. With healthy hearts, strong muscles, lean bodies, and a repertoire of physical skills they can call on for recreation and enjoyment, fit people can maintain their physical and mental well-being throughout their lives.

Choose a Healthy Diet   In addition to being sedentary, many Americans have a diet that is too high in calories, fat, and added sugars and too low in fiber and complex carbohydrates. This diet is linked to a number of chronic diseases, including heart disease, stroke, and certain kinds of cancer. A healthy diet promotes wellness in both the short and long term. It provides necessary nutrients and sufficient energy without also providing too much of the dietary substances linked to diseases.

Maintain a Healthy Body Weight   Overweight and obesity are associated with a number of disabling and potentially fatal conditions and diseases, including heart disease, cancer, and diabetes. Healthy body weight is an important part of wellness—but short-term dieting is not part of a fit and well lifestyle. Maintaining a healthy body weight requires a lifelong commitment to regular exercise, a healthy diet, and effective stress management.

Manage Stress Effectively   Many people cope with stress by eating, drinking, or smoking too much. Others don't deal with it at all. In the short term, inappropriate stress management can lead to fatigue, sleep disturbances, and other unpleasant symptoms. Over longer periods of time, poor management of stress can lead to less efficient functioning of the immune system and increased susceptibility to disease. There *are* effective ways to handle stress, and learning to incorporate them into daily life is an important part of a fit and well lifestyle.

Avoid Use of Tobacco and Other Drugs and Use Alcohol Wisely, If at All   Tobacco use is associated with 6 of the top 10 causes of death in the United States; it kills more Americans each year than any other behavioral or environmental factor (see Table 1-2). A hundred years ago, before cigarette smoking was widespread, lung cancer was considered a rare disease. Today, with nearly 25% of the American population smoking, lung cancer is the most common cause of cancer death among both men and women and one of the leading causes of death overall.

Excess alcohol consumption is linked to 5 of the top 10 causes of death. It is an especially important factor in death and disability among young people through its association with **unintentional injuries** (such as car crashes and drownings) and violence. Illegal drug use is responsible for an additional 20,000 deaths each year in the United States.

Protect Yourself from Disease and Injury   The most effective way of dealing with disease and injury is to prevent them. Many of the lifestyle strategies discussed here—being physically active, managing body weight, and so on—help protect you against chronic illnesses. In addition, specific steps can be taken to avoid infectious diseases, particularly those that are sexually transmitted.

physical fitness   The ability of the body to respond or adapt to the demands and stress of physical effort.   **TERMS**

unintentional injury   An injury that occurs without harm being intended.

Regular physical activity improves physical and mental health in the following ways:

- Reduces the risk of dying prematurely from all causes
- Reduces the risk of dying from heart disease
- Reduces the risk of developing diabetes
- Reduces the risk of developing high blood pressure
- Helps reduce blood pressure in people who already have high blood pressure
- Reduces the risk of developing colon cancer
- Reduces feelings of depression and anxiety
- Helps control weight, develop lean muscle, and reduce body fat

- Helps build and maintain healthy bones, muscles, and joints
- Helps older adults become stronger and better able to move about without falling
- Promotes psychological well-being

(The changes and benefits that occur in response to physical activity are discussed in Chapters 2–6.)

SOURCE: U.S. Department of Health and Human Services. 1996. *Physical Activity and Health: A Report of the Surgeon General*. Department of Health and Human Services, Centers for Disease Control and Prevention, National Center for Chronic Disease Prevention and Health Promotion.

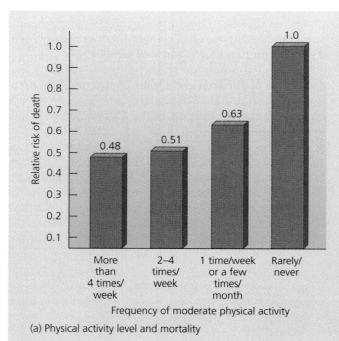

(a) Physical activity level and mortality

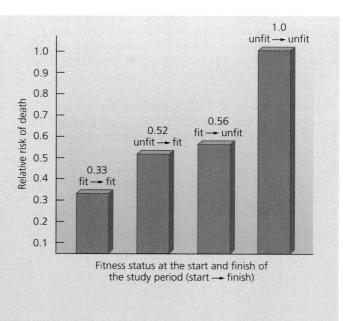

(b) The effects of changes in fitness status on mortality rates

VITAL STATISTICS

Figure 1-3 Physical activity, physical fitness, and mortality. Many long-term research studies have clearly shown the benefits of regular physical activity. (a) A study that followed more than 40,000 postmenopausal women for 7 years found a strong relationship between physical activity and relative risk of death: the more frequent the activity, the lower the relative risk of death. (b) A study of more than 9500 men that tracked changes in fitness level for periods of 1–18 years found that fitness level was closely tied to risk of death: The lowest death rate was seen in men who were physically fit at the start and end of the study period; the highest death rate was in men who were unfit throughout the study. Men who improved from unfit to fit during the study experienced a 44% reduction in mortality risk relative to men who remained unfit. SOURCES: Kushi, L. H., et al. 1997. Physical activity and mortality in postmenopausal women. *Journal of the American Medical Association* 277(16): 1287–1292. Blair, S. N., et al. 1995. Changes in physical fitness and all-cause mortality: A prospective study of healthy and unhealthy men. *Journal of the American Medical Association* 273(14):1093–1098

When it comes to striving for wellness, most differences among people are insignificant. We all need to exercise, eat well, and manage stress. We need to know how to protect ourselves from heart disease, cancer, sexually transmitted diseases, and injuries.

But some of our differences—differences among us both as individuals and as members of groups—do have implications for wellness. Some of us, for example, have grown up eating foods that increase our risk of obesity or heart disease. Some of us have inherited predispositions for certain health problems, such as osteoporosis or high cholesterol levels. These health-related differences among individuals and groups can be biological—determined genetically—or cultural—acquired as patterns of behavior through daily interactions with our family, community, and society. Many health conditions are a function of biology and culture combined.

When we talk about wellness issues as they relate to diverse populations, we face two related dangers. The first is the danger of stereotyping, of talking about people as groups rather than as individuals. The second is that of overgeneralizing, of ignoring the extensive biological and cultural diversity that exists among people who may be grouped together because of their gender, socioeconomic status, or ethnicity. Every person is an individual with her or his own unique genetic endowment as well as unique experiences in life. However, many of these influences are shared with others of similar genetic and cultural backgrounds. Information about group similarities relating to wellness issues can be useful; for example, it can alert people to areas that may be of special concern for them and their families.

Wellness-related differences among groups can be identified and described along several different dimensions, including the following:

- *Gender.* Men and women have different life expectancies and different incidences of many diseases, including heart disease, cancer, and osteoporosis. They also differ in body composition and certain aspects of physical performance.

- *Socioeconomic status.* People with low income levels have higher rates of many conditions and diseases, including overweight, alcohol and drug abuse, heart disease, and HIV infection.

- *Ethnicity.* A genetic predisposition for a particular health problem can be linked to ethnicity as a result of each ethnic group's relatively distinct history. Diabetes is more prevalent among individuals of Native American or Latino heritage, for example, and African Americans have higher rates of hypertension. Ethnic groups may also vary in other ways that relate to wellness: traditional diets; patterns of family and interpersonal relationships; and attitudes toward using tobacco, alcohol, and other drugs, to name just a few.

These are just some of the "dimensions of diversity"—differences among people and groups that are associated with different wellness concerns. Other factors, too, such as age, educational attainment, and disability, can present challenges as an individual strives for wellness. In this book, topics and issues relating to wellness that affect different American populations are given special consideration in boxes labeled Dimensions of Diversity. All of these discussions are designed to deepen our understanding of the concepts of wellness and vitality in the context of ever-growing diversity.

These diseases are preventable through responsible sexual behavior, another component of a fit and well lifestyle.

Unintentional injuries are the leading cause of death for people age 45 and under, but they, too, can be prevented. Learning and adopting safe, responsible behaviors is also part of a fit and well lifestyle.

Other important behaviors in a fit and well lifestyle include developing meaningful relationships, planning ahead for successful aging, becoming knowledgable about the health care system, and acting responsibly in relation to the environment. Lab 1-1 will help you evaluate your behaviors as they relate to wellness.

The Role of Other Factors in Wellness

Of course, behavior isn't the only factor involved in good health. Heredity, the environment, and access to adequate health care are other important influences. These factors can interact in ways that raise or lower the quality of a person's life and the risk of developing particular diseases. For example, a sedentary lifestyle combined with a ge-

netic predisposition for diabetes can greatly increase a person's risk for developing the disease. If this person also lacks adequate health care, he or she is much more likely to suffer dangerous complications from diabetes and have a lower quality of life. (For a discussion of how different factors affect people as members of groups, see the box "Wellness Issues for Diverse Populations.")

But in many cases, behavior can tip the balance toward health even if heredity or environment is a negative factor. Breast cancer, for example, can run in families, but it also may be associated with overweight and a sedentary lifestyle. A woman with a family history of breast cancer is less likely to die from the disease if she controls her weight, exercises, performs regular breast self-exams, and consults with her physician about mammograms. By taking appropriate action, this woman can influence the effects of heredity on her health.

National Wellness Goals

You may think of health and wellness as personal concerns, goals that you strive for on your own for your own

TABLE 1-3	Selected Healthy People 2000 Objectives		
Objective		Estimate of Current Status	Goal
Increase the proportion of people age 6 and over who engage regularly, preferably daily, in light to moderate physical activity for at least 30 minutes per day.		24% (5 times/week) 17% (7 times/week)	30% 30%
Increase the consumption of fruits and vegetables.		4 servings/day	5 servings/day
Reduce the prevalence of overweight among people age 20 and over.		35%	20%
Reduce the proportion of people age 18 and over who experience adverse health effects from stress each year.		39.2%	Less than 35%
Reduce the prevalence of cigarette smoking among people age 18 and over.		26%	15%
Reduce the proportion of college students engaging in recent occasions of heavy drinking of alcoholic beverages.		40%	32%
Increase the proportion of sexually active, unmarried people who used a condom at last sexual intercourse.		25%	50%
Increase the use of helmets by bicyclists.		17.6%	50%

SOURCES: U.S. Department of Health and Human Services. 1990. *Healthy People 2000: National Health Promotion and Disease Prevention Objectives.* Washington, D.C.: U.S. Government Printing Office, DHHS Pub. (PHS) 91-50212. National Center for Health Statistics. 1997. *Healthy People 2000 Review, 1997.* Hyattsville, Md.: Public Health Service, DHHS Pub. (PHS) 98-1256.

benefit. But the U.S. government also has a vital interest in the health of all Americans. A healthy population is the nation's greatest resource, the source of its vigor and wealth. Poor health, in contrast, drains the nation's resources and raises national health care costs. As the embodiment of our society's values, the federal government also has a humane interest in people's health.

The U.S. government's national Healthy People initiative seeks to prevent unnecessary disease and disability and to achieve a better quality of life for all Americans. Healthy People reports, published first in 1980 and revised every decade, include national health goals based on 10-year agendas. Each report includes both broad goals—such as increasing the span of healthy life for all Americans and reducing health disparities among special populations within our society—and specific, measurable targets in many different priority areas that relate to wellness (physical activity, nutrition, and so on). Healthy People targets serve as the basis for national monitoring and tracking of health status, health risks, and use of preventive services. They encompass individual actions as well as larger-scale changes in environmental and medical services.

Examples of individual health promotion objectives from *Healthy People 2000,* as well as estimates of how we are tracking toward the goals, appear in Table 1-3. (For information on the Healthy People initiative and the development of *Healthy People 2010* objectives, contact the Healthy People office or Web sites listed in the For More Information section at the end of the chapter.) As you can see, the objectives are tied closely to the wellness lifestyle described in this chapter. The principal topics covered in

this book parallel the priority concerns of the Healthy People initiative, and the approach of *Fit and Well* is based on the initiative's premise that personal responsibility is a key to achieving wellness.

REACHING WELLNESS THROUGH LIFESTYLE MANAGEMENT

The picture drawn here of a fit and well lifestyle may seem complex and out of reach to you right now. Many people fall into a lifestyle that puts them at risk. Some aren't aware of the damage they're doing, others don't want to or know how to change, and still others want to change but can't get started. These are all real problems, but they aren't insurmountable. If they were, there would be no ex-smokers, recovering alcoholics, or people who have successfully lost excess body weight. People can and do make difficult changes in their lives.

Taking big steps toward wellness may at first seem like too much work, but as you make progress, it gets easier. At first you'll be rewarded with a greater sense of control over your life, a feeling of empowerment, higher self-esteem, and more joy. These benefits will encourage you to make further improvements. Over time, you'll come to know what wellness feels like—more energy; greater vitality; deeper feelings of curiosity, interest, and enjoyment; and a higher quality of life.

This section introduces the general process of behavior change and highlights the decisions and challenges you'll face at each stage. For additional help and advice, work through the activities in the Behavior Change Workbook at the end of the text.

Getting Serious About Your Health

Before you can start changing a wellness-related behavior, you have to know that the behavior is problematic and that you *can* change it. To make good decisions, you need information about relevant topics and issues. You also need knowledge about yourself—how you relate to the wellness lifestyle described in this chapter and what strengths you can draw on to change your behavior and improve your health. While knowledge is a necessary ingredient, it isn't usually enough to make you act. Millions of smokers stick to their habit, for example, even though they know it's bad for their health.

Many people start to consider changing a behavior when they get help from others. An observation from a friend, family member, or physician can help you see yourself as others do and may get you thinking about your behavior in a new way. For example, Jason has been getting a lot of stomachaches lately. His girlfriend, Anna, notices other changes as well and suggests that the stress of classes plus a part-time job and serving as president of the school radio station might be causing some of Jason's problems. Jason never thought much about trying to control the stressors in his life, but with encouragement from Anna he starts noticing what events trigger stress for him.

Landmark events can also get you thinking about behavior change. A birthday, the birth of a child, or the death of someone close to you can be a powerful motivator for thinking seriously about behaviors that affect wellness. New information can also help you get started. As you read this text, you may find yourself reevaluating some of your wellness-related behaviors. This could be a great opportunity to make healthful changes that will stay with you for the rest of your life.

What Does It Take to Change?

As we all know, change doesn't just happen because we want it to. Some people are able to change and grow fairly easily, whereas others get stuck in problem behaviors for years. What are the secrets of moving toward wellness?

Motivation   Once you recognize that you have an unhealthy behavior, you may consider changing it. But before you can change, you need strong motivation to do so. Although some people are motivated by long-term goals, such as avoiding a disease that may hit them in 20 or 30 years, most are more likely to be moved to action by shorter-term, more personal goals. Looking better, being more popular, doing better in school, getting a good job, improving at a sport, and increasing self-esteem are common sources of motivation.

You can strengthen your motivation by raising your consciousness about your problem behavior. This will enable you to focus on the negatives of the behavior and imagine the consequences if you don't make a change. At the same time, you can visualize the positive results of changing your behavior. Ask yourself: What do I want for myself, now and in the future?

For example, Ruby has never worried much about her smoking because the problems associated with it seem so far away. But lately she's noticed her performance on the volleyball team isn't as good as it used to be. Over the summer she visited her aunt, who has chronic emphysema from smoking and can barely leave her bed. Ruby knows she wants to have children and a career as a teacher someday, and seeing her aunt makes her wonder if her smoking habit could make it difficult for her to reach these goals. She starts to wonder whether her smoking habit is worth the short- and long-term sacrifices.

Social pressures can also increase the motivation to make changes. In Ruby's case, anti-smoking ordinances make it impossible for her to smoke in her dorm and in many public places. The inconvenience of finding a place to smoke—and pressure from her roommate, who doesn't like the smoky smell of Ruby's clothes in their room—add to Ruby's motivation to quit.

Locus of Control   When you start thinking about changing a health behavior, a big factor in your eventual success is whether or not you believe you can change. Who do you believe is controlling your life? Is it your parents, friends, or school? Is it "fate"? Or is it you?

Locus of control refers to the figurative "place" a person designates as the source of responsibility for the events in his or her life. People who believe they are in control of their own lives are said to have an internal locus of control. Those who believe that factors beyond their control—heredity, friends and family, the environment, fate, luck, or other outside forces—are more important in determining the events of their lives are said to have an external locus of control. Most people are not purely "internalizers" or "externalizers"; their locus of control changes in response to the situation.

For lifestyle management, an internal locus of control is an advantage because it reinforces motivation and commitment. An external locus of control can sabotage efforts to change behavior. For example, if you believe you are destined to die of breast cancer because your mother died from the disease, you may view monthly breast self-exams and regular checkups as a waste of time. In contrast, an internal locus of control is an advantage. If you believe you can take action to reduce your hereditary risk of

locus of control   The figurative "place" where a person locates the source of responsibility for the events in his or her life.

breast cancer, you will be motivated to follow guidelines for early detection of the disease.

People who tend to have an external locus of control can learn to view the events in their lives differently. Examine your attitudes carefully. If you find yourself attributing too much influence to outside forces, gather more information about your wellness-related behaviors. List all the ways that making lifestyle changes will improve your health. If you believe you'll succeed, and if you recognize and accept that you are in charge of your life, you're on your way to wellness.

Choosing a Target Behavior

The worst thing you can do is try to change everything at once—quit smoking, give up high-fat foods, eat a good breakfast, start jogging, plan your study time better, avoid drugs, get enough sleep. Overdoing it leads to burnout. Concentrate on one behavior that you want to change, your **target behavior,** and work on it systematically. Start with something simple, like substituting olive oil for butter in your diet or low-fat milk for whole milk. Or concentrate on getting to sleep by 10:00 P.M. Working on even one behavior change will make high demands on your energy.

Developing a Behavior Change Plan

Once you are committed to making a change, it's time to put together a plan of action. Your key to success is a well-thought-out plan that sets goals, anticipates problems, and includes rewards.

1. Monitor Your Behavior and Gather Data   Begin by keeping careful records of the behavior you wish to change (your target behavior) and the circumstances surrounding it. Keep these records in a health journal, a notebook in which you write the details of your behavior along with observations and comments. Note exactly what the activity was, when and where it happened, what you were doing, and what your feelings were at the time. In a journal for a weight-loss plan, for example, you would typically record how much food you ate, the time of day, the situation, the location, your feelings, and how hungry you were (Figure 1-4). If your goal is to start an exercise program, use your journal to track your daily activities to determine how best to make time for your workouts. Keep your journal for a week or two to get some solid information about the behavior you want to change.

2. Analyze the Data and Identify Patterns   After you have collected data on the behavior, analyze the data to identify patterns. When are you most likely to overeat? What events trigger your appetite? Perhaps you are especially hungry at midmorning or when you put off eating dinner until 9:00. Perhaps you overindulge in food and drink when you go to a particular restaurant or when you're with certain friends. Note the connections between your feelings and such external cues as time of day, location, situation, and the actions of others around you. Do you always think of having a cigarette when you read the newspaper? Do you always bite your fingernails when you're studying?

3. Set Specific Goals   It's a good idea to break your ultimate goal down into a few small steps. Your plan will seem less overwhelming and more manageable, increasing the chances that you'll stick to it. You'll also build in more opportunities to reward yourself (discussed in step 4), as well as milestones you can use to measure your progress.

If you plan to lose 30 pounds, for example, you'll find it easier to take off 10 pounds at a time. If you want to start an exercise program, begin by taking 10- to 15-minute walks a few times per week. Then gradually increase the amount of exercise you do. Take easier steps first and work up to harder steps.

4. Devise a Strategy or Plan of Action   As you write in your health journal, you gather a lot of information about your target behavior—the times it typically occurs; the situations in which it usually happens; the ways sight, smell, mood, situation, and accessibility trigger it. You can probably trace the chain of events that leads to the behavior and perhaps also identify points along the way where making a different choice would mean changing the behavior.

MODIFY YOUR ENVIRONMENT   You can be more effective in changing behavior if you control the environmental cues that provoke it. This might mean not having cigarettes or certain foods or drinks in the house, not going to parties where you're tempted to overindulge, or not spending time with particular people, at least for a while. If you always get a candy bar at a certain vending machine, change your route so you don't pass by it. If you always end up taking a coffee break and chatting with friends when you go to the library to study, choose a different place to study, such as your room.

It's also helpful to control other behaviors or habits that are linked to the target behavior. You may give in to an urge to eat when you have a beer (alcohol increases the appetite) or watch TV. Try substituting other activities for habits that are linked with your target behavior, such as exercising to music instead of plopping down in front of the TV. Or, if possible, put an exercise bicycle in front of the set and burn calories while watching your favorite show.

TERMS   **target behavior**   An isolated behavior selected as the basis for a behavior change program.

Date _____ November 5 _____   Day   M (TU) W   TH   F   SA   SU

Time of day	M/S	Food eaten	Cals.	H	Where did you eat?	What else were you doing?	How did someone else influence you?	What made you want to eat what you did?	Emotions and feelings?	Thoughts and concerns?
7:30	M	1 C Crispix cereal 1/2 C skim milk coffee, black 1 C orange juice	110 40 — 120	3	dorm cafeteria	reading newspaper	eating w/ friends, but I ate what I usually eat	I always eat cereal in the morning	a little keyed up & worried	thinking about quiz in class today
10:30	S	1 apple	90	1	library	studying	alone	felt tired & wanted to wake up	tired	worried about next class
12:30	M	1 C chili 1 roll 1 pat butter 1 orange 2 oatmeal cookies 1 soda	290 120 35 60 120 150	2	cafeteria terrace	talking	eating w/ friends; we decided to eat at the cafeteria	wanted to be part of group	excited and happy	interested in hearing everyone's plans for the weekend

M/S = Meal or snack   H = Hunger rating (0–3)

Figure 1-4   Sample health journal entries.

You can change the cues in your environment so they trigger the new behavior you want instead of the old one. Tape a picture of a cyclist speeding down a hill on your TV screen. Leave your exercise shoes in plain view. Put a chart of your progress in a special place at home to make your goals highly visible and inspire you to keep going. When you're trying to change a strong habit, small cues can play an important part in keeping you on track.

REWARD YOURSELF   A second powerful way to affect your target behavior is to set up a reward system that will reinforce your efforts. Most people find it difficult to change longstanding habits for rewards they can't see right away. Giving yourself instant, real rewards for good behavior will help you stick with a plan to change your behavior.

Carefully plan your reward payoffs and what they will be. In most cases, rewards should be collected when you reach specific objectives or subgoals in your plan. For example, you might treat yourself to a movie after a week of avoiding extra snacks. Don't forget to reward yourself for good behavior that is consistent and persistent—if you simply stick with your program week after week. Decide on a reward after you reach a certain goal or mark off the sixth week or month of a valiant effort. Write it down in your health journal and remember it as you follow your plan—especially when the going gets rough.

Make a list of your activities and favorite events to use as rewards. They should be special, inexpensive, and preferably unrelated to food or alcohol. You might treat yourself to a concert, a ball game, a new CD, a long-distance phone call to a friend, a day off from studying for a long hike in the woods—whatever is rewarding to you.

INVOLVE THE PEOPLE AROUND YOU   Rewards and support can also come from family and friends. Tell them about your plan, and ask for their help. Encourage them to be active, interested participants. Ask them to support you when you set aside time to go running or avoid second helpings at Thanksgiving dinner. You may have to remind them not to do things that make you "break training" and not to be hurt if you have to refuse something when they forget. Getting encouragement, support, and praise from important people in your life can powerfully reinforce the new behavior you're trying to adopt.

5. Make a Personal Contract   Once you have set your goals and developed a plan of action, make your plan into a personal contract. A serious personal contract—one that commits your word—can result in a higher chance of follow-through than a casual, offhand promise. Your contract can help prevent procrastination by specifying the important dates and can also serve as a reminder of your personal commitment to change.

Your contract should include a statement of your goal and your commitment to reaching it. Include details of your plan: the date you'll begin, the steps you'll use to measure your progress, the concrete strategies you've

Many actions and behaviors are shaped by cues in the environment. For these softball players, easy access to a vending machine selling fruit, rather than candy, makes it more likely that they will choose a healthy snack.

developed for promoting change, and the date you expect to reach your final goal. Have someone—preferably someone who will be actively helping you with your program—sign your contract as a witness.

A Sample Behavior Change Plan Let's take the example of Michael, who wants to break a longstanding habit of eating candy and chips every afternoon and evening. Michael begins by keeping track of his snacking in a journal. He discovers that he always buys candy or a bag of chips at the snack bar on campus between two of his afternoon classes. In the evenings, he eats several candy bars or a large bag of chips while he studies at home.

Next, Michael sets specific goals. He sets a start date and decides to break his plan into two parts. He will begin by cutting out his afternoon snack of candy or chips. Once he successfully reaches this goal, he'll concentrate on his evening snacking. He decides to allow 3 weeks for each half of his behavior change plan.

Michael decides to make several changes in his behavior to help control his urges to buy and eat candy and chips. He plans to bring a healthy snack, such as an apple or orange, to eat between his afternoon classes. He decides to avoid going near the snack bar; instead, he'll spend his between-classes break taking a walk around campus or reading in the student union. To help break his evening habit, he decides to study at the library instead of at home; when he's at home, he'll try studying in a different room. He also plans to stock the refrigerator with healthy snacks. Finally, Michael decides on some rewards he'll give himself when he meets his goals, choosing things he likes that aren't too expensive.

After Michael has thought through his plan to stop snacking on candy and chips, he's ready to create and sign a behavior change contract. He decides to enlist one of his housemates as a witness to his contract; he also asks his housemate to check on his progress and offer encouragement (Figure 1-5). Once Michael has signed his contract, he's ready to take action.

Putting Your Plan into Action

The starting date has arrived, and you are ready to put your plan into action. This stage requires commitment, the resolve to stick with the plan no matter what temptations you encounter. Remember all the reasons you have to make the change—and remember that *you* are the boss.

Use all your strategies to make your plan work. Substitute behaviors are often very important—go for a walk after class instead of eating a bag of chips. Make sure your environment is change-friendly by keeping cues that trigger the problem behavior to a minimum.

Social support can make a big difference as you take action. Try to find a buddy who wants to make the same changes you do. You can support and encourage each other, as well as exchange information and motivation. For example, an exercise buddy can provide companionship and encouragement for times when you might be tempted to skip that morning jog. Or you and a friend can watch to be sure that you both have only one alcoholic beverage at a party.

Let the people around you know about your plan, and enlist their support in specific ways. Perhaps you know people who have reached the goal you are striving for; they could be role models or mentors for you. Talk to them about what strategies worked for them.

Use your health journal to keep track of how well you are doing in achieving your ultimate goal. Record your daily activities and any relevant details, such as how far you walked or how many calories you ate. Each week, chart your progress on a graph and see how it compares to the subgoals on your contract. You may want to track more than one behavior, such as the time you spend exercising each week and your weight.

If you aren't making progress, analyze your plan to see what might be causing the problem. Possible barriers to success are listed in the section "Staying with It," along with suggestions for addressing them. Once you've identified the problem, revise your plan. Refer to the box

My Personal Contract for Giving Up Snacking on Candy and Chips

I agree to stop snacking on candy and chips twice every day. I will begin my program on __10/4__ and plan to reach my final goal by __11/15__. I have divided my program into two parts, with two separate goals. For each step in my program, I will give myself the reward listed.

1. I will stop having candy or chips for an afternoon snack on __10/4__.
(Reward: _new CD_____)
2. I will stop having candy or chips for an evening snack on __10/25__.
(Reward: _Concert_____)

My plan for stopping my snacking includes the following strategies:
1. _Avoid snack bar by taking a walk or reading at student union._
2. _Eating healthy snacks instead of candy and chips._
3. _Studying at the library instead of at home._

I understand that it is important for me to make a strong personal effort to make this change in my behavior. I sign this contract as an indication of my personal commitment to reach my goal.

Michael Cook   9/28

Witness: _Katie Lim_   9/28

Figure 1-5 A sample behavior change contract.

"Maximizing Your Chances of Success" for additional suggestions.

Be sure to reward yourself for your successes by treating yourself as specified in your contract. And don't forget to give yourself a pat on the back—congratulate yourself, notice how much better you look or feel, and feel good about how far you've come and how you've gained control of your behavior.

Staying with It

As you continue with your program, don't be surprised when you run up against obstacles; they're inevitable. In fact, it's a good idea to expect problems and give yourself time to step back, see how you're doing, and make some changes before going on. If your program is grinding to a halt, identify what is blocking your progress. It may come from one of these sources.

Social Influences Take a hard look at the reactions of the people you're counting on, and see if they're really supporting you. If they come up short, connect and network with others who will be more supportive.

A related trap is trying to get your friends or family members to change *their* behaviors. The decision to make a major behavior change is something people come to only after intensive self-examination. You may be able to influence someone by tactfully providing facts or support, but that's all. Focus on yourself. If you succeed, you may become a role model for others.

Levels of Motivation and Commitment You won't make real progress until an inner drive leads you to the stage of change at which you are ready to make a personal commitment to the goal. If commitment is your problem, you may need to wait until the behavior you're dealing with makes your life more unhappy or unhealthy; then your desire to change it will be stronger. Or you may find that changing your goal will inspire you to keep going. If you really want to change but your motivation comes and goes, look at your support system and at your own level of confidence. Building these up may be the key to pushing past a barrier. For more ideas, refer to Activity 9 in the Behavior Change Workbook at the end of the text.

Choice of Techniques and Level of Effort If your plan is not working as well as you thought it would, make changes where you're having the most trouble. If you've lagged on your running schedule, for example, maybe it's because you don't like running. An aerobics class might suit you better. There are many ways to move toward your goal. Or you may not be trying hard enough. You do have to push toward your goal. If it were easy, you wouldn't need to have a plan.

Stress Barrier If you've hit a wall in your program, look at the sources of stress in your life. If the stress is temporary, such as catching a cold or having a term paper due, you may want to wait until it passes before strengthening your efforts. If the stress is ongoing, find healthy ways to manage it, such as taking a half-hour walk after lunch. You

- *Make your efforts cost-effective and time-effective.* Be sure your new behavior has a real and lasting value for you personally. Be realistic about the amount of time and energy you can put into it. Choose a strategy or approach that works for you. For example, many activities—from walking to bicycle racing—lead to physical fitness; for long-term success, you need to choose one that you enjoy and that fits smoothly into your schedule.

- *Find a buddy.* A buddy can provide support, encouragement, and motivation. The fear of letting your buddy down makes it less likely that you'll take a day off, and in a crisis, your buddy can help overcome an urge to slip (and vice versa). If you can't find a buddy who shares your goal from among your friends, family members, and classmates, try joining a group such as Weight Watchers for a ready-made set of buddies.

- *Prepare for problem situations.* If you know in advance that you're going to be in a situation that will trigger your target

behavior, rehearse what you'll do. If you don't want to drink too much at a party, decide on your drink limit ahead of time, and switch to a soft drink when you reach your limit.

- *Expect success.* Change your ideas about yourself as you change your behavior. Drop your old self-image and start thinking of yourself in a new way—as a jogger, a non-smoker, a person in control.

- *Realize that lasting change takes time.* Major life changes involve giving up a familiar and comfortable part of your life in exchange for something new and unknown. They happen one day at a time, with lots of ups and downs.

- *Forgive and forget.* If you slip—miss a workout or eat a bag of candy—focus on discovering what triggered the slip and how to deal with it next time. Don't waste time blaming yourself. Keeping up your self-esteem will help you stay with your plan; negative feelings will get in your way.

may even want to make stress management your highest priority for behavior change (see Chapter 10).

Procrastinating, Rationalizing, and Blaming Try to detect the games you might be playing with yourself so that you can stop them. If you're procrastinating ("It's Friday already; I might as well wait until Monday to begin"), break your plan down into still smaller steps that you can accomplish one day at a time. If you're rationalizing or making excuses ("I wanted to go swimming today, but I wouldn't have had time to wash my hair afterward"), remember that when you "win" by deceiving yourself, it's not much of a victory. If you're wasting time blaming yourself or others ("Everyone in that class talks so much that I don't get a chance to speak"), recognize that blaming is a way of taking your focus off the real problem and denying responsibility for your actions. Try refocusing by taking a positive attitude and renewing your determination to succeed.

Getting Outside Help

Outside help is often needed for changing behavior that may be too deeply rooted for a self-management approach. Alcohol and other drug addictions, excessive overeating, and other conditions or behaviors that put you at a serious health risk fall into this category; so do behaviors that interfere with your ability to function. Many communities have programs to help with these problems—Weight Watchers, Alcoholics Anonymous, Smoke Enders, and Coke Enders, for example.

On campus, you may find courses in physical fitness, stress management, and weight control. The student health center or campus counseling center may also be a source of assistance. Many communities offer a wide vari-

ety of low-cost services through adult education, school programs, health departments, and private agencies. Consult the yellow pages, your local health department, or the United Way; the latter often sponsors local referral services. Whatever you do, don't be stopped by a problem when you can tap into resources to help you solve it.

Being Fit and Well for Life

Your first attempts at making behavior changes may never go beyond the project stage. Those that do may not all succeed. But as you experience some success, you'll start to have more positive feelings about yourself. You may discover physical activities you enjoy; you may encounter new situations and meet new people. Perhaps you'll surprise yourself by accomplishing things you didn't think were possible—breaking a nicotine habit, competing in a race, climbing a mountain, developing a lean, muscular body. Most of all, you'll discover the feeling of empowerment that comes from taking charge of your health (see the box "Ten Warning Signs of Wellness").

Once you've started, don't stop. Assume that health improvement is forever. Take on the easier problems first, and then use what you learn to tackle more difficult problems later. Periodically review what you've accomplished to make sure you don't fall into old habits. And keep informed about the latest health news and trends. Research is constantly providing new information that directly affects daily choices and habits.

This book will introduce you to the main components of a fit and well lifestyle, show you how to assess your current health status, and help you put together a program that will lead to wellness. You can't control every aspect of your health—there are too many unknowns in life for that to be possible. But you can create a lifestyle that

Ten Warning Signs of Wellness

1. The persistent presence of a support network.

2. Chronic positive expectations; the tendency to frame events in a constructive light.

3. Episodic outbreaks of joyful, happy experiences.

4. A sense of spiritual involvement.

5. A tendency to adapt to changing conditions.

6. Rapid response and recovery of stress response systems to repeated challenges.

7. An increased appetite for physical activity.

8. A tendency to identify and communicate feelings.

9. Repeated episodes of gratitude and generosity.

10. A persistent sense of humor.

SOURCE: Ten warning signs of good health. 1996. *Mind/Body Health Newsletter* 5(1). Reprinted by permission.

minimizes your health risks and maximizes your enjoyment of life and well-being. You can take charge of your health in a dramatic and meaningful way. *Fit and Well* will show you how.

SUMMARY

- Wellness is the ability to live life fully, with vitality and meaning. Wellness is dynamic and multidimensional; it incorporates physical, emotional, intellectual, spiritual, interpersonal and social, and environmental dimensions.

- As chronic diseases have become the leading causes of death in the United States, people have recognized that they have greater control over, and greater responsibility for, their health than ever before.

- Behaviors that promote wellness include being physically active; choosing a healthy diet; maintaining a healthy body weight; managing stress effectively; avoiding use of tobacco and other drugs and using alcohol wisely, if at all; and protecting oneself from disease and injury.

- Although heredity, environment, and health care all play roles in wellness and disease, behavior can mitigate their effects.

- Knowledge about topics in wellness and about yourself is necessary to begin making changes in behavior. Observations by others and landmark events can help get people started on change.

- Strong motivation to change and an internal locus of control are keys to successful behavior change. It is best to concentrate on one target behavior at a time.

- A specific plan for change can be developed by (1) monitoring behavior by keeping a journal, (2) analyzing the recorded data, (3) setting specific goals, (4) devising strategies for modifying the environment, rewarding yourself, and involving others, and (5) making a personal contract.

- To start and maintain a behavior change program you need commitment, a well-developed and man-

ageable plan, social support, and a system of rewards. It is also important to monitor the progress of your program, revising it as necessary.

- Obstacles sometimes come in the form of unsupportive people, a low level of motivation or commitment, inappropriate techniques, too much stress, and procrastinating, rationalizing, and blaming. Taking advantage of outside resources can help.

FOR MORE INFORMATION

Books

Hunt, P., and M. Hillsdon. 1996. *Changing Eating and Exercise Behaviour.* London: Blackwell Science. *A guide to using behavior modification techniques to change eating and exercise habits.*

Prochaska, J. O., J. C. Norcross, and C. C. DiClemente. 1994. *Changing for Good: The Revolutionary Program That Explains the Six Stages of Change and Teaches You How to Free Yourself from Bad Habits.* New York: Morrow. *Outlines the authors' model of behavior change and offers suggestions and advice for each stage of change.*

Sobel, D. S., and R. Ornstein. 1996. *The Healthy Mind, Healthy Body Handbook.* Los Altos, Calif.: DR$_x$. *Presents concrete strategies for changing behavior, staying well, managing common health problems, and becoming a better health consumer.*

Newsletters

Consumer Reports on Health, P.O. Box 56360, Boulder, CO 80323.

Harvard Health Letter, P.O. Box 420300, Palm Coast, FL 32142 (http://www.countway.harvard.edu/publications/Health_Publications).

Harvard Men's Health Watch, P.O. Box 420099, Palm Coast, FL 32142.

Harvard Women's Health Watch, P.O. Box 420234, Palm Coast, FL 32142.

Healthline, 830 Menlo Ave., Suite 100, Menlo Park, CA 94025 (http://www.healthline.com).

HealthNews, P.O. Box 52924, Boulder, CO 80322 (http://www.onhealth.com).

Mayo Clinic Health Letter, P.O. Box 53889, Boulder, CO 80322.

Mind/Body Health, P.O. Box 381069, Boston, MA 02238.

University of California at Berkeley Wellness Letter, P.O. Box 420148, Palm Coast, FL 32142 (http://magazines.enews.com/magazines/ucbwl).

Organizations, Hotlines, and Web Sites

The Internet addresses (also called uniform resource locators, or URLs) listed here were accurate at the time of publication. However, Internet information changes rapidly. If a site has moved and there is no link to the new URL, you can use a search engine to locate the new site.

Centers for Disease Control and Prevention. Through phone, fax, and the Internet, the CDC provides a wide variety of information, including materials on HIV infection, national health statistics, and governmental nutrition recommendations.

  404-332-4555 (CDC Infoline)

  http://www.cdc.gov

CNN/Health. Provides recent news on a wide variety of health topics.

  http://www.cnn.com/HEALTH

Go Ask Alice. Sponsored by the health education and wellness program at Columbia University Health Service, this Web site provides a searchable, interactive service in which professional and peer educators answer student questions about stress, sexuality, fitness, and many other health-related topics.

  http://www.goaskalice.columbia.edu

Healthfinder. A gateway to online publications, Web sites, support and self-help groups, and agencies and organizations that produce reliable health information.

  http://www.healthfinder.gov

Healthy People 2000/Healthy People 2010. Provide information on Healthy People objectives and priority areas.

  202-205-8583

  http://odphp.osophs.dhhs.gov/pubs/hp2000

  http://web.health.gov/healthypeople

Mayo Health O@sis. Sponsored by the Mayo Clinic, the site provides daily news and articles on a wide range of health topics.

  http://www.mayohealth.org

National Health Information Center (NHIC). An organization that helps put consumers and health professionals in touch with the organizations that are best able to provide answers to health-related questions. Provides information on over 100 organizations and an extensive list of toll-free numbers.

  800-336-4797

  http://nhic-nt.health.org

National Women's Health Information Center. Provides information and answers to frequently asked questions.

  800-994-WOMAN

  http://www.4woman.org

University of Wisconsin, Stevens Point Wellness Links. Includes links to the top 100 wellness sites; organized by topic.

  http://wellness.uwsp.edu/CollHlth/sites.htm

Yahoo/Health. A Web site and search engine that includes a directory of hundreds of health-related Web sites, covering a wide range of topics.

  http://www.yahoo.com/health

Your Health Daily. Provides health and fitness information from the *New York Times.*

  http://nytsyn.com/med

SELECTED BIBLIOGRAPHY

American Cancer Society. 1998. *Cancer Facts and Figures—1998.* Atlanta: American Cancer Society.

American Heart Association. 1998. *1998 Heart and Stroke Statistical Update* (retrieved January 25, 1998; http://www.americanheart.org/scientific/HSstats98/index.html).

Blair, S. N., et al. 1996. Influences of cardiorespiratory fitness and other precursors on cardiovascular disease and all-cause mortality in men and women. *Journal of the American Medical Association* 276(3): 205–210.

Booth, F. W., and B. S. Tseng. 1995. America needs to exercise for health. *Medicine and Science in Sports and Exercise* 27:462–465.

Douglas, K. A., et al. 1997. Results from the 1995 National College Health Risk Behavior Survey. *Journal of American College Health* 46(2): 55–56.

Fuller, P. R., et al. 1998. Effects of a personalized system of skill acquisition and an educational program in the treatment of obesity. *Addictive Behavior* 23(1): 97–100.

Grace, T. W. 1997. Health problems of college students. *Journal of American College Health* 45(6): 243–250.

Hunink, M. G. M., et al. 1997. The recent decline in mortality from coronary heart disease, 1980–1990. *Journal of the American Medical Association* 277(7): 535–542.

Koff, E., and C. L. Bauman. 1997. Effects of wellness, fitness, and sport skills programs on body image and lifestyle behaviors. *Perceptual and Motor Skills* 84(2): 555–562.

Lee, I. M., C. C. Hsieh, and R. S. Paffenbarger. 1995. Exercise intensity and longevity in men. The Harvard Alumni Health Study. *Journal of the American Medical Association* 273(15): 1179–1184.

Narayan, K. M., et al. 1998. Randomized clinical trial of lifestyle interventions in Pima Indians: A pilot study. *Diabetic Medicine* 15(1): 66–72.

National Center for Health Statistics. 1997. *Healthy People 2000 Review 1997.* Hyattsville, Md.: Public Health Service, DHHS Pub. (PHS) 98-1256.

Ni, M. C., B. M. Margetts, and V. M. Speller. 1997. Applying the stages-of-change model to dietary change. *Nutrition Reviews* 55(1 Pt. 1): 10–16.

Nieman, D. C. 1999. *Exercise Testing and Prescription: A Health-Related Approach,* 4th ed. Mountain View, Calif.: Mayfield.

Parsons, J. T., A. W. Siegel, and J. H. Cousins. 1997. Late adolescent risk-taking: Effects of perceived benefits and perceived risks on behavioral intentions and behavioral changes. *Journal of Adolescence* 20(4): 381–392.

Reif, C. J., and A. B. Elster. 1998. Adolescent preventive services. *Primary Care* 25(1): 1–21.

U.S. Bureau of the Census. 1997. *Resident Population of the United States: Estimates by Sex, Race, and Hispanic Origin, with Median Age* (retrieved April 9, 1997; http://www.census.gov/population/estimates/nation/intfile3-1.txt).

U.S. Department of Health and Human Services. 1997. *Health, United States, 1996–97.* Washington, D.C.: U.S. Government Printing Office, DHHS Pub. (PHS) 96-1232.

U.S. Department of Health and Human Services. 1996. *Healthy People 2000 Midcourse Review and 1995 Revisions.* Washington, D.C.: U.S. Government Printing Office, DHHS Pub. (PHS).

Basic Principles of Physical Fitness

2

LOOKING AHEAD

After reading this chapter, you should be able to answer these questions about physical fitness:

- How much exercise is recommended for developing health and fitness?

- What are the components of physical fitness, and how does each one affect wellness?

- What is the goal of physical training, and what are the basic principles of training?

- What principles are involved in designing a well-rounded exercise program? What kinds of activities should be included?

- What steps can be taken to make an exercise program safe, effective, and successful?

Any list of the benefits of physical activity is impressive. A physically active lifestyle helps you generate more energy, control your weight, manage stress, and boost your immune system. It provides psychological and emotional benefits, contributing to your sense of competence and well-being. It offers protection against heart disease, diabetes, high blood pressure, osteoporosis, cancer, and even premature death. Exercise increases your physical capacity so that you are better able to meet the challenges of daily life with energy and vigor. Although people vary greatly in the levels of physical fitness and performance they can ultimately achieve, the benefits of regular physical activity are available to everyone. (For more on the benefits of exercise, see the box "A Runner's Rationale.")

This chapter provides an overview of physical fitness. It explains how lifestyle physical activity and more formal exercise programs contribute to wellness. It describes the components of fitness, the basic principles of physical training, and the essential elements of a well-rounded exercise program. Chapters 3–6 provide an in-depth look at each of the elements of a fitness program; Chapter 7 will help you put all these elements together into a complete, personalized program.

PHYSICAL ACTIVITY AND EXERCISE FOR HEALTH AND FITNESS

Despite the many benefits of an active lifestyle, levels of physical activity have declined in recent years and remain low for all populations of Americans (Table 2-1). More than 60% of U.S. adults do not engage in recommended amounts of physical activity; 25% are not active at all. In the summer of 1996, the U.S. Surgeon General published *Physical Activity and Health*, a landmark report designed to reverse these trends and get Americans moving. The report summarized current knowledge about the relationship between physical activity and health; its major findings included the following:

- People of all ages benefit from regular physical activity.

- People can obtain significant health benefits by including a moderate amount of physical activity on most, if not all, days of the week. Through a modest increase in daily activity, most Americans can improve their health and quality of life.

- Additional health benefits can be gained through greater amounts of physical activity. People who can maintain a regular regimen of more vigorous or longer-duration activity are likely to obtain even greater benefits.

Evidence is growing that simply becoming more physically active may be the single most important lifestyle change for promoting health and well-being.

VITAL STATISTICS

TABLE 2-1	*Adults Who Regularly Engage in Physical Activity*	
	Moderate Intensity[a]	High Intensity[b]
Overall	20.1%	14.4%
Sex		
Men	21.5	12.9
Women	18.9	15.8
Ethnicity		
White	20.8	15.3
Black	15.2	9.4
Hispanic (Latino)	20.1	11.9
Education		
Less than 12 years	15.6	8.2
12 years	17.8	11.5
13–15 years	22.7	14.9
16 or more years	23.5	21.9
Income		
Less than $10,000	17.6	9.0
$10,000–$19,999	18.7	10.8
$20,000–$34,999	20.3	14.2
$35,000–$49,999	20.9	16.3
$50,000 or more	23.5	20.5
Geographic region		
Northeast	20.2	13.8
North Central	18.2	13.7
South	19.0	13.8
West	24.0	16.8

[a]Adults who engage in moderate-intensity physical activity five or more times per week for at least 30 minutes per session.
[b]Adults who engage in high-intensity physical activity three or more times per week for at least 20 minutes per session.

SOURCE: U.S. Department of Health and Human Services. 1996. *Physical Activity and Health: A Report of the Surgeon General.* Atlanta, Ga.: U.S. Department of Health and Human Services.

cally active may be the single most important lifestyle change for promoting health and well-being.

Physical Activity on a Continuum

Physical activity can be defined as any movement of the body that is carried out by the muscles and requires energy to produce. Different types of physical activity can be arranged on a continuum based on the amount of energy they require. Quick, easy movements such as standing up or walking down a hallway require little energy or effort; more intense, sustained activities such as cycling 5 miles or running in a race require considerably more.

The term **exercise** is usually used to refer to a subset of physical activity—planned, structured, repetitive movement of the body designed specifically to improve or maintain physical fitness. As discussed in Chapter 1, physical

Much of the attention surrounding exercise focuses on its benefits for physical health. But for many exercisers, improved health and longevity are only part of the reason they begin and continue to train. In this selection, long-time Runner's World *columnist George Sheehan highlights the diverse and interconnected nature of the wellness benefits of exercise.*

When I lecture, I often begin with a short film on running. The opening scene is the start of the Boston Marathon. Thousands of runners stream toward the camera, while the narrator remarks that these marathoners are only the visible elite of millions of runners now surging along the world's roads and filling its parks. "The nonrunner watches," he says, "and wonders— *why?*"

The audience almost always laughs at that question. To the people in the film, running is normal; to those in my audience, running—especially marathon running—is a mystery. When the film ends and the lights go on, I ascend the stage and address the question, Why do people run?

My answer is direct: Their lives depend upon it. People begin running for any number of motives, but we stick to it for one basic reason—to find out who we really are. Running or some other form of exercise is essential in the drive to become and perpetuate the ultimate self, because finding out who we are means finding out what our limits are—and we have to *test* ourselves to do that.

I run because my life in all its aspects depends upon it. The length of my life, certainly; the hours in my day, just as surely. The person I am, my productivity, my creativity, my pursuit of happiness—all are conditioned and determined by my hours on the road.

Most non-exercisers are unaware of this global, whole-life effect of athletic training. The experts—physicians, psychologists, sociologists, teachers, even philosophers—carve out discrete territories in which they operate. They focus on certain parts of our lives, but not life in its totality—not Life with a capital *L.*

The physician tells me that my lifespan is related to my lifestyle. When I began running, my coronary risk factors practically disappeared. I stopped smoking, my weight returned to what it had been in college, and my blood pressure didn't rise as I got older. Running also added hours to my day. My physical work capacity is far greater than it was when I was 38 years old and (presumably) in my prime. Clearly, my body benefits from fitness.

But my mind does, too. The psychologist tells me that. The negative feelings—anxiety and depression, anger and hostility—are all reduced by training. While these destructive feelings diminish, constructive ones such as self-esteem and self-confidence rise.

And the public me benefits also: The sociologist argues that my professional success is linked to the fitness I earn from running. It is no longer simply survival of the fittest, it is also success to the fittest. Fit people occupy the upper echelons in education, position, and salary.

The educator views my running and racing as a laboratory where I learn about such things as sacrifice and solitude, courage and cooperation, victory and defeat. And the philosopher reminds me that creative thinking requires the inner and outer solitude that running confers.

So it goes: Each specialist sees the role of exercise through the prism of that particular specialty. I explain this fragmentation to the audience, and then I tell them that no one piece of the puzzle is enough. Each of these experts sees only a bit of me. But I am not a cholesterol level, I am not a Rorschach profile. I am not an ergometer reading or an IQ. I am a physician, a student, a problem solver. I am also a parent, a sibling, a lover, a friend.

But none of these entirely defines me. "I absolutely deny," wrote D. H. Lawrence, "that I am a soul, or a body or an intelligence, or a nervous system or a bunch of glands, or any of the rest of the bits of me. The whole is greater than the sum of my parts. . . . I am a total living human being."

I look out over the audience and ask them, "Are you content with this total living person you are now?" American writer Lewis Mumford once remarked that today might be a fair sample of eternity. If so, who you are today would be the eternal you, the final product of your years on earth. If this were your last day, would you be satisfied?

There it is—my *why* of running, my reason for exercise—no less than the creation of the human being I become. [1986]

Runner's World, January 1995. Reprinted with the permission of the estate of George Sheehan.

---

fitness is the ability of the body to adapt to the demands of physical effort—to perform moderate-to-vigorous levels of physical activity without becoming overly tired. Levels of fitness depend on such physiological factors as the heart's ability to pump blood and the size of muscle fibers. To develop fitness, a person must perform a sufficient amount of physical activity to stress the body and cause long-term physiological changes. The precise type and amount of activity required to develop fitness will be discussed in greater detail later in the chapter. For our purposes in this section, it is important to know that only some types of physical activity—what is commonly referred to as exercise—will develop fitness. This distinction is important for setting goals and developing a program.

Lifestyle Physical Activity for Health Promotion
The Surgeon General's report recommends that all Americans

physical activity Any movement of the body that is carried   **TERMS**
out by the skeletal muscles and that requires energy to produce.

exercise Planned, structured, repetitive movement of the body designed to improve or maintain physical fitness.

Washing and waxing a car for 45–60 minutes **Less Vigorous, More Time**
Washing windows or floors for 45–60 minutes
Playing volleyball for 45 minutes
Playing touch football for 30–45 minutes
Gardening for 30–45 minutes
Wheeling self in wheelchair for 30–40 minutes
Walking 1¾ miles in 35 minutes (20 min/mile)
Basketball (shooting baskets) for 30 minutes
Bicycling 5 miles in 30 minutes
Dancing fast (social) for 30 minutes
Pushing a stroller 1½ miles in 30 minutes
Raking leaves for 30 minutes
Walking 2 miles in 30 minutes (15 min/mile)
Water aerobics for 30 minutes
Swimming laps for 20 minutes
Wheelchair basketball for 20 minutes
Basketball (playing a game) for 15–20 minutes
Bicycling 4 miles in 15 minutes
Jumping rope for 15 minutes
Running 1½ miles in 15 minutes (10 min/mile)
Shoveling snow for 15 minutes
Stairwalking for 15 minutes **More Vigorous, Less Time**

Figure 2-1   Examples of moderate amounts of physical activity.
A moderate amount of physical activity is roughly equivalent to physical activity that uses approximately 150 calories of energy per day, or 1000 calories per week. Some activities can be performed at various intensities; the suggested durations correspond to expected intensity of effort.   SOURCE: U.S. Department of Health and Human Services. 1996. *Physical Activity and Health. A Report of the Surgeon General: At-A-Glance.* Washington, D.C.: U.S. Department of Health and Human Services.

The Surgeon General recommends that all Americans accumulate at least 30 minutes of moderate-intensity activity on most days of the week. Yard work is one of many household chores that can contribute to your daily total of physical activity.

include a moderate amount of physical activity on most, preferably all, days of the week. The report suggests a goal of 150 calories per day, or about 1000 calories per week, expended in physical activity. Because energy expenditure is a function of both the intensity and the duration of the activity, the same amount of activity can be obtained in longer sessions of moderately intense activities as in shorter sessions of more strenuous activities. Thus, 30 minutes of brisk walking or raking leaves is equivalent to 15 minutes of running or shoveling snow. Examples of moderate physical activities are given in Figure 2-1.

In this lifestyle approach to physical activity, the daily total of activity can be accumulated in multiple short bouts—for example, two 10-minute bicycle rides to and from class and a brisk 15-minute walk to the post office. People can choose activities that they find enjoyable and that fit into their daily routine; everyday tasks at school, work, and home can be structured to contribute to the daily activity total (see the box "Becoming More Active" for suggestions). In addition to recommending moderate-intensity physical activity, the Surgeon General's report recommends that people perform resistance training (exercising against an opposing force such as a weight) at least twice per week to build and maintain muscular strength.

By increasing lifestyle physical activity in accordance with the guidelines given in the Surgeon General's report, people can expect to significantly improve their health and well-being. If all the Americans who are now completely sedentary were to adopt a more active lifestyle, there would be enormous benefit to the public's health and to individual well-being. Such a program may not, however, increase physical fitness.

Exercise Programs to Develop Physical Fitness   The Surgeon General's report also summarized the benefits of more formal exercise programs. It concluded that people can obtain even greater health benefits by increasing the duration and intensity of activity. Thus a person who engages in a structured, formal exercise program designed to measurably improve physical fitness will obtain even greater improvements in quality of life and greater reductions in disease and mortality risk. Chapters 3–7 provide specific guidelines for developing an exercise program that will develop total fitness.

How Much Physical Activity Is Enough?

The Surgeon General's report has generated controversy among researchers. Some experts feel that people get most of the health benefits of an exercise program simply by becoming more active over the course of the day. Others feel that the lifestyle approach sets too low of an activity goal; they argue that people should exercise long enough and intensely enough to improve their body's capacity for exercise—that is, to improve physical fitness. More research is needed to clarify the health effects of moderate-intensity vs. high-intensity exercise and continuous vs. intermittent exercise. However, there is probably truth in both of these positions.

Regular physical activity, regardless of intensity, makes you healthier and can help protect you from many chronic diseases. However, exercising at low intensities does little to improve physical fitness. While you get

- Take the stairs instead of the elevator or escalator.
- Walk to the mailbox, post office, store, bank, or library whenever possible.
- Park your car a mile or even just a few blocks from your destination, and walk briskly.
- Do at least one chore every day that requires physical activity: wash the windows or your car, clean your room or house, mow the lawn, rake the leaves.
- Take study or work breaks to avoid sitting for more than 30 minutes at a time. Get up and walk around the library, your office, or your home or dorm; go up and down a flight of stairs.

- Stretch when you stand in line or watch TV.
- When you take public transportation, get off one stop down the line and walk to your destination.
- Go dancing instead of to a movie.
- Walk to visit a neighbor or friend rather than calling him or her on the phone. Go for a walk while you chat.
- Put your remote controls in storage; when you want to change TV or radio stations, get up and do it by hand.
- Seize every opportunity to get up and walk around. Move more and sit less.

many of the health benefits of exercise by simply being more active, you obtain even more benefits when you are physically fit. In addition to long-term health benefits, fitness also significantly contributes to quality of life. Fitness can give you freedom—freedom to move your body the way you want. Fit people have more energy and better body control. They can enjoy a more active lifestyle—cycling, hiking, skiing, and so on—than their more sedentary counterparts. Even if you don't like sports, you need physical energy and stamina in your daily life and for many nonsport leisure activities—visiting museums, playing with children, gardening, and so on.

Where does this leave you? Most experts agree that some physical activity is better than none, but that more—as long as it does not result in injury—is probably better than some. At the very least, strive to become more active and meet the goal set by the Surgeon General's report of using about 150 calories per day in physical activity—the equivalent of about 30 minutes of moderate-intensity activity such as brisk walking (see Figure 2-1). Choose to be active whenever you can—walk to class, mow the lawn, wash your car, climb the stairs, work in the garden, quit using all your remote control devices. And for even better health and well-being, participate in a structured exercise program that develops physical fitness. Any increase in physical activity will contribute to your health and well-being, now and in the future.

Next, let's take a closer look at the components of physical fitness and the basic principles of fitness training.

HEALTH-RELATED COMPONENTS OF PHYSICAL FITNESS

Physical fitness has many components, some related to general health and others related more specifically to particular sports or activities. The five components of fitness most important for health are cardiorespiratory endurance, muscular strength, muscular endurance, flexibility, and body composition (proportion of fat to fat-free weight). Health-related fitness contributes to your capacity to enjoy life, helps your body withstand physical and psychological challenges, and protects you from chronic disease.

Cardiorespiratory Endurance

Cardiorespiratory endurance is the ability to perform prolonged, large-muscle, dynamic exercise at moderate-to-high levels of intensity. It depends on such factors as the ability of the lungs to deliver oxygen from the environment to the bloodstream, the heart's capacity to pump blood, the ability of the nervous system and blood vessels to regulate blood flow, and the capability of the body's chemical systems to use oxygen and process fuels for exercise.

When levels of cardiorespiratory fitness are low, the heart has to work very hard during normal daily activities and may not be able to work hard enough to sustain high-intensity physical activity in an emergency. As cardiorespiratory fitness improves, the heart begins to function more efficiently. It doesn't have to work as hard at rest or during low levels of exercise. The heart pumps more blood per heartbeat, resting heart rate slows down, blood volume increases, blood supply to the tissues improves, the body is better able to cool itself, and resting blood pressure decreases. A healthy heart can better withstand the strains of everyday life, the stress of occasional emergencies, and the wear and tear of time. Endurance training also improves

cardiorespiratory endurance The ability of the body to perform prolonged, large-muscle, dynamic exercise at moderate-to-high levels of intensity.   **TERMS**

Cardiorespiratory endurance is a key component of health-related fitness. These stationary cyclists are conditioning their hearts and lungs as well as gaining many other health benefits.

the functioning of the chemical systems, particularly in the muscles and liver, thereby enhancing the body's ability to use energy supplied by food.

Cardiorespiratory endurance is a central component of health-related fitness because the functioning of the heart and lungs is so essential to overall good health. A person can't live very long or very well without a healthy heart. Low levels of cardiorespiratory fitness are linked with heart disease, the leading cause of death in the United States.

Muscular Strength

Muscular strength is the amount of force a muscle can produce with a single maximum effort. Strong muscles are important for the smooth and easy performance of everyday activities, such as carrying groceries, lifting boxes, and climbing stairs, as well as for emergency situations. They help keep the skeleton in proper alignment, preventing back and leg pain and providing the support necessary for good posture. Muscular strength has obvious importance in recreational activities. Strong people can hit a tennis ball harder, kick a soccer ball farther, and ride a bicycle uphill more easily. Muscle tissue is an important element of overall body composition. Greater muscle mass means a higher rate of **metabolism** and faster energy use. Maintaining strength and muscle mass is vital for healthy aging. Older people tend to lose muscle cells, and many of the remaining muscle cells become nonfunctional because they lose their attachment to the nervous system. Strength training helps maintain muscle mass and function and possibly helps decrease the risk of osteoporosis in older people, which greatly enhances their quality of life and prevents life-threatening injuries.

Muscular Endurance

Muscular endurance is the ability to sustain a given level of muscle tension—that is, to hold a muscle contraction for a long period of time or to contract a muscle over and over again. Muscular endurance is important for good posture and for injury prevention. For example, if abdominal and back muscles can't hold the spine correctly, the chances of low-back pain and back injury are increased. Muscular endurance helps people cope with the physical demands of everyday life and enhances performance in sports and work. It is also important for most leisure and fitness activities.

Flexibility

Flexibility is the ability to move the joints through their full range of motion. Although range of motion isn't a significant factor in everyday activities for most people, inactivity causes the joints to become stiffer with age. Stiffness often causes older people to assume unnatural body postures that can stress joints and muscles. Stretching exercises can help ensure a healthy range of motion for all major joints.

Body Composition

Body composition refers to the relative amounts of **fat-free mass** (muscle, bone, and water) and fat in the body. Healthy body composition involves a high proportion of fat-free mass and an acceptably low level of body fat, adjusted for age and gender. A person with excessive body fat is more likely to experience a variety of health problems, including heart disease, high blood pressure, stroke, joint problems, diabetes, gallbladder disease, cancer, and back pain. The best way to lose fat is through a lifestyle that includes a sensible diet and exercise. The best way to add muscle mass is through weight training, also known as strength or resistance training.

In addition to these five health-related components of physical fitness, physical fitness for a particular sport or activity might include any or all of the following: coordination, speed, reaction time, agility, balance, and skill. Sport-specific skills are best developed through practice. The skill and coordination needed to play basketball, for example, are developed by playing basketball.

PRINCIPLES OF PHYSICAL TRAINING

The human body is very adaptable. The greater the demands made on it, the more it adjusts to meet the demands. Over time, immediate, short-term adjustments translate into long-term changes and improvements. When breathing and heart rate increase during exercise, for example, the heart gradually develops the ability to pump more blood with each beat. Then, during exercise, it doesn't have to beat as fast to meet the cells' demands for oxygen. The goal of **physical training** is to bring about these long-term changes and improvements in the body's functioning. Although people differ in the maximum levels of physical fitness and performance they can achieve through training, the wellness benefits of exercise are available to everyone (see the box "Fitness and Disability").

Particular types and amounts of exercise are most effective in developing the various components of fitness. To put together an effective exercise program, a person should first understand the basic principles of physical training. Important principles are specificity, progressive overload, reversibility, and individual differences.

Specificity

To develop a particular fitness component, exercises must be performed that are specifically designed for that component. This is the principle of **specificity**. Weight training, for example, develops muscular strength, not cardiorespiratory endurance or flexibility. Specificity also applies to the skill-related fitness components—to improve at tennis, you must practice tennis—and to the different parts of the body—to develop stronger arms, you must exercise your arms. A well-rounded exercise program includes exercises geared to each component of fitness, to different parts of the body, and to specific activities or sports.

Progressive Overload

The body adapts to the demands of exercise by improving its functioning. When the amount of exercise (also called overload or stress) is progressively increased, fitness continues to improve. This is the principle of **progressive overload.**

The amount of overload is very important. Too little exercise will have no effect on fitness (although it may improve health); too much may cause injury. For every type of exercise, there is a training threshold at which fitness benefits begin to occur, a zone within which maximum fitness benefits occur, and an upper limit of safe training (Figure 2-2). The amount of exercise needed depends on the individual's current level of fitness, his or her fitness goals, and the component being developed. A novice, for example, might experience fitness benefits from jogging a mile in 10 minutes, but this level of exercise would cause no physical adaptations in a trained distance runner. Beginners should start at the lower end of the fitness benefit zone; fitter individuals will make more rapid gains by exercising at the higher end of the fitness benefit zone.

The amount of overload needed to maintain or improve a particular level of fitness is determined in terms of three dimensions: exercise frequency (how often), intensity (how hard), and duration (how long).

Frequency Developing fitness requires regular exercise. Optimum exercise frequency, expressed in number of days per week, varies with the component being developed and the individual's fitness goals. For most people, a frequency of 3–5 days per week for cardiorespiratory endurance exercise and 2–3 days per week for resistance and flexibility training is appropriate for a general fitness program.

TERMS

muscular strength The amount of force a muscle can produce with a single maximum effort.

metabolism The sum of all the vital processes by which food energy and nutrients are made available to and used by the body.

muscular endurance The ability of a muscle or group of muscles to remain contracted or to contract repeatedly for a long period of time.

flexibility The range of motion in a joint or group of joints; flexibility is related to muscle length.

body composition The relative proportion of fat-free mass (muscle, bone, and water) and fat in the body.

fat-free mass The nonfat component of the human body, consisting of skeletal muscle, bone, and water.

physical training The performance of different types of activities that cause the body to adapt and improve its level of fitness.

specificity The training principle according to which the body adapts to the particular type and amount of stress placed on it.

progressive overload The training principle according to which increasing amounts of stress are placed on the body, causing adaptations that improve fitness.

Physical fitness and athletic achievement are not limited to the able-bodied. People with disabilities can also attain high levels of fitness and performance, as shown by the elite athletes who compete in the Paralympics. The premier event for athletes with disabilities, the Paralympics is held in the same year and city as the Olympics. Participants include people with cerebral palsy, people with visual impairments, paraplegics, quadriplegics, and others. They compete in wheelchair races and wheelchair basketball, tandem cycling, in which a blind cyclist pedals with a sighted athlete, and other events. The performance of these skilled athletes makes it clear that people with disabilities can be active, healthy, and extraordinarily fit.

Paralympians point out that able-bodied athletes and athletes with disabilities have two important things in common: both are striving for excellence, and both can serve as role models. Currently, some 34–43 million Americans are estimated to have chronic, significant disabilities. Some disabilities are the result of injury, such as spinal cord injuries sustained in car crashes. Others result from illness, such as the blindness that sometimes occurs as a complication of diabetes or the joint stiffness that accompanies arthritis. And some disabilities are present at birth, as in the case of congenital limb deformities.

Exercise and physical activity are as important for people with disabilities as for able-bodied individuals—if not *more* important. Being active helps prevent secondary conditions that may result from prolonged inactivity, such as circulatory or muscular problems. It also provides an emotional boost that helps support a positive attitude. Currently, about 10% of people with disabilities engage in regular vigorous activity and 27% engage in moderate activity.

People with disabilities don't have to be Olympians to participate in sports and lead an active life. Depending on the nature of the disability, numerous options exist, including tennis, basketball, cycling, swimming, and running. Some fitness centers offer modified aerobics, mild exercise in warm water, and other exercises adapted for people with disabilities.

For those who prefer to get their exercise at home, special workout videos are available. Most of these videos are produced by hospitals and health associations and are geared to specific disabilities. For example, there are workout videos designed especially for people with arthritis; for individuals with hearing impairments (instructors both speak and sign); for women who have had breast surgery and need to strengthen arm, shoulder, and back muscles; for people who use wheelchairs; and many others. Some videos are designed so that both able-bodied people and people with disabilities can participate.

If you want to try one of these videos or participate in some form of adapted physical activity, check with your physician about what's appropriate for you. Remember that no matter what your level of ability or disability, it's possible to make exercise an integral part of your life.

SOURCES: U.S. Department of Health and Human Services. 1996. *Physical Activity and Health: A Report of the Surgeon General.* Atlanta, Ga.: U.S. Department of Health and Human Services. Nemeth, M. 1992. Willing and able. *Maclean's,* 7 September. Silver, M. 1990. All the right moves. *U.S. News & World Report,* 12 December.

Intensity Fitness benefits occur when a person exercises harder than his or her normal level of activity. The appropriate exercise intensity varies with each fitness component. To develop cardiorespiratory endurance, for example, a person must raise his or her heart rate above normal; to develop muscular strength, a person must lift a heavier weight than normal; to develop flexibility, a person must stretch muscles beyond their normal length. The intensity required to develop each fitness component is discussed in detail in Chapters 3–5. In general, the intensity required to improve fitness is greater than that needed to obtain health benefits from lifestyle physical activity.

Duration If fitness benefits are to occur, exercise sessions must last for an extended period of time. For cardiorespiratory endurance exercise, a total duration of 20–60 minutes is recommended; exercise can take place in a single session or in multiple bouts that last 10 or more minutes. The intensity of exercise affects the total duration required to obtain fitness benefits. For high-intensity exercise such as running, for example, a total duration at the low end of the range—20–30 minutes—is appropriate. For more-moderate-intensity exercise, such as walking, a longer duration—perhaps 45–60 minutes—is required. High-intensity exercise poses a greater risk of injury than lower-intensity exercise, so if you are a nonathletic adult, it's probably best to emphasize lower-to-moderate-intensity activity of longer duration.

For muscular strength, muscular endurance, and flexibility, similar amounts of time are advisable, but these exercises are more commonly organized in terms of a specific number of repetitions of particular exercises. For resistance training, for example, a recommended program includes 1 or more sets of 8–12 repetitions of 8–10 different exercises that work the major muscle groups.

Reversibility

Fitness is a reversible adaptation. The body adjusts to lower levels of physical activity the same way it adjusts to higher levels. This is the principle of **reversibility.** When a person stops exercising, up to 50% of fitness improvements are lost within 2 months. If a training schedule must be curtailed temporarily, fitness improvements are best maintained if exercise intensity is kept constant and frequency and/or duration is reduced.

Individual Differences

Anyone watching the Olympics, a professional football game, or a tennis championship match can readily see that from a physical standpoint, we are not all created

Figure 2-2 **Amount of exercise for improving physical fitness.**

equal. There are large individual differences in our ability to improve fitness and perform and learn sports skills. Some people are able to run longer distances, or lift more weight, or kick a soccer ball more skillfully than others will ever be able to, no matter how much they train. There are limits on the adaptability—the potential for improvement—of any human body. The body's ability to transport and use oxygen, for example, can be improved by only about 15–30% through training. An endurance athlete must therefore inherit a large metabolic capacity in order to reach competitive performance levels.

However, an individual doesn't have to be an Olympic sprinter to experience health benefits from running. Physical training improves fitness regardless of heredity. For the average person, the body's adaptability is enough to achieve all fitness goals. An improvement of 15–30% in oxygen consumption can mean the difference between lifelong health and the development of a chronic disease.

DESIGNING YOUR OWN EXERCISE PROGRAM

Physical training works best when you have a plan. The plan helps you make gradual but steady progress toward your goals in all five areas of health-related fitness. The basic idea of a workout or training session is to introduce a stress powerful enough to cause adaptation but not so severe as to cause injury.

Assessment

The first step in creating a successful fitness program is to assess your current level of physical activity and fitness for each of the five health-related fitness components. The

results of the assessment tests will help you set specific fitness goals and plan your fitness program. Lab 2-1 gives you the opportunity to assess your current overall level of activity and determine if it is appropriate. Assessment tests in Chapters 3, 4, 5, and 6 will help you evaluate your cardiorespiratory endurance, muscular strength, muscular endurance, flexibility, and body composition.

Setting Goals

The ultimate goal of every health-related fitness program is the same—wellness that lasts a lifetime. Is this goal inspiring enough to motivate you to begin and stay with a program of regular exercise? Think carefully about your goals and your reasons for exercising. You may want to exercise to improve your body composition, have more energy, or lower your blood pressure; you may want to be able to run a 10K road race or ski a more advanced slope; or you may just want to feel better about yourself.

Whatever your goals, they must be important enough to you to keep you motivated. Studies have shown that exercising for yourself, rather than for the impression you think you'll make on others, is more likely to lead to long-lasting commitment. After you complete the assessment tests in Chapters 3–6, you will be able to set goals directly related to each fitness component, such as working toward a 3-mile jog or doing 20 push-ups. First, though, think carefully about your overall goals, and be clear about why you are starting a program.

reversibility The training principle according to which fitness improvements are lost when demands on the body are lowered.

TERMS

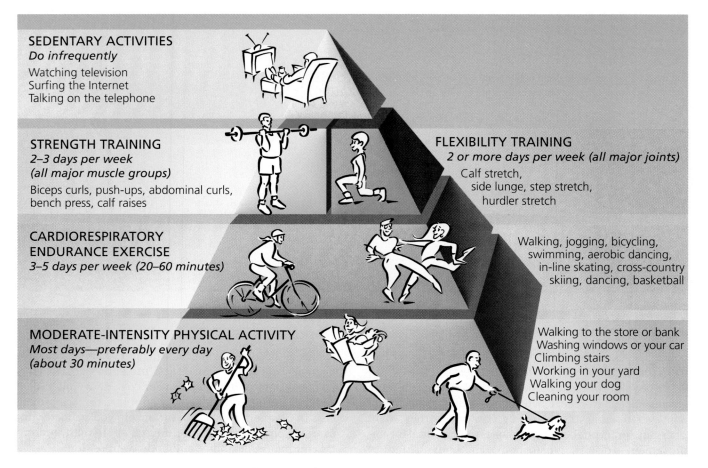

SEDENTARY ACTIVITIES
Do infrequently
Watching television
Surfing the Internet
Talking on the telephone

STRENGTH TRAINING
2–3 days per week
(all major muscle groups)
Biceps curls, push-ups, abdominal curls, bench press, calf raises

FLEXIBILITY TRAINING
2 or more days per week (all major joints)
Calf stretch,
side lunge, step stretch,
hurdler stretch

CARDIORESPIRATORY ENDURANCE EXERCISE
3–5 days per week (20–60 minutes)

Walking, jogging, bicycling, swimming, aerobic dancing, in-line skating, cross-country skiing, dancing, basketball

MODERATE-INTENSITY PHYSICAL ACTIVITY
Most days—preferably every day
(about 30 minutes)

Walking to the store or bank
Washing windows or your car
Climbing stairs
Working in your yard
Walking your dog
Cleaning your room

Figure 2-3   Physical activity pyramid.   Similar to the Food Guide Pyramid, this physical activity pyramid is designed to help people become more active. If you are currently sedentary, begin at the bottom of the pyramid and gradually increase the amount of moderate-intensity physical activity in your life. If you are already moderately active, begin a formal exercise program that includes cardiorespiratory endurance exercise, flexibility training, and strength training to help you develop all the health-related components of fitness.

Choosing Activities for a Balanced Program

An ideal fitness program combines a physically active lifestyle with a systematic exercise program to develop and maintain physical fitness. This overall program is illustrated in the physical activity pyramid shown in Figure 2-3. If you are currently sedentary, your goal is to start at the bottom of the pyramid and gradually increase the amount of moderate-intensity physical activity in your daily life. Appropriate activities include brisk walking, climbing stairs, yard work, and washing your car. You don't have to exercise vigorously, but you should experience a moderate increase in your heart and breathing rates. As described earlier, your activity time can be broken up into small blocks over the course of a day. The time it takes to walk to the library, climb a flight of stairs five times, and clean the house can quickly add up to 30 or more minutes of moderate activity.

The next two levels of the pyramid illustrate parts of a formal exercise program. The American College of Sports Medicine has established guidelines for creating an exercise program that will develop physical fitness (Table 2-2). A balanced program includes activities to develop all the health-related components of fitness.

- *Cardiorespiratory endurance* is developed by activities that involve continuous rhythmic movements of large muscle groups. Walking, jogging, cycling, swimming, and aerobic dance (also referred to as group exercise) are all good activities for developing endurance. Choose activities that you enjoy and that are convenient. Many popular leisure activities can develop endurance, including in-line skating, dancing, and backpacking. Start-and-stop activities such as tennis, racquetball, and soccer can also develop endurance if one's skill level is sufficient to enable periods of continuous play. Training for cardiorespiratory endurance is discussed in Chapter 3.

TABLE 2-2   *Exercise Recommendations for Healthy Adults*

Exercise to Develop and Maintain Cardiorespiratory Endurance and Body Composition

Mode of activity	Any activity that uses large muscle groups, can be maintained continuously, and is rhythmical and aerobic in nature; for example, walking-hiking, running-jogging, cycling-bicycling, cross-country skiing, group exercise (aerobic dance), rope skipping, rowing, stairclimbing, swimming, skating, and endurance game activities.
Frequency of training	3–5 days per week.
Intensity of training	55/65–90% of maximum heart rate or 40/50–85% of maximum oxygen uptake reserve. The lower intensity values (55–64% of maximum heart rate and 40–49% of maximum oxygen uptake reserve) are most applicable to individuals who are quite unfit.*
Duration of training	20–60 total minutes of continuous or intermittent (in sessions lasting 10 or more minutes) aerobic activity. Duration is dependent on the intensity of activity; thus, lower-intensity activity should be conducted over a longer period of time (30 minutes or more). Lower-to-moderate-intensity activity of longer duration is recommended for the nonathletic adult.

Exercise to Develop and Maintain Muscular Strength and Endurance, Flexibility, and Body Composition

Resistance training	One set of 8–10 exercises that condition the major muscle groups should be performed 2–3 days per week. Most people should complete 8–12 repetitions of each exercise; for older and more frail people (approximately 50–60 years of age and above), 10–15 repetitions with a lighter weight may be more appropriate. Multiple-set regimens may provide greater benefits if time allows.
Flexibility training	Stretches for the major muscle groups should be performed a minimum of 2–3 days per week; at least four repetitions, held for 10–30 seconds, should be completed.

*Instructions for calculating target heart rate intensity for cardiorespiratory endurance exercise are presented in Chapter 3.

SOURCE: American College of Sports Medicine. 1998. Position Stand: The Recommended Quantity and Quality of Exercise for Developing and Maintaining Cardiorespiratory and Muscular Fitness, and Flexibility in Healthy Adults. *Medicine and Science in Sports and Exercise* 30(6): 975–991.

- *Muscular strength and endurance* can be developed through resistance training—training with weights or performing calisthenic exercises such as push-ups and sit-ups. Training for muscular strength and endurance is discussed in Chapter 4.
- *Flexibility* is developed by stretching the major muscle groups, regularly and with proper technique. Flexibility is discussed in Chapter 5.
- *Healthy body composition* can be developed by combining a sensible diet and a program of regular exercise. Endurance exercise is best for reducing body fat; resistance training builds muscle mass, which helps increase metabolism (the rate of energy expenditure). Body composition is discussed in Chapter 6.

There are as many different fitness programs as there are individuals. Consider the following examples:

- Maggie is a person whose life revolves around sports. She's been on softball teams and swim teams, and now she's on her college varsity soccer team. She follows a rigorous exercise regimen established by her soccer coach. Soccer practice is from four to six afternoons a week. It begins with warm-ups, drills, and practice in

specific skills, and it ends with a scrimmage and then a jog around the soccer field. Games are every Saturday. Maggie likes team sports, but she also enjoys exercising alone, so she goes on long bicycle rides whenever she can fit them in. She can't imagine what it would be like not to be physically active every day.

- Maria is a busy young mother of twins. To keep in shape, she joined a health club with a weight room, exercise classes, and child care. Every Monday, Wednesday, and Friday morning, she takes the twins to the club and attends the 7:00 "wake-up" low-impact aerobics class. The instructor leads the class through warm-ups; a 20-minute aerobic workout; exercises for the arms, abdomen, buttocks, and legs; stretches; and a relaxation exercise. Maria is exhilarated and ready for the rest of the day before 9:00 A.M.

- Tom is an engineering student with a lot of studying to do and an active social life as well. For exercise, he plays tennis three times a week. He likes to head for the courts around 6:00 P.M., when most people are eating dinner. He warms up for 10 minutes by practicing his forehand and backhand against a backboard and

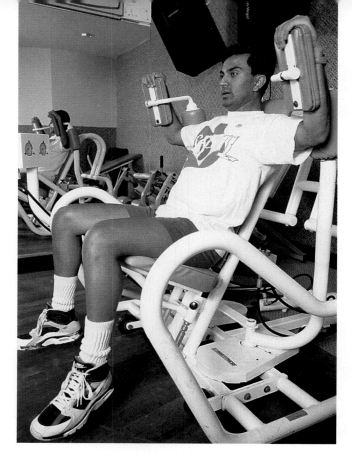

An important principle of exercising is to train the way you want your body to change. By working out on weight training equipment, this young man is increasing the strength and definition of specific muscles and improving the overall appearance of his body.

then plays a hard, fast game with his regular partner for 45 minutes to an hour. Afterwards, he does some stretching exercises while his muscles are still warm. Then he showers and gets ready for dinner. Twice a week he works out at the gym, with particular attention to keeping his arms strong and his shoulders limber. On Saturday nights, he goes dancing with friends.

Each of these people has worked an adequate or more-than-adequate fitness program into their busy daily routine. Chapter 7 contains guidelines to help you choose activities and put together a complete exercise program that suits your goals and preferences.

What about the tip of the activity pyramid? Although sedentary activities are often unavoidable—attending class, studying, working in an office, and so on—many people choose inactivity over activity during their leisure time. Change sedentary patterns by becoming more active whenever you can. Move more and sit less.

Guidelines for Training

The following guidelines will make your exercise program more effective and successful.

• *Train the way you want your body to change.* Stress your body such that it adapts in the desired direction.

To have a more muscular build, lift weights. To be more flexible, do stretching exercises. To improve performance in a particular sport, practice that sport or the movements used in it.

• *Train regularly.* Consistency is the key to improving fitness. Adaptations to exercise are reversible; fitness improvements are lost if too much time is allowed to pass between exercise sessions.

• *Get in shape gradually.* An exercise program can be divided into three phases: the beginning phase, during which the body adjusts to the new type and level of activity; the progress phase, during which fitness is increased; and the maintenance phase, in which the targeted level of fitness is maintained over the long term (Figure 2-4). When beginning a program, it is critical to start slowly to give your body time to adapt to the stress of exercise. As you progress, increase duration and frequency before increasing intensity. If you train too much or too intensely, you are more likely to suffer injuries or become **overtrained,** a condition characterized by lack of energy, aching muscles and joints, and decreased physical performance. Injuries and overtraining slow down an exercise program and impede motivation. The goal is not to get in shape as quickly as possible but to gradually become and remain physically fit. When you reach your desired level of fitness, maintain it by exercising regularly.

• *Warm up before exercising, and cool down afterward.* Warming up decreases the chances of injury by helping the body gradually progress from rest to activity. A warm-up should include low-intensity movements similar to those used in the activity that will follow. Stretching exercises are also often recommended. Cooling down after exercise is important for restoring circulation to its normal resting condition. Cool down by continuing to exercise but at a lower level of intensity.

• *Listen to your body.* Don't exercise if it doesn't feel right. Sometimes you need a few days of rest to recover enough to train with the intensity required for improving fitness. On the other hand, you can't train sporadically either. If you listen to your body and it always tells you to rest, you won't make any progress. You have to work to improve fitness, so try to maintain a structured —but flexible—workout program.

• *Try training with a partner.* Training partners can motivate and encourage each other through hard spots and help each other develop proper exercise techniques. Training with a partner can make exercising seem easier and more fun.

• *Train your mind.* This is one of the most difficult skills to acquire, but it is critical for achieving and maintaining fitness. Becoming fit requires commitment, discipline, and patience. These qualities come from understanding the importance of exercise and having clear

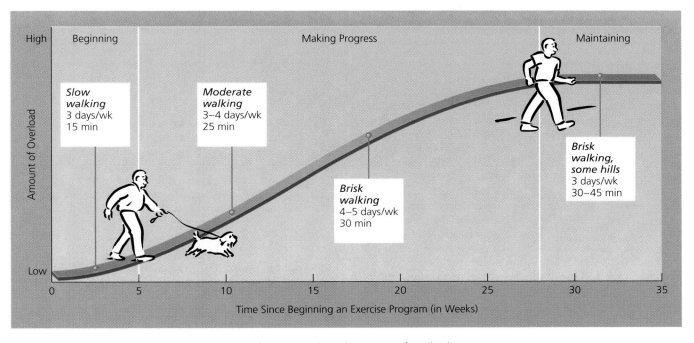

Figure 2-4 Phases of an exercise program. This figure shows how the amount of overload is increased gradually over time in a sample walking program. Regardless of the activity chosen, it is important that an exercise program begin slowly and progress gradually. Once a person achieves the desired level of fitness, she or he can maintain it by exercising at least 3 days per week.   SOURCE: Progression data from American College of Sports Medicine. 1995. *Guidelines for Exercise Testing and Prescription,* 5th ed. Baltimore, Md.: Williams and Wilkins.

and reachable goals. Use the lifestyle management techniques discussed in Chapter 1 to keep your program on track. Believe in yourself and your potential—and you *will* achieve your goals!

• *Keep your exercise program in perspective.* As important as physical fitness is, it is only part of a well-rounded life. You have to have time for work and school, family and friends, relaxation and hobbies. Some people become overinvolved in exercise and neglect other parts of their lives. They think of themselves as runners, dancers, swimmers, or triathletes rather than as people who participate in those activities. Balance and moderation are the key ingredients of a fit and well life.

• Regular, moderate activity on most days of the week substantially contributes to good health. Even if you do not participate in a formal, vigorous exercise program, you can get many of the health benefits of exercise by becoming more active during the day. If you are already physically active, you will benefit even more by increasing the intensity or duration of your activity.

• The five components of physical fitness most important for health are cardiorespiratory endurance, muscular strength, muscular endurance, flexibility, and body composition.

• Physical training is the process of bringing about long-term improvements in the body's functioning through exercise. Four important principles of training are specificity, progressive overload, reversibility, and individual differences.

• Progressive overload is quantified in terms of frequency, intensity, and duration of exercise.

• Individual differences mean that people will vary in the maximum level of fitness or performance they can achieve. However, every person is capable of reaching personal fitness goals.

• Important steps in designing an exercise program include assessing your current level of fitness, setting realistic goals, and choosing activities that develop all the components of fitness.

overtraining   A condition caused by training too much or too intensely, characterized by lack of energy, decreased physical performance, fatigue, depression, aching muscles and joints, and susceptibility to injury.   **TERMS**

COMMON QUESTIONS ANSWERED

Is exercise safe for me? People of any age who are not at high risk for serious health problems can safely exercise at a moderate intensity (60% or less of maximum heart rate) without a prior medical evaluation. (See Chapter 3 for a discussion of maximum heart rate.) Likewise, if you are male and under 40 or female and under 50 and in good health, exercise is probably safe for you. If you are over these ages or have health problems (especially high blood pressure, heart disease, muscle or joint problems, or obesity), see your physician before starting a vigorous exercise program. The Canadian Society for Exercise Physiology has developed a questionnaire called PAR-Q to help determine exercise safety. This questionnaire is included in Lab 2-2. Completing it should alert you to any potential problems you may have. If a physician isn't sure whether exercise is safe for you, he or she may recommend an **exercise stress test** to see whether you develop symptoms of heart disease during exercise. For most people, however, it's far safer to exercise than to remain sedentary.

You must also consider your physical safety when exercising. If you ride a bicycle or run on public streets, wear clothing that can be seen easily. Bicyclists should always wear helmets. Even though you may have the right-of-way, give cars plenty of leeway; in a collision, a car will usually sustain less damage than a bicycle or your unprotected body. Don't train in isolated areas unless you're with a friend. Exercising alone, you could easily be injured or become a crime victim. (See Appendix A for more information on personal safety.)

Where can I get help and advice about exercise? Because fitness is essential to a wellness lifestyle, you need to learn as much as you can about exercise. One of the best places to get help is an exercise class. There, expert instructors can help you learn the basics of training and answer your questions. Read articles by credible experts in fitness magazines. Because of competition among publications, these magazines include articles by leading experts in exercise science written at a layperson's level.

A qualified personal trainer can also be helpful in getting you started in an exercise program or a new form of training. Make sure this person has proper qualifications, such as a college degree in exercise physiology or physical education or ACSM certification. Don't seek out a person for advice simply because he or she looks fit.

Should I follow my exercise program if I'm sick? If you have a mild head cold or feel one coming on, it is probably OK to exercise moderately. Just begin slowly and see how you feel. However, if you have symptoms of a more serious illness—fever, swollen glands, nausea, extreme tiredness, muscle aches—wait until you have fully recovered before resuming your exercise program. Continuing to exercise while suffering from an illness more serious than a cold can compromise your recovery and may even be dangerous.

How can I fit my exercise program into my day? Good time management is an important skill in creating and maintaining an exercise program. Choose a regular time to exercise, preferably the same time every day. Don't tell yourself you'll exercise "sometime during the day" when you have free time—that free time may never come. Schedule your workout, and make it a priority. Include alternative plans in your program to account for circumstances like bad weather or vacations.

You don't have to work on all fitness components in the same exercise session. You can jog and stretch in one session and lift weights in another. The important thing is to have a regular schedule. (You'll have the chance to develop strategies for successful time management in the Behavior Change Workbook at the end of the text.)

Where can I work out? Identify accessible and pleasant places to work out. For running, find a field or park with a soft surface. For swimming, find a pool that's open at times convenient for you. For cycling, find an area with minimal traffic and air pollution. Make sure the place you exercise is safe and convenient.

If you join a health club or fitness center, choose one close to your home or place of work. You'll be less likely to go to the club if it's farther away. Choose a club with an atmosphere that fits with your personality and offers the activities you want. For guidelines, refer to the box "Choosing a Fitness Center."

- Guidelines that can make an exercise program more effective include training the way you want your body to change, training regularly, getting in shape gradually, warming up and cooling down, maintaining a structured but flexible program, training with a partner, training your mind, and keeping exercise in perspective.

TERMS **exercise stress test** A test usually administered on a treadmill or cycle ergometer that involves analysis of the changes in electrical activity in the heart from an electrocardiogram (EKG or ECG) taken during exercise. Used to determine if any heart disease is present and to assess current fitness level.

FOR MORE INFORMATION

Books

American College of Sports Medicine. 1995. *ACSM's Guidelines for Exercise Testing and Prescription*, 5th ed. Baltimore: Williams & Wilkins. *Includes the ACSM guidelines for safety of exercising, a basic discussion of exercise physiology, and information about fitness testing and prescription.*

American College of Sports Medicine. 1998. *ACSM Fitness Book*, 2d ed. Champaign, Ill.: Human Kinetics. *A brief, easy-to-use guide to creating a successful fitness program.*

Burke, E., and E. Burke. 1996. *Complete Home Fitness Handbook*. Champaign, Ill.: Human Kinetics. *A comprehensive exercise plan for people who want to exercise at home.*

If you're thinking of becoming a member of a health club or fitness center, the following guidelines will help you make a final choice.

1. Does the center provide programs that are appropriate for you and at convenient times? You may wish to consult with a physician about your specific exercise needs.

2. Ask members and former members about the operation, services, staff, and programs.

3. Visit the club at the time of day when you plan to use it. Are the classes crowded, or are there long lines for the equipment you plan to use?

4. Check the atmosphere of the club. Are personnel well trained, friendly, enthusiastic, attentive, and well informed? Do instructors have special training? Is there a fitness supervisor who has a degree in exercise science or certification from the ACSM or another recognized organization?

5. Observe the facility. Is it clean, well ventilated, and properly maintained? Is the equipment in good condition? Is there shock-absorbent flooring for aerobics workouts? Is safety information provided for using weight machines? Are dressing rooms and showers available and clean?

6. Find out about the different types of memberships and payment plans the club offers. Ask for a short-term trial membership. Don't be rushed into signing a long-term contract. Before signing any contract, ask for a few days to think it over; a reputable facility will let you consider joining without applying pressure.

7. Read the contract carefully before signing, or get a knowledgeable person to read it. Be sure you understand the provisions and agreements. Don't hesitate to ask questions.

8. Understand what happens if you wish to cancel the membership. What type of refund policy does the club have?

9. Find out if the club will suspend your membership temporarily when you're on vacation or unable to exercise for another reason.

10. Find out how long the club has been in your area. The longer the better, and if under the same management, that's another plus. Beware of new clubs offering "pre-opening" membership discounts.

11. Find out if the club belongs to the Association of Physical Fitness Centers or the International Racquet Sports Association. These trade associations have established standards to help protect consumer health, safety, and rights. You can also check with the Better Business Bureau to see if any complaints have been filed against the club.

In addition, be wary of promotion gimmicks and high-pressure sales techniques. Be alert to practices such as special reduced prices, free visits, reservation forms, and guarantees of fitness improvements or weight loss. Get all the facts before making a decision. If you feel any excessive amount of pressure, leave or at least ask for more time. Under no circumstances should you feel badgered, embarrassed, or threatened. You want to find a facility that you feel comfortable with and that meets your needs.

SOURCES: Health Clubs: The right choice for you? 1996. *Consumer Reports*, January, 27–30; Cornacchia, H. 1994. How to choose a fitness center. *Healthline*, April. Krucoff, C. 1989. Joining the club. *Washington Post Health*, 5 September, 20.

Diamond, J. 1996. *Exercises for Airplanes: (And Other Confined Spaces)*. New York: Excalibur. *A guide to exercising in airplanes and confined spaces, such as the office.*

Farquhar, J. W. 1996. *Fresh Start: The Stanford Medical School Health and Fitness Program.* San Francisco: KQED. *An excellent guide to exercising for health and prevention of disease.*

Nieman, D. C. 1999. *Exercise Testing and Prescription: A Health-Related Approach,* 4th ed. Mountain View, Calif.: Mayfield. *Comprehensive discussions of fitness testing, exercise and disease, nutrition and physical performance, and exercise prescription.*

Rippe, J. M., and M. A. Waite. 1996. *Fit over Forty: A Revolutionary Plan to Achieve Lifelong Physical and Spiritual Health and Well-Being.* New York: William Morrow. *A sensible approach to incorporating exercise into a wellness lifestyle.*

U.S. Department of Health and Human Services. 1996. *Physical Activity and Health: A Report of the Surgeon General.* Department of Health and Human Services. (Also available online: http://www.cdc.gov/nccdphp/sgr/sgr.htm) *Provides a summary of the evidence for the benefits of physical activity as well as all the recent recommendations.*

Journals

ACSM Health and Fitness Journal (401 West Michigan Street, Indianapolis, IN 46202; http://www.wwilkins.com/esources/journdex/FIT/index.html)

Physician and Sportsmedicine (4530 W. 77th Street, Minneapolis, MN 55435; many of the articles are also available online at http://www.physsportsmed.com)

Organizations, Hotlines, and Web Sites

American Alliance for Health, Physical Education, Recreation, and Dance (AAHPERD). A professional organization dedicated to promoting quality education programs to improve the health and fitness of Americans.
800-213-7193
http://www.aahperd.org

American College of Sports Medicine (ACSM). Provides brochures, publications, and audio- and videotapes on the positive effects of exercise.
317-637-9200
http://www.acsm.org/sportsmed

American Council on Exercise (ACE). Promotes exercise and fitness for all Americans; the Web site features fact sheets on many consumer topics, including choosing shoes, cross-training, steroids, and getting started on an exercise program.

800-529-8227 (Consumer Fitness Hotline)

http:/www.acefitness.org

American Medical Association/Personal Trainer. Includes a fitness assessment and guidelines for creating a safe, effective program for developing the health-related components of fitness.

http://www.ama-assn.org/insight/gen_hlth/trainer

Balance Magazine. An online health and fitness magazine with practical advice for exercisers.

http://www.hyperlink.com/balance

Disabled Sports USA. Provides sports and recreation services to people with physical or mobility disorders.

301-217-0960

http://www.nas.com/~dsusa

Fitness Management Magazine's Fitness World. Includes current issues of the magazine, information about exercise books and videos, news highlights related to exercise, and answers to frequently asked questions.

http://www.fitnessworld.com

Fitness Partner Connection Jumpsite. A resource of fitness-related information on the Internet.

http://primusweb.com/fitnesspartner

Fitness-Related Web Sites. Includes many links to helpful fitness- and health-related sites.

http://www.montana.com/Stafford/fitnesslinks.html

Internet's Fitness Resource. Provides extensive links to sites about general fitness, specific activities, and fitness equipment.

http://www.netsweat.com

Melpomene Institute. Provides information about physical activity and health for women.

612-642-1951

http://www.melpomene.org

Physical Activity & Health Network. Provides resources and links on the relationship between physical activity and health.

http://www.pitt.edu/~pahnet

Worldguide Health and Fitness Forum. Provides information on anatomy, cardiorespiratory endurance exercise, strength training, nutrition, and sports medicine.

http://www.worldguide.com/Fitness/hf.html

SELECTED BIBLIOGRAPHY

American College of Sports Medicine. 1998. ACSM Position Stand: The Recommended Quantity and Quality of Exercise for Developing and Maintaining Cardiorespiratory and Muscular Fitness, and Flexibility in Healthy Adults. *Medicine and Science in Sports and Exercise* 30(6):975–991.

American College of Sports Medicine. 1995. *ACSM's Guidelines for Exercise Testing and Prescription,* 5th ed. Baltimore: Williams & Wilkins.

Brooks, G. A., T. D. Fahey, and T. P. White. 1996. *Exercise Physiology: Human Bioenergetics and Its Applications,* 2d ed. Mountain View, Calif.: Mayfield.

Coogan, P. F., et al. 1997. Physical activity in usual occupation and risk of breast cancer (United States). *Cancer Causes Control* 8:626–631.

Folsom, A. R., et al. 1997. Physical activity and incidence of coronary heart disease in middle-aged women and men. *Medicine and Science in Sports and Exercise* 29:901–909.

Haapanen, N., et al. 1997. Association of leisure time physical activity with the risk of coronary heart disease, hypertension and diabetes in middle-aged men and women. *International Journal of Epidemiology* 26:739–747.

How far should you go to stay fit: The battle between tough and tame. 1997. *U.S. News & World Report,* 10 November, 95–96.

Hyperthermia and dehydration-related deaths associated with intentional rapid weight loss in three collegiate wrestlers. 1998. *Morbidity and Mortality Weekly Report* 47(6): 105–108.

Kujala, U. M., et al. 1998. Relationship of leisure-time physical activity and mortality: The Finnish twin cohort. *Journal of the American Medical Association* 279(6): 440–444.

Kushi, L. H., et al. 1997. Physical activity and mortality in post-menopausal women. *Journal of the American Medical Association* 277(16): 1287–1292.

Lee, I. M., C. C. Hsieh, and R. S. Paffenbarger. 1995. Exercise intensity and longevity in men. The Harvard Alumni Health Study. *Journal of the American Medical Association* 273(15): 1179–1184.

Lee, I. M., et al. 1997. Physical activity and risk of colon cancer: The Physicians' Health Study (United States). *Cancer Causes Control* 8:568–574.

McInnis, K. J., S. Hayakawa, and G. J. Balady. 1997. Cardiovascular screening and emergency procedures at health clubs and fitness centers. *American Journal of Cardiology* 80: 380–383.

National Center for Chronic Disease Prevention and Health Promotion, Centers for Disease Control and Prevention. 1997. Guidelines for school and community programs to promote lifelong physical activity among young people. *Journal of School Health* 67:202–219.

National Institutes of Health. 1996. *Physical Activity and Cardiovascular Health.* National Institutes of Health Consensus Development Conference Statement, December 18–20, 1995 (retrieved March 10, 1996; http://text.nlm.gov/nih/cdc/www/101.html).

Nattiv, A., J. C. Puffer, and G. A. Green. 1997. Lifestyles and health risks of collegiate athletes: A multi-center study. *Clinical Journal of Sports Medicine* 7:262–272.

Nieman, D. C. 1997. Moderate exercise boosts the immune system: Too much exercise can have the opposite effect. *ACSM's Health and Fitness Journal* 1(5): 14–19.

Pate, R. R., et al. 1995. Physical activity and public health: A recommendation from the Centers for Disease Control and Prevention and the American College of Sports Medicine. *Journal of the American Medical Association* 273(5): 402–407.

Roos, R. J. 1997. The Surgeon General's report: A prime resource for exercise advocates. *The Physician and Sportsmedicine* 25(4): 122–132.

Sacco, R. L., et al. 1998. Leisure-time physical activity and ischemic stroke risk: The Northern Manhattan Stroke Study. *Stroke* 29(2): 380–387.

U.S. Department of Health and Human Services. 1996. *Physical Activity and Health: A Report of the Surgeon General.* Atlanta, Ga.: U.S. Department of Health and Human Services, Centers for Disease Control and Prevention, National Center for Chronic Disease Prevention and Health Promotion.

Cardiorespiratory Endurance

3

LOOKING AHEAD

After reading this chapter, you should be able to answer these questions about cardiorespiratory endurance:

• How does the body produce the energy it needs for exercise?

• What are the major effects and benefits of cardiorespiratory endurance exercise?

• How is cardiorespiratory endurance measured and assessed?

• How do type, intensity, duration, and frequency of exercise affect the development of cardiorespiratory endurance?

• What elements go into a successful cardiorespiratory fitness program?

• What are the best ways to prevent and treat exercise injuries?

C ardiorespiratory endurance—the ability of the body to perform prolonged, large-muscle, dynamic exercise at moderate-to-high levels of intensity—is a key health-related component of fitness. As explained in Chapter 2, a healthy cardiorespiratory system is essential to high levels of fitness and wellness.

This chapter reviews the short- and long-term effects and benefits of cardiorespiratory endurance exercise. It then describes several tests that are commonly used to assess cardiorespiratory fitness. Finally, it provides guidelines for creating your own cardiorespiratory endurance program, one that is geared to your current level of fitness and built around activities you enjoy.

BASIC PHYSIOLOGY OF CARDIORESPIRATORY ENDURANCE EXERCISE

A basic understanding of the body processes involved in cardiorespiratory endurance exercise can help you design a safe and effective fitness program. In this section, we'll take a brief look at how the cardiorespiratory system functions and how the body produces the energy it needs to respond to the challenge of physical activity.

The Cardiorespiratory System

The cardiorespiratory system picks up and transports oxygen, nutrients, and other key substances to the organs and tissues that need them; it also picks up waste products and carries them to where they can be used or expelled. The cardiorespiratory system consists of the heart, the blood vessels, and the respiratory system (Figure 3-1).

The Heart The heart is a four-chambered, fist-sized muscle located just beneath the ribs under the left breast. Its role is to pump oxygen-poor blood to the lungs and oxygenated (oxygen-rich) blood to the rest of the body. Blood actually travels through two separate circulatory systems: The right side of the heart pumps blood to the lungs in what is called **pulmonary circulation,** and the left side pumps blood through the rest of the body in **systemic circulation.**

Waste-carrying, oxygen-poor blood enters the right upper chamber, or **atrium,** of the heart through the **venae cavae,** the largest veins in the body (Figure 3-2). As the right atrium fills, it contracts and pumps blood into the right lower chamber, or **ventricle,** which, when it contracts, pumps blood through the pulmonary artery into the lungs. There, blood picks up oxygen and discards carbon dioxide. Cleaned, oxygenated blood then flows from the lungs through the pulmonary veins into the left atrium. As this chamber fills, it contracts and pumps blood into the powerful left ventricle, which pumps it

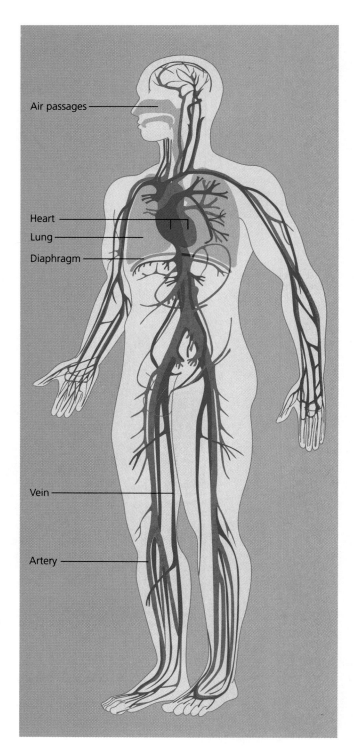

Figure 3-1 The cardiorespiratory system.

through the **aorta,** the body's largest artery, to be fed into the rest of the body's blood vessels.

The period of the heart's contraction is called **systole;** the period of relaxation is called **diastole.** During systole, the atria contract first, pumping blood into the ventricles;

① Waste-carrying, oxygen-poor blood enters the right atrium from the superior and inferior venae cavae.

Pulmonary artery

Aorta

Superior vena cava

Right lung

③ In the lungs, blood picks up oxygen and discards carbon dioxide; it then flows through the pulmonary veins into the left atrium.

Left lung

Right atrium

Pulmonary vein

Left atrium

② Blood flows from the right atrium into the right ventricle; from there it is pumped through the pulmonary arteries into the lungs.

④ Oxygen-rich blood flows from the left atrium into the left ventricle; from there it is pumped through the aorta into the rest of the body's blood vessels.

Left ventricle

Right ventricle

Inferior vena cava

Figure 3-2   Circulation in the heart.

a fraction of a second later, the ventricles contract, pumping blood to the lungs and the body. During diastole, blood flows into the heart. A person weighing 150 pounds has about 5 quarts of blood, which are circulated about once every minute.

The heartbeat—the split-second sequence of contractions of the heart's four chambers—is controlled by electrical impulses. These signals originate in a bundle of specialized cells in the right atrium called the pacemaker. Unless it is speeded up or slowed down by the brain in response to such stimuli as danger or exhaustion, the heart produces electrical impulses at a steady rate.

The Blood Vessels   Blood vessels are classified by size and function. **Veins** carry blood to the heart; **arteries** carry it away from the heart. Veins have thin walls, but arteries have thick elastic walls that enable them to expand and relax with the volume of blood being pumped through them. After leaving the heart, the aorta branches into smaller and smaller vessels. The smallest arteries branch still further into **capillaries**, tiny vessels only one cell thick. The capillaries deliver oxygen and nutrient-rich blood to the tissues and receive oxygen-poor, waste-carrying blood. From the capillaries, this blood empties into small veins and then into larger veins that return it to the heart to repeat the cycle.

Blood pumped through the heart doesn't reach its cells, so the heart has its own network of arteries, veins, and capillaries. Two large vessels, the right and left coronary arteries, branch off the aorta and supply the heart muscle with oxygenated blood. Blockage of a coronary artery is a leading cause of heart attacks (see Chapter 11).

The Respiratory System The **respiratory system** supplies oxygen to the body and carries off carbon dioxide, a waste product of body processes. Air passes in and out of the lungs as a result of pressure changes brought about by the contraction and relaxation of the diaphragm and rib muscles; the lungs expand and contract about 12–20 times a minute. As air is inhaled, it passes through the nasal passages, the throat, larynx, trachea (windpipe), and bronchi into the lungs. The lungs consist of many branching tubes that end in tiny, thin-walled air sacs called **alveoli.**

Carbon dioxide and oxygen are exchanged between alveoli and capillaries in the lungs. Carbon dioxide passes from blood cells into the alveoli, where it is carried up and out of the lungs (exhaled). Oxygen from inhaled air is passed from the alveoli into blood cells; these oxygen-rich blood cells then return to the heart and are pumped throughout the body. Oxygen is an important component of the body's energy-producing system, so the cardiorespiratory system's ability to pick up and deliver oxygen is critical for the functioning of the body—at rest and during exercise.

Energy Production

Metabolism is the sum of all the chemical processes necessary to maintain the body. Energy is required to fuel vital body functions—to build and break down tissue, contract muscles, conduct nerve impulses, regulate body temperature, and so on. The rate at which your body uses energy—its metabolic rate—depends on your level of activity. At rest, you have a low metabolic rate; if you stand up and begin to walk, your metabolic rate increases. If you jog, your metabolic rate may increase more than 800% above its resting level. Olympic-caliber distance runners can increase their metabolic rate by a whopping 2000% or more.

Energy from Food The body converts chemical energy from food into substances that cells can use as fuel. These fuels can be used immediately or stored for later use. The body's ability to store fuel is critical, because if all the energy from food were released immediately, much of it would be wasted.

The three classes of energy-containing nutrients in food are carbohydrates, fats, and proteins. During digestion, most carbohydrates are broken down into the simple sugar **glucose.** Some glucose remains circulating in the blood ("blood sugar"), where it can be used as a quick source of fuel to produce energy. Glucose may also be converted to **glycogen** and stored in the liver, muscles, and kidneys. If glycogen stores are full and the body's immediate need for energy is met, the remaining glucose is converted to fat and stored in the body's fatty tissues. Excess energy from dietary fat is also stored as body fat. Protein in the diet is used primarily to build new tissue, but it can be broken down for energy or incorporated into fat stores. Glucose, glycogen, and fat are important fuels for the production of energy in the cells; protein is used for energy only when other fuels are lacking. (See Chapter 8 for more on the other roles of carbohydrate, fat, and protein in the body.)

ATP: The Energy "Currency" of Cells The basic form of energy used by cells is **adenosine triphosphate,** or **ATP.** When a cell needs energy, it breaks down ATP, a process that releases energy in the only form the cell can use directly. Cells store a small amount of ATP; when they need more, they create it through chemical reactions that utilize the body's stored fuels—glucose, glycogen, and fat. When you exercise, your cells need to produce more energy. Consequently, your body mobilizes its stores of fuel to increase ATP production.

TERMS

respiratory system The lungs, air passages, and breathing muscles; supplies oxygen to the body and carries off carbon dioxide.

alveoli Tiny air sacs in the lungs through whose walls gases such as oxygen and carbon dioxide diffuse in and out of blood.

glucose A simple sugar that circulates in the blood and can be used by cells to fuel ATP production.

glycogen A complex carbohydrate stored principally in the liver and skeletal muscles; the major fuel source during most forms of intense exercise.

adenosine triphosphate (ATP) Energy source for cellular processes.

immediate energy system Energy system that supplies energy to muscle cells through the breakdown of cellular stores of ATP and creatine phosphate.

nonoxidative (anaerobic) energy system Energy system that supplies energy to muscle cells through the breakdown of muscle stores of glucose and glycogen; also called the *anaerobic system* or the *lactic acid system* because chemical reactions take place without oxygen and produce lactic acid.

anaerobic Occurring in the absence of oxygen.

lactic acid A metabolic acid resulting from the metabolism of glucose and glycogen; an important source of fuel for many tissues of the body, its accumulation may produce fatigue.

oxidative (aerobic) energy system Energy system that supplies energy to cells through the breakdown of glucose, glycogen, fats, and amino acids; also called the *aerobic system* because chemical reactions require oxygen.

aerobic Dependent on the presence of oxygen.

TABLE 3-1	Characteristics of the Body's Energy Systems		
	Energy System*		
	Immediate	Nonoxidative	Oxidative
Duration of activity for which system predominates	0–10 seconds	10 seconds–2 minutes	>2 minutes
Intensity of activity for which system predominates	High	High	Low to moderately high
Rate of ATP production	Immediate, very rapid	Rapid	Slower but prolonged
Fuel	Adenosine triphosphate (ATP), creatine phosphate (CP)	Muscle stores of glycogen and glucose	Body stores of glycogen, glucose, fat, and protein
Oxygen used?	No	No	Yes
Sample activities	Weight lifting, picking up a bag of groceries	400-meter run, running up several flights of stairs	1500-meter run, 30-minute walk, standing in line for a long time

*For most activities, all three systems contribute to energy production; the duration and intensity of the activity determine which system predominates.

SOURCE: Adapted from Brooks, G. A., T. D. Fahey, and T. P. White. 1996. *Exercise Physiology: Human Bioenergetics and Its Applications,* 2d ed. Mountain View, Calif.: Mayfield.

Exercise and the Three Energy Systems

The muscles in your body have three energy systems by which they can create ATP and fuel cellular activity. These systems utilize different fuels and chemical processes, and they perform different, specific functions during exercise (Table 3-1).

The Immediate Energy System The **immediate energy system** provides energy rapidly but for only a short period of time. It is used to fuel activities that last for about 10 or fewer seconds—examples in sport include weight lifting and shot-putting; examples in daily life include rising from a chair or picking up a bag of groceries. The components of this energy system include existing cellular ATP stores and creatine phosphate (CP), a chemical that cells can use to make ATP. CP levels are depleted rapidly during exercise, so the maximum capacity of this energy system is reached within a few seconds. Cells must then switch to the other energy systems to restore levels of ATP and CP. (Without adequate ATP, muscles will stiffen and become unusable.)

The Nonoxidative (Anaerobic) Energy System The **nonoxidative energy system** is used at the start of an exercise session and for high-intensity activities lasting for about 10 seconds to 2 minutes, such as the 400-meter run. During daily activities, this system may be called on to help you run to catch a bus or dash up several flights of stairs. The nonoxidative energy system creates ATP by breaking down glucose and glycogen. This system doesn't require oxygen, which is why it is sometimes referred to as the **anaerobic** system. The capacity of this system to produce energy is limited, but it can generate a great deal of ATP in a short period of time. For this reason, it is the most important energy system for very intense exercise.

There are two key limiting factors for the nonoxidative energy system. First, the body's supply of glucose and glycogen is limited. Once these are depleted, a person may experience fatigue and dizziness, and judgment may be impaired. (The brain and nervous system rely on carbohydrates as fuel and must have a continuous supply to function properly.) Second, the nonoxidative system results in the production of **lactic acid.** Although lactic acid is an important fuel for the body, it releases substances called hydrogen ions that are thought to interfere with metabolism and muscle contraction, thereby causing fatigue. During heavy exercise, such as sprinting, the body produces large amounts of lactic acid and hydrogen ions, and muscles fatigue rapidly. Fortunately, exercise training increases the body's ability to cope with these substances.

The Oxidative (Aerobic) Energy System The **oxidative energy system** is used during any physical activity that lasts longer than about 2 minutes, such as distance running, swimming, hiking, or even standing in line for a long time. The oxidative system requires oxygen to generate ATP, which is why it is considered an **aerobic** process. The oxidative system cannot produce energy as quickly as the other two systems, but it can supply energy for much longer periods of time. It provides energy during most daily activities.

In the oxidative energy system, ATP production takes place in cellular structures called **mitochondria.** Because mitochondria can use carbohydrates (glucose and glycogen) or fats to produce ATP, the body's stores of fuel for this system are much greater than those for the other two energy systems. The actual fuel used depends on the intensity and duration of exercise and on the fitness status of the individual. Carbohydrates are favored during intense exercise, fats for lower-intensity activities. During a prolonged exercise session, carbohydrates are the predominant fuel at the start of the workout, but fat utilization increases over time. Fit individuals use a greater proportion of fat as fuel, an important adaptation because glycogen depletion is one of the limiting factors for the oxidative energy system. Thus, by being able to use more fat as fuel, a fit individual can exercise for a longer duration before glycogen is depleted and muscles become fatigued.

Oxygen is another limiting factor. The oxygen requirement of this energy system is proportional to the intensity of exercise—as intensity increases, so does oxygen consumption. There is a limit to the body's ability to increase the transport and use of oxygen; this limit is referred to as **maximal oxygen consumption,** or $\dot{V}O_{2max}$. $\dot{V}O_{2max}$ is determined partly by genetics and partly by fitness status. It depends on many factors, including the capacity of blood to carry oxygen, the rate at which oxygen is transported to the tissues, and the amount of oxygen that cells extract from the blood. $\dot{V}O_{2max}$ determines how intensely a person can perform endurance exercise and for how long, and it is considered the best overall measure of the capacity of the cardiorespiratory system. (The assessment tests described later in the chapter are designed to help you predict your $\dot{V}O_{2max}$.)

The Energy Systems in Combination Your body typically uses all three energy systems when you exercise. The intensity and duration of the activity will determine which system predominates. For example, when you play tennis, you use the immediate energy system when hitting the ball, but you replenish cellular energy stores using the nonoxidative and oxidative systems. When cycling, the oxidative system predominates. However, if you must suddenly exercise very intensely—ride up a steep hill, for example—the other systems become important because the oxidative system is unable to supply ATP fast enough to sustain high-intensity effort.

Physical Fitness and Energy Production Physically fit people can increase their metabolic rate substantially, generating the energy needed for powerful or sustained exercise. People with lower levels of fitness cannot respond to exercise in the same way. Their bodies are less capable of delivering oxygen and fuel to exercising muscles; they are also less able to cope with lactic acid and other substances produced during intense physical activity. Because of this, they fatigue more rapidly—their legs hurt and they breathe heavily walking up a flight of stairs, for example. Regular physical training can substantially improve the body's ability to produce energy and meet the challenges of increased physical activity.

For many sports, one energy system will be most important. For weight lifters, for example, it is the immediate energy system; for sprinters, the nonoxidative system; and for endurance runners, the oxidative system. In designing an exercise program, focus on the energy system most important to your goals. Because improving the functioning of the cardiorespiratory system is critical to overall wellness, endurance exercise that utilizes the oxidative energy system—activities performed at moderate to high intensities for a prolonged duration—is a key component of any health-related fitness program.

Cardiorespiratory endurance exercise helps the body become more efficient and better able to cope with physical challenges. It also lowers risk for many chronic diseases. Let's take a closer look at the physiological adaptations and long-term benefits of regular endurance exercise.

Improved Cardiorespiratory Functioning

At rest, a healthy cardiorespiratory system has little difficulty keeping pace with the body's need for oxygen, fuel, and waste removal. During exercise, however, the demands on the system increase dramatically as metabolic rate goes up. The principal cardiorespiratory responses to exercise include the following:

- Increased cardiac output. More blood is pumped by

TERMS **mitochondria** Intracellular structures containing enzymes used in the chemical reactions that convert the energy in food to a form the body can use.

maximal oxygen consumption, expressed as $\dot{V}O_{2max}$ The highest rate of oxygen consumption an individual is capable of during maximum physical effort, reflecting the body's ability to transport and use oxygen; measured in milliliters used per minute for each kilogram of body weight.

blood pressure The force exerted by the blood on the walls of the blood vessels; created by the pumping action of the heart. Blood pressure increases during systole and decreases during diastole.

free radicals Highly reactive compounds that can damage cells by taking electrons from key cellular components such as DNA or the cell membrane; produced by normal metabolic processes and through exposure to environmental factors, including sunlight.

the heart each minute because both heart rate and stroke volume (the amount of blood pumped with each beat) go up. Increased cardiac output speeds the delivery of oxygen and fuel and the removal of waste products.

- Increased ventilation (rate and depth of breathing).
- Increased blood flow to active skeletal muscles and to the heart; constant or slightly increased blood flow to the brain.
- Increased blood flow to the skin and increased sweating. The chemical reactions that produce energy for exercise release heat, which must be dissipated to maintain a safe body temperature.
- Decreased blood flow to the stomach, intestines, liver, and kidneys, resulting in reduced activity in the gastrointestinal tract and reduced urine output.

All of these changes help the body respond to the challenge of exercise in the short term. When performed regularly, endurance exercise also causes more permanent adaptations. It improves the functioning of the heart, the ability of the cardiorespiratory system to carry oxygen to the body's tissues, and the capacity of the cells to take up and use oxygen. These improvements reduce the effort required to carry out everyday activities and make the body better able to respond to physical challenges.

Endurance training enhances the health of the heart by maintaining or increasing its blood and oxygen supply, decreasing work and oxygen demand of the heart, and increasing the function of the heart muscle. The trained heart is more efficient and subject to less stress. It pumps more blood per beat, so heart rate is lower at rest and during exercise. The resting heart rate of a fit person is often 10–20 beats per minute lower than that of a sedentary person; this translates into as many as 10 million fewer beats in the course of one year. Improved heart efficiency results because endurance training improves heart contraction strength, increases heart cavity size (in young adults), and increases blood volume so that the heart pushes more blood into the circulation system during each of its contractions. Training also tends to reduce **blood pressure,** so the heart does not have to work as hard when it contracts.

Improved Cellular Metabolism

Regular endurance exercise also improves metabolism at the cellular level. It increases the number of capillaries in the muscles so that they can be supplied with more oxygen and fuel. It also trains the muscles to make the most of available oxygen and fuel so that they work more efficiently. Exercise increases the size and number of mitochondria in muscle cells, thereby increasing the energy capacity of the cells. Endurance training also helps in energy production by preventing glycogen depletion and increasing the muscles' ability to use lactic acid and fat as fuels.

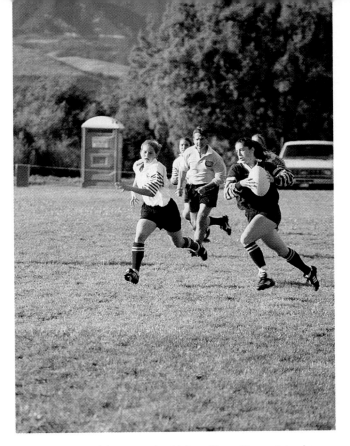

Exercise offers both long-term health benefits and immediate pleasures. Many popular sports and activities, including rugby, develop cardiorespiratory endurance.

Fitness programs that best develop metabolic efficiency are characterized by both long-duration, moderately intense endurance exercise and brief periods of more intense effort. For example, climbing a small hill while jogging or cycling introduces the kind of intense exercise that leads to more efficient use of lactic acid and fats. (As described earlier, activities of different intensities utilize different energy systems and will cause different adaptations.)

Regular exercise may also help protect your cells from chemical damage. Many scientists believe that aging and some chronic diseases are linked to cellular damage caused by **free radicals.** Training activates antioxidant enzymes that prevent free radical damage to cell structures, thereby enhancing health. (See Chapter 8 for more on free radicals and antioxidants.) Training also improves the functional stability of cells and tissues by improving the regulation of salts and fluids in the cells. This is particularly important in the heart, where instability can lead to cardiac arrest and death.

Reduced Risk of Chronic Disease

Regular endurance exercise lowers your risk of many chronic, disabling diseases. It can also help people with those diseases improve their health.

Cardiovascular Disease A sedentary lifestyle is one of the five major risk factors for **cardiovascular disease (CVD)** (see Chapter 11). The other factors are smoking, unhealthy cholesterol levels, high blood pressure, and obesity. People who are sedentary have CVD death rates significantly higher than those of fit individuals.

Endurance exercise has a positive effect on levels of fats in the blood. High concentrations of blood fats such as cholesterol and triglycerides are linked to cardiovascular disease because they contribute to the formation of fatty deposits on the lining of arteries. If one of the coronary arteries, which supply oxygenated blood to the heart, becomes blocked by such a deposit, the result is a heart attack; blockage of a cerebral artery can cause a stroke.

Cholesterol is carried in the blood by **lipoproteins,** which are classified according to size and density. Cholesterol carried by low-density lipoproteins (LDLs) tends to stick to the walls of arteries. High-density lipoproteins (HDLs), on the other hand, pick up excess cholesterol in the bloodstream and carry it back to the liver for excretion from the body. High LDL levels and low HDL levels are associated with a high risk of CVD. High levels of HDL and low levels of LDL are associated with lower risk. More information about cholesterol and heart disease is provided in Chapter 11. For our purposes in this chapter, it is important to know only that endurance exercise influences blood fat levels in a positive way—by increasing HDL and decreasing triglycerides (and possibly LDL)—thereby reducing the risk of CVD.

Regular exercise tends to reduce high blood pressure, a contributing factor in diseases such as **coronary heart disease,** stroke, kidney failure, and blindness. It also helps prevent obesity and diabetes, both of which contribute to CVD.

Cancer Some studies have shown a relationship between increased physical activity and a reduction in a person's risk of all types of cancer, but these findings are not conclusive. There is strong evidence that exercise reduces the risk of colon cancer and promising data that it reduces the risk of cancer of the breast and reproductive organs in women. Exercise may decrease the risk of colon cancer by speeding the movement of food through the gastrointestinal tract (quickly eliminating potential carcinogens), enhancing immune function, and reducing blood fats. The protective mechanism in the case of reproductive system cancers is less clear, but physical activity during the high school and college years may be particularly important for preventing breast cancer later in life.

Diabetes Recent studies have shown that regular exercise helps prevent the development of the most common form of diabetes (see Chapter 6 for more on diabetes). Exercise burns excess sugar and makes cells more sensitive to the hormone insulin, which is involved in the regulation of blood sugar levels. Obesity is a key risk factor for diabetes, and exercise helps keep body fat at healthy levels. For people who have diabetes, physical activity is an important part of treatment.

Osteoporosis A special benefit of exercise, especially for women, is protection against osteoporosis, a disease that results in loss of bone density and poor bone strength. Weight-bearing exercise helps build bone during the teens and twenties. People with denser bones can better endure the bone loss that occurs with aging. With stronger bones and muscles and better balance, fit people are less likely to experience debilitating falls and bone fractures. (See Chapter 8 for more on osteoporosis.)

Better Control of Body Fat

Too much body fat is linked to a variety of health problems, including cardiovascular disease, cancer, and diabetes. Healthy body composition can be difficult to achieve and maintain because a diet that contains all essential nutrients can be relatively high in calories, especially for someone who is sedentary. Excess calories are stored in the body as fat. Regular exercise increases daily calorie expenditure so that a healthy diet is less likely to lead to weight gain. Endurance exercise burns calories directly and, if intense enough, continues to do so by raising resting metabolic rate for several hours following an exercise session. A higher metabolic rate means that a person can consume more calories without gaining weight.

Endurance exercise can also help maintain or increase metabolic rate by helping people maintain a high proportion of fat-free mass: The more muscle mass, the higher the metabolic rate. Strength training, discussed in Chapter 4, is even more effective at building muscle mass than endurance training. (Energy balance and the role of exercise in improving body composition are discussed in detail in Chapter 6.)

TERMS **cardiovascular disease (CVD)** Disease of the heart and blood vessels.

lipoproteins Substances in blood, classified according to size, density, and chemical composition, that transport fats.

coronary heart disease Heart disease caused by the buildup of fatty deposits on the arteries that supply oxygen to the heart; also called *coronary artery disease.*

epinephrine A hormone secreted in response to stress that stimulates the heart, makes carbohydrates available in the liver and muscles, and releases fat from fat cells.

norepinephrine A stress hormone with many of the same effects as epinephrine.

endorphins Substances resembling morphine that are secreted by the brain and that decrease pain, suppress fatigue, and produce euphoria.

neurotransmitters Brain chemicals that transmit nerve impulses.

Exercise and the Mind

If you've ever gone for a long, brisk walk after a hard day's work, you know how refreshing exercise can be. Exercise can improve mood, stimulate creativity, clarify thinking, relieve anxiety, and provide an outlet for anger or aggression. But why does exercise make you feel good? Does it simply take your mind off your problems? Or does it cause a physical reaction that affects your mental state?

Current research indicates that exercise triggers many physical changes in the body that can alter mood. Scientists are now trying to explain how and why exercise affects the mind. One theory has to do with the physical structure of the brain. The area of the brain responsible for the movement of muscles is near the area responsible for thought and emotion. As muscles work vigorously, the resulting stimulation in the muscle center of the brain may also stimulate the thought and emotion center, producing improvements in mood and cognitive functions.

Other researchers suggest that exercise stimulates the release of **endorphins,** chemicals in the brain that can suppress fatigue, decrease pain, and produce euphoria. The "runner's high" often experienced after running several miles may be due to an increased production of endorphins.

A third area of research focuses on changes in brain activity during and after exercise. One change is an increase in alpha brain-wave activity. Alpha waves indicate a highly relaxed state; meditation also induces alpha wave activity. A second change is an alteration in the levels of **neurotransmitters,** brain chemicals that increase alertness and reduce stress.

Higher levels of neurotransmitters may explain how exercise improves mild to moderate cases of depression. Researchers have found that cardiorespiratory endurance exercise can be as effective as psychotherapy in treating depression, and even more effective when used in conjunction with other therapies. In addition to boosting neurotransmitter activity, exercise provides a distraction from stressful stimuli, enhances self-esteem, and may provide an opportunity for positive social interactions.

Although most people don't associate exercise with mental skills, physical activity has been shown to have positive effects on cognitive functioning in both the short term and the long term. Exercise improves alertness and memory and can help you perform cognitive tasks at your peak level. Exercise may also help boost creativity. In a study of college students, those who ran regularly or took aerobic dance classes scored significantly higher on standard psychological tests of creativity than sedentary students. Over the long term, exercise can slow and possibly even reverse certain age-related declines in cognitive performance, including slowed reaction time and loss of short-term memory and nonverbal reasoning skills.

The message from all this research is that exercise is a critical factor in developing *all* the dimensions of wellness, not just physical health. Even moderate exercise like walking briskly a few times per week can significantly improve your well-being. A lifetime of physical activity can leave you with a healthier body and a sharper, happier, more creative mind.

Improved Immune Function

Exercise can have either positive or negative effects on the immune system, the physiological processes that protect us from disease. Moderate endurance exercise boosts immune function, whereas excessive training (overtraining) depresses it. Physically fit people get fewer colds and upper respiratory tract infections than people who are not fit. In addition to regular exercise, the immune system can be strengthened by eating a well-balanced diet rich in whole grains, fruits, vegetables, and low-fat dairy and meat products; managing stress; and getting 7–8 hours of sleep every night.

Improved Psychological and Emotional Well-Being

Most people who participate in regular endurance exercise experience social, psychological, and emotional benefits. Performing physical activities provides proof of skill mastery and self-control, thus enhancing self-image. Recreational sports provide an opportunity to socialize, have fun, and strive to excel.

Endurance exercise also provides protection against the effects of stress that have been linked to poor cardiorespiratory health. Psychological stress causes increased secretion of **epinephrine** and **norepinephrine,** the so-called fight-or-flight hormones, which are thought to speed the buildup of fatty deposits in the arteries. Excessive hostility and anger are also associated with the risk of heart disease. Endurance exercise decreases the secretion of hormones triggered by emotional stress. It can diffuse hostility and alleviate depression and anxiety by providing an emotional outlet and inducing feelings of relaxation (see the box "Exercise and the Mind"). Regular exercise can also relieve sleeping problems.

Refer to the box "Benefits of Cardiorespiratory Endurance Exercise" for a summary of specific physiological benefits. As cardiorespiratory fitness is developed, these benefits translate into both physical and emotional well-being and a much lower risk of chronic disease.

ASSESSING CARDIORESPIRATORY FITNESS

The body's ability to maintain a level of exertion (exercise) for an extended period of time is a direct reflection of cardiorespiratory fitness. It is determined by the body's abil-

Cardiorespiratory System

Cardiorespiratory endurance exercise tends to increase the following:

- Heart size
- Stroke volume (the amount of blood pumped per beat)
- Total blood volume
- Number of red blood cells
- Blood concentration of high-density lipoproteins (HDLs)
- Capillary density (associated with the increased ability of cells to extract oxygen from blood)
- Overall efficiency of the delivery of oxygen to the tissues ($\dot{V}O_{2max}$)
- Blood flow to active muscles during exercise

Cardiorespiratory endurance exercise tends to decrease the following:

- Resting heart rate and heart rate at different workloads
- Concentrations of epinephrine and norepinephrine during exercise
- Blood levels of triglycerides and possibly low-density lipoproteins (LDLs)
- Blood pressure
- Platelet stickiness (a factor in coronary artery disease)

Skeletal Muscles

Cardiorespiratory endurance exercise tends to increase the following:

- Amount of stored glycogen
- Number and size of mitochondria (the energy-producing parts of cells)
- Myoglobin content (aids in the delivery of oxygen to the mitochondria)
- Capacity to use fat and lactic acid as fuel

Other Benefits

Cardiorespiratory endurance exercise tends to increase or maintain the following:

- Fat-free mass
- Density and strength of bones, ligaments, and tendons
- Sensitivity to insulin (helps prevent Type 2 diabetes)
- Ability to exercise during hot weather
- Performance in sports, recreational activities, and work
- Feelings of well-being
- Self-concept

Cardiorespiratory endurance exercise tends to decrease the following:

- Total body fat
- Strain associated with stress
- Anxiety and depression
- Risk of death from coronary artery disease, colon cancer, and some types of reproductive cancers (women)

---

ity to take up, distribute, and use oxygen during physical activity. As explained earlier, the best quantitative measure of cardiorespiratory endurance is maximal oxygen consumption, expressed as $\dot{V}O_{2max}$, the amount of oxygen the body uses when a person reaches maximum ability to supply oxygen during exercise (measured in milliliters of oxygen used per minute for each kilogram of body weight). Maximal oxygen consumption can be measured precisely in an exercise physiology laboratory through analysis of the air a person inhales and exhales when exercising to a level of exhaustion (maximum intensity). This procedure can be expensive and time-consuming, making it impractical for the average person.

Four Assessment Tests

Fortunately, several simple assessment tests provide reasonably good estimates of maximal oxygen consumption (within ±10–15% of the results of a laboratory test).

Four methods are described here and presented in Lab 3-1: a 1-mile walk test, a 3-minute step test, a 1.5-mile run-walk test, and the Åstrand-Rhyming cycle ergometer test. To assess yourself, choose among these methods based on your access to equipment, your current physical condition, and your own preference. Don't take any of these tests without checking with your physician if you are ill or have any of the risk factors for exercise discussed in Chapter 2 and Lab 2-2. Table 3-2 lists the fitness prerequisites and cautions recommended for each test.

You'll get more accurate results from these tests if you avoid strenuous activity the day of the test; avoid caffeine, which can affect heart rate; and don't smoke or eat a heavy meal for up to 3 hours before the test. Record your test results in Lab 3-1, and then use the appropriate formula to calculate your maximal oxygen consumption.

The 1-Mile Walk Test   The 1-mile walk test estimates your level of cardiorespiratory fitness (maximal oxygen

TABLE 3-2	Fitness Prerequisites and Cautions for the Cardiorespiratory Endurance Assessment Tests

Note: The conditions for exercise safety given in Chapter 2 apply to all fitness assessment tests. If you answered yes to any question on the PAR-Q in Lab 2-2, see your physician before taking any assessment test. If you experience any unusual symptoms while taking a test, stop exercising, and discuss your condition with your instructor.

Test	Fitness Prerequisites/Cautions
1-mile walk test	Recommended for anyone who meets the criteria for safe exercise. Can be used by individuals who cannot perform other tests because of low fitness level or injury.
3-minute step test	If you suffer from joint problems in your ankles, knees, or hips or are significantly overweight, check with your physician before taking this test.
1.5-mile run-walk test	Recommended for people who are healthy and at least moderately active. If you have been sedentary, you should participate in a 4- to 8-week walk-run program before taking the test. Don't take this test in extremely hot or cold weather if you aren't used to exercising under those conditions.
Åstrand-Rhyming test	Recommended for people who are healthy and at least moderately active. It can be taken by people with some joint problems because body weight is supported by the cycle.

consumption) based on the amount of time it takes you to complete 1 mile of brisk walking and your exercise heart rate at the end of your walk; age, gender, and body weight are also considered. A fast time and a low heart rate indicate a high level of cardiorespiratory endurance.

The 3-Minute Step Test   The rate at which the pulse returns to normal after exercise is also a good measure of cardiorespiratory capacity; heart rate remains lower and recovers faster in people who are more physically fit. For the step test, you step continually at a steady rate for 3 minutes and then monitor your heart rate during recovery.

The 1.5-Mile Run-Walk Test   The 1.5-mile run-walk test is considered one of the best indirect measures of cardiorespiratory capacity. Oxygen consumption increases with speed in distance running; a fast time on this test indicates high maximal oxygen consumption.

The Åstrand-Rhyming Cycle Ergometer Test   A cycle ergometer measures power output, the amount of resistance the cycle exerts against a person's pedaling. A higher power output means the cyclist is applying more pressure—that is, pedaling harder or faster. The Åstrand-Rhyming test estimates maximal oxygen consumption from the exercise heart rate reached after pedaling a cycle ergometer for 6 minutes at a constant rate and resistance. A low exercise heart rate after pedaling at a high power output indicates a high maximal oxygen consumption.

Monitoring Your Heart Rate

Each time your heart beats, it pumps blood into your arteries; this surge of blood causes a pulse that you can feel by holding your fingers against an artery. Counting your pulse to determine your exercise heart rate is a key part of most assessment tests for maximal oxygen consumption. Heart rate can also be used to monitor exercise intensity during a workout. (Intensity is described in more detail in the next section.)

The two most common sites for monitoring heart rate are the carotid artery in the neck and the radial artery in the wrist. To take your pulse, press your index and middle fingers gently on the correct site. You may have to shift position several times to find the best position to feel your pulse. Don't use your thumb to check your pulse; it has a pulse of its own that can confuse your count. Be careful not to push too hard, particularly when taking your pulse in the carotid artery (strong pressure on this artery may cause a reflex that slows the heart rate).

Heart rates are usually assessed in beats per minute (bpm). But counting your pulse for an entire minute isn't practical when you're exercising. And because heart rate slows rapidly when you stop exercising, it can give inaccurate results. It's best to do a shorter count—10 seconds—and then multiply the result by 6 to get your heart rate in beats per minute. The same procedure can be used to take someone else's pulse, as in the cycle ergometer test.

Interpreting Your Score

Once you've completed one or more of the assessment tests, use Table 3-3 to determine your level of cardiorespiratory fitness. Find the row that corresponds to your age and gender, and then find the category that contains your score for maximal oxygen consumption. For example, a 19-year-old female with a maximal oxygen consumption score of 36 ml/kg/min would be classified as

A pulse count can be used to determine exercise heart rate. The pulse can be taken at the carotid artery in the neck (left) or at the radial artery in the wrist (right).

TABLE 3-3	Cardiorespiratory Fitness Classification					
	Maximal Oxygen Consumption (ml/kg/min)					
	Very Poor	*Poor*	*Fair*	*Good*	*Excellent*	*Superior*
Women						
Age: 18–29	Below 30.6	30.6–33.7	33.8–36.6	36.7–40.9	41.0–46.7	Above 46.7
30–39	Below 28.7	28.7–32.2	32.3–34.5	34.6–38.5	38.6–43.8	Above 43.8
40–49	Below 26.5	26.5–29.4	29.5–32.2	32.3–36.2	36.3–40.9	Above 40.9
50–59	Below 24.3	24.3–26.8	26.9–29.3	29.4–32.2	32.3–36.7	Above 36.7
60 and over	Below 22.8	22.8–24.4	24.5–27.1	27.2–31.1	31.2–37.4	Above 37.4
Men						
Age: 18–29	Below 37.1	37.1–40.9	41.0–44.1	44.2–48.1	48.2–53.9	Above 53.9
30–39	Below 35.4	35.4–38.8	38.9–42.3	42.4–46.7	46.8–52.4	Above 52.4
40–49	Below 33.0	33.0–36.7	36.8–39.8	39.9–44.0	44.1–50.3	Above 50.3
50–59	Below 30.2	30.2–33.7	33.8–36.6	36.7–40.9	41.0–47.0	Above 47.0
60 and over	Below 26.5	26.5–30.1	30.2–33.5	33.6–38.0	38.1–45.1	Above 45.1

SOURCE: Based on norms from the Cooper Institute for Aerobics Research, Dallas, Texas; used with permission.

having fair cardiorespiratory fitness. You can see from Table 3-3 that there are differences in ratings for $\dot{V}O_{2max}$ between men and women; for more on this disparity, see the box "Gender Differences in Cardiorespiratory Endurance."

You can monitor the progress of your fitness program by repeating the cardiorespiratory assessment test(s) from time to time. Because your $\dot{V}O_{2max}$ score will vary somewhat for different types of tests, always compare scores for the *same* test.

DEVELOPING A CARDIORESPIRATORY ENDURANCE PROGRAM

Cardiorespiratory endurance exercises are best for developing the type of fitness associated with good health, so they should serve as the focus of your exercise program.

To create a successful endurance exercise program, you must set realistic goals; choose suitable activities; set your starting frequency, intensity, and duration of exercise at appropriate levels; remember to warm up and cool down; and adjust your program as your fitness improves.

Setting Goals

You can use the results of cardiorespiratory fitness assessment tests to set a specific oxygen consumption goal for your cardiorespiratory endurance program. Your goal should be high enough to ensure a healthy cardiorespiratory system, but not so high that it will be impossible to achieve. Scores in the fair and good ranges for maximal oxygen consumption suggest good fitness; scores in the excellent and superior ranges indicate a high standard of physical performance. You can also set more general goals, such as lowering your risk for diabetes or being able to hike 5 miles.

Research has shown that there are significant differences in the average levels of cardiorespiratory endurance, as measured by maximal oxygen consumption, for men and women. When expressed in absolute terms, maximal oxygen consumption is about 40% higher in men. When this is adjusted for body weight, as it is in Table 3-3, the difference drops to 20%—a smaller difference, but still significant.

Several factors are believed to contribute to this difference. Males tend to be larger than females, and they have larger hearts, in both size and volume. This means that their hearts pump more blood with each beat (stroke volume), thereby delivering more oxygenated blood to working muscles. Females tend to have higher heart rates during exercise, but this higher rate does not entirely compensate for their lower stroke volume.

Men have relatively higher concentrations of hemoglobin in their blood than women. Hemoglobin is a blood protein that transports oxygen throughout the body; higher hemoglobin levels translate into a higher maximal oxygen consumption. Men have higher levels of androgens (steroid hormones), which stimulate their bodies to produce more hemoglobin. And menstrual blood loss contributes to lower hemoglobin levels among women.

Differences in body composition also affect maximal oxygen consumption. Men tend to have relatively more muscle mass, while women's bodies have a higher percentage of fat. (Body composition is discussed in greater detail in Chapter 6.) This additional muscle mass gives men more strength and power in both absolute and relative terms, and it raises maximal oxygen consumption. The relationship between maximal oxygen consumption and fat-free mass is so strong that when $\dot{V}O_{2max}$ is expressed in terms of fat-free weight instead of total body weight, the gender difference in maximal oxygen consumption drops to about 10%.

One area in which there is no difference between the sexes is in the benefits of training. Both men and women can improve their maximal oxygen consumption by up to 15–30%. Physical activity is critical for the health and wellness of everyone.

SOURCE: Adapted from Brooks, G. A., T. D. Fahey, and T. P. White. 1996. *Exercise Physiology: Human Bioenergetics and Its Applications*, 2d ed. Mountain View, Calif.: Mayfield.

Choosing Sports and Activities

As mentioned in Chapter 2, cardiorespiratory endurance exercises include activities that involve the rhythmic use of large muscle groups for an extended period of time, such as jogging, walking, cycling, aerobic dancing (group exercise), cross-country skiing, and swimming. Start-and-stop sports, such as tennis and racquetball, also qualify, as long as you have enough skill to play continuously and intensely enough to raise your heart rate to target levels. Cardiorespiratory fitness ratings of many common activities are listed in the box "Activities and Sports for Developing Cardiorespiratory Endurance."

Having fun is a strong motivator; select a physical activity that you enjoy, and it will be easier to stay with your program. Exercising with a friend can also be helpful as a motivator. Consider whether you prefer competitive or individual sports, or whether starting something new would be best. Other important considerations are access to facilities, expense, and the time required to achieve an adequate skill level and workout.

Determining Frequency of Training

To build cardiorespiratory endurance, you should exercise 3–5 days per week. Beginners should start with 3 and work up to 5 days per week. Training more than 5 days per week can lead to injury and isn't necessary for the typical person on an exercise program designed to promote wellness. Training fewer than 3 days per week

makes it difficult to improve your fitness (unless exercise intensity is very high) or to use exercise to lose weight. In addition, you risk injury because your body never gets a chance to fully adapt to regular exercise training.

Determining Intensity of Training

Intensity is the most important factor in achieving training effects. You must exercise intensely enough to stress your body so that fitness improves. Two methods of monitoring exercise intensity are described below; choose the method that works best for you. Be sure to make adjustments in your intensity levels for environmental or individual factors. For example, on a hot and humid day or on your first day back to your program after an illness, you should decrease your intensity level.

Target Heart Rate Zone One of the best ways to monitor the intensity of cardiorespiratory endurance exercise is to measure your heart rate. It isn't necessary to exercise at your maximum heart rate to improve maximal oxygen consumption. Fitness adaptations occur at lower heart rates with a much lower risk of injury.

According to the American College of Sports Medicine, your **target heart rate zone**—rates at which you should

target heart rate zone The range of heart rates that should **TERMS** be reached and maintained during cardiorespiratory endurance exercise to obtain training effects.

Activities and Sports for Developing Cardiorespiratory Endurance

The potential of an activity to develop cardiorespiratory endurance depends primarily on the intensity, duration, and frequency of training. The ratings given here are general guidelines.

High Potential

Aerobic dance
Backpacking
Badminton (singles)
Basketball
Bicycling
Cross-country skiing
Cross-country skiing machine
Field hockey
Frisbee, ultimate
Handball (singles)
Hiking
Hockey, ice and roller
In-line skating
Jogging and running
Karate

Lacrosse
Outdoor fitness trails
Racquetball (singles)
Rope skipping
Rowing
Rugby
Soccer
Squash (singles)
Stationary cycling
Step aerobics
Swimming
Tennis (singles)
Treadmill
Walking
Water Polo
Wrestling

Medium Potential

Ballet
Ballroom dancing
Baseball (pitcher and catcher)
Canoeing and kayaking
Cheerleading
Fencing
Folk and square dancing
Football, touch
Horseback riding
Judo
Modern dance
Popular dancing
Rock climbing
Skating, ice and roller
Skiing, alpine

Slide boarding
Surfing
Synchronized swimming
Table tennis
Volleyball
Water aerobics
Water skiing

Low Potential

Archery
Bowling
Golf (riding cart)
Sailing
Weight training
Yoga

exercise to experience cardiorespiratory benefits—is between 65% and 90% of your maximum heart rate. To calculate your target heart rate zone, follow these steps:

1. Estimate your maximum heart rate (MHR) by subtracting your age from 220, or have it measured precisely by undergoing an exercise stress test in a physician's office, hospital, or sports medicine laboratory.

2. Multiply your MHR by 65% and 90% to calculate your target heart rate zone.

For example, a 19-year-old would calculate her target heart rate zone as follows:

MHR = 220 − 19 = 201
65% training intensity = 0.65 × 201 = 131 bpm
90% training intensity = 0.90 × 201 = 181 bpm

To gain fitness benefits, the young woman in our example would have to exercise at an intensity that raises her heart rate to between 131 and 181 bpm.

Use Lab 3-2 to determine your target heart rate zone. If you have been sedentary, start by exercising at the lower end of your target heart rate range (65% training intensity) for at least 4–6 weeks. Fast and significant gains in maximal oxygen consumption can be made by exercising closer to the top of the range, but you may increase your risk of injury and overtraining. You *can* achieve significant health benefits by exercising at the bottom of your target range, so don't feel pressured into exercising at an unnecessarily intense level. If you exercise at a lower intensity, you can increase the duration or frequency of training to obtain as much benefit to your health, as long

as you are above the 65% training threshold. (For people with a very low initial level of fitness, a lower training intensity, 55–64% of maximum heart rate, may be sufficient to achieve improvements in maximal oxygen consumption, especially at the start of an exercise program.)

By monitoring your heart rate, you will always know if you are working hard enough to improve, not hard enough, or too hard. To monitor your heart rate during exercise, count your pulse while you're still moving or immediately after you stop exercising. Count beats for 10 seconds, and then multiply that number by 6 to see if your heart rate is in your target zone. If the young woman in our example were aiming for 144 bpm, she would want a 10-second count of 24 beats.

Ratings of Perceived Exertion The second way to monitor intensity is to monitor your perceived level of exertion. Repeated pulse counting during exercise can become a nuisance if it interferes with the activity. As your exercise program progresses, you will probably become familiar with the amount of exertion required to raise your heart rate to target levels. In other words, you will know how you feel when you have exercised intensely enough. If this is the case, you can use the scale of **ratings of perceived exertion (RPE)** shown in Figure 3-3 to monitor the intensity of your exercise session without checking your pulse.

To use the RPE scale, select a rating that corresponds to your subjective perception of how hard you are exercising when you are training in your target heart rate zone. If your target zone is about 135–155 bpm, exercise in-

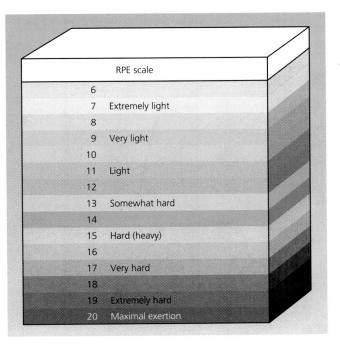

RPE scale	
6	
7	Extremely light
8	
9	Very light
10	
11	Light
12	
13	Somewhat hard
14	
15	Hard (heavy)
16	
17	Very hard
18	
19	Extremely hard
20	Maximal exertion

Figure 3-3   Ratings of perceived exertion.

tensely enough to raise your heart rate to that level, and then associate a rating—for example, "somewhat hard" or "hard" (14 or 15)—with how hard you feel you are working. To reach and maintain intensity in future workouts, exercise hard enough to reach what you feel is the same level of exertion. You should periodically check your RPE against your target heart rate zone to make sure it's correct. Research has shown RPE to be an accurate means of monitoring exercise intensity, and you may find it more convenient than pulse counting.

Determining Duration of Training

A total duration of 20–60 minutes is recommended; exercise can take place in a single session or in multiple bouts lasting 10 or more minutes. The total duration of exercise depends on its intensity. To improve cardiorespiratory endurance during a low-to-moderate-intensity activity such as walking or slow swimming, you should exercise for 45–60 minutes. For high-intensity exercise performed at the top of your target heart rate zone, a duration of 20 minutes is sufficient. Some studies have shown that 5–10 minutes of extremely intense exercise (greater than 90% of maximal oxygen consumption) improves cardiorespiratory endurance. However, training at this intensity, particularly during high-impact activities, increases the risk of injury. Also, because of the discomfort of high-intensity exercise, you are more likely to discontinue your exercise program. Longer-duration, low-to-moderate-intensity activities generally result in more gradual gains in maximal oxygen consumption. You

should start off with less-vigorous activities and only gradually increase intensity.

Warming Up and Cooling Down

It's important to warm up before every session of cardiorespiratory endurance exercise and to cool down afterward. Because the body's muscles work better when their temperature is slightly above resting level, warming up enhances performance and decreases the chance of injury. It gives the body time to redirect blood to active muscles and the heart time to adapt to increased demands. Warming up also helps spread **synovial fluid** throughout the joints, which helps protect their surfaces from injury.

As mentioned in Chapter 2, a warm-up session should include low-intensity movements similar to those in the activity that will follow. Low-intensity movements include walking slowly before beginning a brisk walk, hitting forehands and backhands before a tennis match, and running a 12-minute mile before progressing to an 8-minute one. Some experts also recommend including stretching exercises in your warm-up; however, it's best to stretch after your body temperature has been elevated by the active part of the warm-up (see Chapter 5).

Cooling down after exercise is important for returning the body to a nonexercising state. A cool-down, consisting of 5–10 minutes of reduced activity, should follow every workout to allow heart rate, breathing, and circulation to return to normal. Stretching exercises can be part of a cool-down.

The general pattern of a safe and successful workout for cardiorespiratory fitness is illustrated in Figure 3-4.

Maintaining Cardiorespiratory Fitness

Although your fitness level will probably improve quickly at the beginning of your fitness program, this rate of progress will probably slow after 4–6 weeks. The more fit you become, the harder you will have to work to improve. But there is a limit. Increasing intensity and duration indefinitely can lead to injury. Once you reach an acceptable level of fitness, maintain it by continuing to exercise at the same intensity at least 3 nonconsecutive days every week.

EXERCISE INJURIES

Even the most careful physically active person can suffer an injury. Most injuries are annoying rather than serious

ratings of perceived exertion (RPE) A system of monitoring exercise intensity based on assigning a number to the subjective perception of target intensity.

synovial fluid Fluid found within many joints that provides lubrication and nutrition to the cells of the joint surface.

TERMS

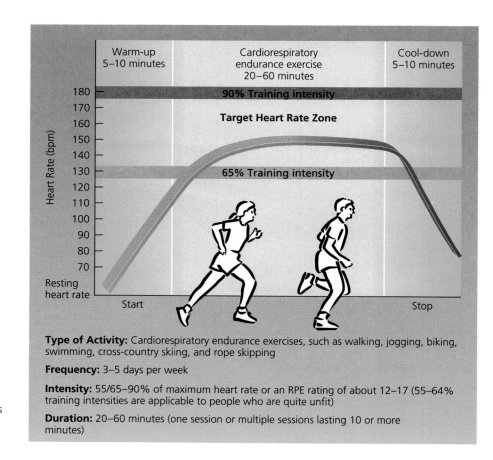

| Warm-up 5–10 minutes | Cardiorespiratory endurance exercise 20–60 minutes | Cool-down 5–10 minutes |

90% Training intensity

Target Heart Rate Zone

65% Training intensity

Heart Rate (bpm): 180 170 160 150 140 130 120 110 100 90 80 70

Resting heart rate

Start   Stop

Type of Activity: Cardiorespiratory endurance exercises, such as walking, jogging, biking, swimming, cross-country skiing, and rope skipping

Frequency: 3–5 days per week

Intensity: 55/65–90% of maximum heart rate or an RPE rating of about 12–17 (55–64% training intensities are applicable to people who are quite unfit)

Duration: 20–60 minutes (one session or multiple sessions lasting 10 or more minutes)

Figure 3-4   A cardiorespiratory endurance workout. Longer-duration exercise at lower intensities can often be as beneficial for promoting health as shorter-duration, high-intensity exercise.

or permanent. However, an injury that isn't cared for properly can escalate into a chronic problem, sometimes serious enough to permanently curtail the activity. It's important to learn how to deal with injuries so they don't derail your fitness program. Strategies for the care of common exercise injuries appear in Table 3-4; some general guidelines are given below.

When to Call a Physician

Some injuries require medical attention. Consult a physician for head and eye injuries, possible ligament injuries, broken bones, and internal disorders such as chest pain, fainting, elevated body temperature, and intolerance to hot weather. Also seek medical attention for ostensibly minor injuries that do not get better within a reasonable amount of time. You may need to modify your exercise program for a few weeks to allow an injury to heal. A knowledgeable physician can often give you important medical advice that will speed healing and get you back to your program sooner.

Managing Minor Exercise Injuries

For minor cuts and scrapes, stop the bleeding and clean the wound. Treat injuries to soft tissue (muscles and joints) immediately with rest and ice packs. Elevate the affected part of the body, and compress it with an elastic

bandage to minimize swelling. Apply ice regularly for 36–48 hours after an injury occurs or until all the swelling is gone. (Don't leave ice on one spot for more than 20 minutes.) Some experts also recommend taking an over-the-counter medication such as aspirin, ibuprofen, or naproxen to decrease inflammation.

Don't apply heat to an injury at first because heat draws blood to the area and increases swelling. After the swelling has subsided, apply either moist heat (hot towels, heat packs, warm water immersion) or dry heat (heating pads) to speed up healing.

To rehabilitate your body, follow the steps listed in the box "Rehabilitation Following a Minor Athletic Injury."

Preventing Injuries

The best method for dealing with exercise injuries is to prevent them. If you choose activities for your program carefully and follow the training guidelines described here and in Chapter 2, you should be able to avoid most types of injuries. Important guidelines for preventing athletic injuries include the following:

- Train regularly, and stay in condition.
- Gradually increase the intensity, duration, or frequency of your workouts.
- Avoid or minimize high-impact activities.
- Get proper rest between exercise sessions.

TABLE 3-4	*Care of Common Exercise Injuries*

Injury	Symptoms	Treatment
Blister	Accumulation of fluid in one spot under the skin	Don't pop or drain it unless it interferes too much with your daily activities. If it does pop, clean the area with antiseptic and cover with a bandage. Do not remove the skin covering the blister.
Bruise (contusion)	Pain, swelling, and discoloration	R-I-C-E: rest, ice, compression, elevation.
Fractures and dislocations	Pain, swelling, tenderness, loss of function, and deformity	Seek medical attention, immobilize the affected area, and apply cold.
Joint sprain	Pain, tenderness, swelling, discoloration, and loss of function	R-I-C-E.
Muscle cramp	Painful, spasmodic muscle contractions	Gently stretch and/or massage the cramped area. Drink fluids if exercising in hot weather.
Muscle soreness or stiffness	Pain and tenderness in the affected muscle	Stretch the affected muscle gently; exercise at a low intensity; apply heat.
Muscle strain	Pain, tenderness, swelling, and loss of strength in the affected muscle	R-I-C-E; apply heat after 36–48 hours if swelling has disappeared. Stretch and strengthen the affected area.
Shin splints	Pain and tenderness on the front of the lower leg; sometimes also pain in the calf muscle	Rest; apply ice to the affected area several times a day and before exercise; wrap with tape for support.
Side stitch	Pain on the side of the abdomen	Decrease the intensity of your workout, or stop altogether; bend over in the direction of the stitch.
Tendinitis	Pain and tenderness of the affected area; loss of use	R-I-C-E; apply heat after 36–48 hours if swelling has disappeared. Stretch and strengthen the affected area.

SOURCES: Adapted from Fahey, T. D., ed. 1986. *Athletic Training Principles and Practice.* Mountain View, Calif.: Mayfield. Pryor, E., and M. G. Kraines. 1996. *Keep Moving! It's Aerobic Dance,* 3d ed. Mountain View, Calif.: Mayfield.

TACTICS AND TIPS   *Rehabilitation Following a Minor Athletic Injury*

1. Reduce the initial inflammation using the R-I-C-E principle:

   Rest: Stop using the injured area as soon as you experience pain. Avoid any activity that causes pain.

   Ice: Apply ice to the injured area to reduce swelling and alleviate pain. Apply ice immediately for 10–20 minutes, and repeat every few hours until the swelling disappears. Let the injured part return to normal temperature between icings, and do not apply ice to one area for more than 20 minutes. An easy method for applying ice is to freeze water in a paper cup, peel some of the paper away, and rub the exposed ice on the injured area. If the injured area is large, you can surround it with several bags of crushed ice or ice cubes; bags of frozen vegetables can also be used. Place a thin towel between the bag and your skin. If you use a cold gel pack, limit application time to 10 minutes.

   Compression: Wrap the injured area firmly with an elastic or compression bandage between icings. If the area starts throbbing or begins to change color, the bandage may be wrapped too tightly. Do not sleep with the wrap on.

   Elevation: Raise the injured area above heart level to decrease the blood supply and reduce swelling. Pillows, books, or a low chair or stool can be used to raise the injured area.

2. After 36–48 hours, apply heat if the swelling has completely disappeared. Immerse the affected area in warm water or apply warm compresses, a hot water bottle, or a heating pad. As soon as it's comfortable, begin moving the affected joints slowly. If you feel pain, or if the injured area begins to swell again, reduce the amount of movement. Continue stretching and moving the affected area until you have regained normal range of motion.

3. Gradually begin exercising the injured area to build strength and endurance. Depending on the type of injury, weight training, walking, and resistance training with a partner can all be effective.

4. Gradually reintroduce the stress of an activity until you can return to full intensity. Don't progress too rapidly or you'll reinjure yourself. Before returning to full exercise participation, you should have a full range of motion in your joints, normal strength and balance among your muscles, normal coordinated patterns of movement (with no injury compensation movements, such as limping), and little or no pain.

Many exercise injuries can be handled by the individual, but serious injuries, such as broken bones and torn ligaments, require medical attention.

- Warm up thoroughly before you exercise, and cool down afterward.
- Achieve and maintain a good level of flexibility.
- Use proper body mechanics when lifting objects or executing sports skills.
- Don't exercise when you are ill or overtrained.
- Use proper equipment, particularly shoes, and choose an appropriate exercise surface. If you exercise on a grass field, soft track, or wooden floor, you are less likely to be injured than on concrete or a hard track.
- Don't return to your normal exercise program until your athletic injuries have healed.

SUMMARY

- The cardiorespiratory system consists of the heart, blood vessels, and respiratory system; it picks up and transports oxygen, nutrients, and waste products.
- Chemical energy from food is used to produce ATP and fuel cellular activities. During exercise, ATP can be produced by the immediate, nonoxidative, and oxidative energy systems; the duration and intensity of the activity determine which energy system predominates. Cardiorespiratory fitness is measured by maximal oxygen consumption ($\dot{V}O_{2max}$).
- Benefits of cardiorespiratory endurance exercise include improved cardiorespiratory functioning; improved cellular metabolism; reduced risk of

chronic diseases, including cardiovascular disease, cancer, diabetes, and osteoporosis; better control of body fat; improved immune function; and improved psychological and emotional well-being.
- Direct measurement of $\dot{V}O_{2max}$ is performed in scientific laboratories. Indirect assessment methods include the 1-mile walk test, the 3-minute step test, the 1.5-mile walk-run test, and the Åstrand-Rhyming cycle ergometer test.
- A successful endurance exercise program sets realistic goals; includes suitable activities; sets starting frequency, intensity, and duration at appropriate levels; includes warm-up and cool-down activities; and is adjusted as fitness improves.
- Intensity of training, the most important factor in achieving cardiorespiratory benefits, can be measured through target heart rate zone and ratings of perceived exertion.
- Serious injuries require medical attention. Application of the R-I-C-E principle (rest, ice, compression, elevation) is appropriate for treating many types of muscle or joint injuries.

FOR MORE INFORMATION

Refer to Chapter 2 for resources on exercise physiology and fitness testing. Additional sources of information and programs include the YMCA and campus or private sports medicine centers for fitness testing; health clubs for places to exercise and training advice; and physical education departments for activity classes.

Books

American Heart Association. 1995. *The Healthy Heart Walking Book.* Indianapolis: Macmillan General Reference. *Includes advice for getting started, building endurance, and maintaining a walking program.*

Edwards, S. 1996. *Sally Edwards' Heart Zone Training: Exercise Smart, Stay Fit and Live Longer.* Holbrook, Mass.: Adams Media. *Describes the use of heart rate and heart rate monitors for the development of fitness; upbeat and motivational.*

Katz, J. 1996. *The All-American Aquatic Handbook: Your Passport to Lifetime Fitness.* Needham Heights, Mass.: Allyn and Bacon. *A guide for people interested in swimming as their primary form of exercise.*

Kusinitz, I., and M. Fine. 1995. *Your Guide to Getting Fit,* 3d ed. Mountain View, Calif.: Mayfield. *Includes assessment tests and a step-by-step guide to developing a cardiorespiratory endurance exercise program.*

Lebow, F., and G. Averbuch, eds. 1997. *The New York Road Runners Club Complete Book of Running and Fitness.* New York: Random House. *A complete guide to running for everyone from the casual jogger to the competitive marathoner.*

Pfeiffer, R. P., and B. C. Mangus. 1998. *Concepts of Athletic Training.* Sudbury, Mass.: Jones and Bartlett. *A comprehensive look at the prevention and treatment of athletic injuries.*

Pryor, E., and M. Kraines. 1997. *Keep Moving! It's Aerobic Dance,*

COMMON QUESTIONS ANSWERED

What kind of clothing should I wear during exercise? Exercise clothing should be comfortable, let you move freely, and allow your body to cool itself. Avoid clothing that constricts normal blood flow or is made from nylon or rubberized fabrics that prevent evaporation of perspiration. Cotton is an excellent material for facilitating the evaporation of sweat. If you sweat heavily when you exercise and find that too much moisture accumulates in cotton clothing, try fabrics containing synthetic materials such as polypropylene that wick moisture away from the skin. Socks made with moisture-wicking compounds may be particularly helpful for people whose feet sweat heavily.

What kind of equipment should I buy? Once you have chosen activities to develop cardiorespiratory fitness, carefully consider what equipment you'll need. Good equipment enhances your enjoyment and decreases your risk of injury. The recent surge of interest in physical activity has been accompanied by a wave of new equipment, but some new products are either overpriced or of poor quality. See the box "Choosing Equipment for Fitness and Sport" for ways to make sound decisions about equipment.

Do I need a special diet for my endurance exercise program? No. For most people, a nutritionally balanced diet contains all the energy and nutrients needed to sustain an exercise program. Don't waste your money on unnecessary vitamins, minerals, and protein supplements. (Chapter 8 has information about putting together a healthy diet.)

Should I drink extra fluids before or during exercise? Yes. your body depends on water to carry out many chemical reactions and to regulate body temperature. Sweating during exercise depletes your body's water supply and can lead to dehydration if fluids aren't replaced. Serious dehydration can cause reduced blood volume, increased heart rate, elevated body temperature, muscle cramps, heat stroke, and even death. Drinking water before and during exercise is important to prevent dehydration and enhance your performance.

Thirst alone isn't a good indication of how much you need to drink because one's sense of thirst is quickly depressed by drinking even small amounts of water. As a rule of thumb, try to drink about 8 ounces of water (more in hot weather) for every 30 minutes of heavy exercise. Bring a water bottle when you exercise so you can replace your fluids while they're being depleted. Water, preferably cold, and diluted carbohydrate drinks are the best fluid replacements. (See Chapter 8 for more on diet and fluid recommendations for active people.)

What is cross-training? Cross-training is a pattern of training in which your program centers on two or more different cardiorespiratory endurance activities. Alternating activities can make your exercise program more fun, but it may slow your development of activity-specific adaptations. For example, if you alternate jogging and tennis, you will probably not develop the coordination, speed, and upper-body strength associated with tennis as quickly as if you just played tennis.

However, if you are quickly bored with a single activity, you'll be more likely to stick with your exercise program if you alternate activities to make it more interesting. Alternating activities may also reduce your risk of some types of injuries.

Is it all right to participate in cardiorespiratory endurance exercise while menstruating? Yes. There is no evidence that exercise during menstruation is unhealthy or that it has negative effects on performance. If you have headaches, backaches, and abdominal pain during menstruation, you may not feel like exercising; for some women, exercise helps relieve these symptoms. Listen to your body, and exercise at whatever intensity is comfortable for you.

Is endurance exercise safe during pregnancy? For most women, there is no reason not to exercise during pregnancy. In the absence of either medical or obstetric complications, pregnant women can continue with an established exercise program and can obtain all the benefits of regular exercise. However, although maternal fitness and a sense of well-being may be enhanced by exercise, no level of exercise during pregnancy has been conclusively demonstrated to be beneficial in improving the outcome of pregnancy.

Consult your physician before continuing or beginning an exercise program. If you were exercising before your pregnancy, you can probably continue with your regular program and modify it as necessary. If you weren't exercising before pregnancy, begin slowly. Throughout pregnancy you should listen to your body and adjust your exercise program to keep it comfortable. Follow the general pattern for cardiorespiratory endurance exercise described in this chapter. Be sure to warm up, cool down, and drink plenty of fluids. General guidelines for exercise during pregnancy from the American College of Obstetricians and Gynecologists are summarized below.

- Exercise regularly (at least three times per week) rather than intermittently.

- Avoid exercise in a supine position—lying on your back—after the first trimester. Research indicates that this position restricts blood flow to the uterus. Also avoid prolonged periods of motionless standing.

- Modify the intensity of your exercise according to how you feel. Stop exercising if you feel fatigued, and don't exercise to exhaustion. You may find that non-weight-bearing exercises such as cycling and swimming are more comfortable than weight-bearing activities in the later months of pregnancy; they also minimize the risk of injury.

- Take care when performing any activity in which balance is important or in which losing balance would prove dangerous. Pregnancy shifts your center of gravity. Also avoid any type of exercise that has the potential for even mild abdominal trauma.

- Eat an adequate diet.

(continued)

- Avoid heat stress, particularly during the first trimester, by drinking an adequate amount of fluids, wearing appropriate clothing, and avoiding exercise in hot and humid weather.

- Resume prepregnancy exercise routines gradually. Many of the changes of pregnancy persist 4–6 weeks postpartum.

- If you experience any unusual symptoms, stop exercising, and consult your physician.

Is it safe to exercise in hot weather?   Prolonged, vigorous exercise can be dangerous in hot and humid weather. Heat from exercise is released in the form of sweat, which cools the skin and the blood circulating near the body surface as it evaporates. The hotter the weather, the more water the body loses through sweat; the more humid the weather, the less efficient the sweating mechanism is at lowering body temperature. If you lose too much water or if your body temperature rises too high, you may suffer from a heat disorder such as heat exhaustion or heat stroke. Use caution when exercising if the temperature is above 80°F or if humidity is above 60%. To exercise safely, watch for the signals of heat disorder, regardless of the weather, and follow the tips given in the box "Exercising in Hot Weather."

Is it safe to exercise in cold weather?   If you dress warmly in layers and don't stay out in very cold temperatures for too long, exercise can be safe even in subfreezing temperatures. Take both the temperature and the wind-chill factor into account when choosing clothing. Dress in layers so you can subtract them as you warm up and add them if you get cold. A substantial amount of heat loss comes from the head and neck, so keep these areas covered. In subfreezing temperatures, protect the areas of your body most susceptible to frostbite—fingers, toes, ears, nose, and cheeks—with warm socks, mittens or gloves, and a cap, hood, or ski mask. Wear clothing that "breathes" and will wick moisture away from your skin to avoid being overheated by trapped perspiration. Warm up thoroughly, and drink plenty of fluids.

Is it safe to exercise in a smoggy city?   Do not exercise outdoors during a smog alert or if air quality is very poor (symptoms of poor air quality include eye and throat irritation and respiratory discomfort). If you have any type of cardiorespiratory difficulty, avoid exertion outdoors when air quality is poor. You can avoid smog and air pollution by exercising in parks, near water (riverbanks, lakeshores, and ocean beaches), or in residential areas with less traffic (areas with stop-and-go traffic will have lower air quality than areas where traffic moves quickly). Air quality is usually better in the early morning and late evening.

TACTICS AND TIPS   *Exercising in Hot Weather*

- Use caution when exercising in extreme heat or humidity (over 80°F and/or 60% humidity).

- Expose yourself gradually to exercise in hot and humid environments; work up slowly to your usual levels of intensity and duration. Use target heart rate to monitor exercise intensity in the heat.

- Exercise in the early morning or evening, when temperatures are lowest.

- Drink a glass or two of fluids before you begin exercising, and drink 4–8 ounces of fluid every 10–15 minutes during exercise (more frequently during high-intensity activities).

- Wear clothing that "breathes," allowing air to circulate and cool the body. Wearing white or light colors will help by reflecting, rather than absorbing, heat. A hat can help keep direct sun off your face. Do not wear rubber, plastic, or other nonporous clothing.

- Rest frequently in the shade.

- Keep a record of your morning body weight to track whether weight lost through sweating is restored.

- Slow down or stop if you begin to feel uncomfortable. Watch for the signs of heat disorders listed below; if they occur, act appropriately.

Problem	Symptoms	Treatment
Heat cramps	Muscle cramps, usually in the muscles most used during exercise.	Stop exercising, drink fluids, and stretch cramped muscles.
Heat exhaustion	Paleness; headache; nausea; fainting; dizziness; profuse sweating; weakness; cold, clammy skin; and a rapid, weak pulse.	Cool the body: Stop exercising, get out of the heat, remove excess clothing, drink cold fluids, and apply cool and/or damp towels to the body.
Heat stroke	Hot, flushed skin (skin may be dry or sweaty); rapid pulse; high body temperature; dizziness; confusion or disorientation; vomiting; diarrhea; unconsciousness.	Get immediate medical attention, and try to lower body temperature: Get out of the heat, remove excess clothing, drink cold fluids, and apply cool and/or damp towels or immerse the body in cold water.

Your choice of exercise equipment often affects your enjoyment, your risk of injury, and the likelihood of your continued participation. Nothing will ruin the joy of an activity more than ill-fitting or defective equipment. Following a few simple principles of equipment selection will greatly enhance your sport and exercise experiences.

Price

Try to purchase the best equipment you can afford. If you shop around, you can often find merchandise of good quality at a discount. Bargains are often available through mail-order companies and discount stores. Look in the back of sports specialty magazines for good prices on items such as tennis rackets, running shoes, and windsurf boards.

Good-quality used equipment can often be purchased at a fraction of the retail price. Used sporting goods shops have become very popular throughout the United States and Canada. Sporting goods are also often listed in newspaper classified ads.

Quality

While price and quality generally go hand in hand, you can often buy good-quality equipment at less than premium prices. Before you invest in a new piece of equipment, investigate it. Ask coaches and instructors if the results are worth the price. Most magazines devoted to individual sports and activities review new equipment. The January 1998 issue of *Consumer Reports* rated several types of home exercise equipment. Don't buy without doing some research. It's also a good idea to buy equipment with a money-back guarantee or a free trial period; if the equipment doesn't meet your expectations, you can return it.

Fit

Equipment that fits properly will enhance your enjoyment and prevent injury. Shoes that pinch your feet will make running unbearable. The wrong size grip on a tennis racket can lead to an elbow injury. When shopping for exercise equipment, take your time and get the help you need to ensure a proper fit.

Intended Use

Many people purchase expensive home exercise equipment, only to have it sit in a corner gathering dust. Before buying an expensive home treadmill, stationary cycle, or stair-climber, try it for several weeks at a local health club or gym. Ask yourself how often you'll actually use the equipment. If you honestly will use it regularly, go ahead and buy a home treadmill or stationary cycle. If you will use a piece of equipment only occasionally, you are better off using one at a gym. Also make sure you have space to use and store it at home. If you really decide you want to own one, buy it for your home.

Also consider how intense your workouts will be. If you intend to push your equipment to the limit, buy a model that can handle the stress. There's nothing more frustrating than a tennis racket that breaks the first time you use it, or a treadmill belt that slips when you try to run fast. While heavy-duty equipment tends to cost more, it may be worth the extra money. But take care not to pay extra for features you don't need.

Your Skill Level

Some equipment is designed for people with superior levels of strength, fitness, and skill. Buying "advanced" equipment can actually diminish your enjoyment of an activity. For example, slalom skis designed for a racer would be extremely difficult for a beginning skier to turn. Shoes designed for competitive marathon runners may have less padding to protect the legs and feet from injury, making them inappropriate for a recreational runner (see Chapter 7 for more on choosing footwear). Buy equipment that is appropriate for your current skill level.

Safety

Don't skimp on safety equipment. For popular sports like in-line skating, failing to buy a helmet and appropriate pads can lead to a serious injury. Check your safety equipment frequently to ensure that it's in good working condition. For example, ski bindings that work perfectly one season may not release properly after sitting in your garage for a year.

3d ed. Mountain View, Calif.: Mayfield. *The fitness principles and techniques every aerobic dancer should know.*

Sharkey, B. J. 1996. *Fitness and Health.* Champaign, Ill.: Human Kinetics. *An excellent guide to fitness and health for people serious about their exercise program.*

Sloane, E. A. 1995. *Sloane's Complete Book of Bicycling,* 5th ed. New York: Simon & Schuster. *A comprehensive guide for beginning and expert cyclists that includes information on equipment selection and maintenance and cycling health and safety.*

YMCA of the USA and T. W. Hanlon. 1995. *Fit for Two: The official YMCA Prenatal Exercise Guide.* Champaign, Ill.: Human Kinetics. *A practical guide to safe exercise during pregnancy.*

Organizations and Web Sites

Aerobics and Fitness Association of America/Your Body. Provides information on exercise, including how to choose an instructor, class, or facility; how to begin a walking program; and how to maintain an exercise program while traveling.

http://www.afaa.com/your_body/yourbody.html

American Heart Association. Provides information on cardiovascular health and disease, including the role of exercise in maintaining heart health and exercise tips for people of all ages.

800-AHA-USA1

http://www.americanheart.org

Dr. Pribut's Running Injuries Page. Provides information about running and many types of running injuries.

http://www.clark.net/pub/pribut/spsport.html

Exploratorium's Science of Cycling. Describes different types of bikes and how muscles work to power a cycle.

http://www.exploratorium.edu/cycling

Franklin Institute Science Museum/The Heart: An Online Exploration. An online museum exhibit with information on the structure and function of the heart, blood vessels, and respiratory system.

http://www.fi.edu/biosci/heart.html

Physician and Sportsmedicine. Provides many articles with easy-to-understand advice about exercise injuries.

http://www.physsportsmed.com

Runner's World Online. Contains a wide variety of information about running, including tips for beginning runners, advice about training, and a shoe buyer's guide.

http://www.runnersworld.com

Yahoo/Recreation. Contains links to many sites with practical advice on many sports and activities.

http://www.yahoo.com/recreation/sports

See also the listings in Chapter 2.

SELECTED BIBLIOGRAPHY

Alessio, H. M., and E. R. Blasi. 1997. Physical activity as a natural antioxidant booster and its effect on a healthy life span. *Research Quarterly in Exercise and Sport* 68(4): 292–302.

American College of Sports Medicine. 1998. ACSM Postition Stand: The Recommended Quantity and Quality of Exercise for Developing and Maintaining Cardiorespiratory and Muscular Fitness, Flexibility in Healthy Adults. *Medicine and Science in Sports and Exercise* 30(6): 975–991.

American College of Sports Medicine. 1995. *Guidelines for Exercise Testing and Prescription,* 5th ed. Baltimore: Williams & Wilkins.

American College of Sports Medicine. 1997. *ACSM's Health/Fitness Facility Standards and Guidelines,* 2d ed. Champaign, Ill.: Human Kinetics.

Araujo, D. 1997. Expecting questions about exercise and pregnancy? *Physician and Sportsmedicine* 25(4): 84–93.

Åstrand, P. O., U. Bergh, and A. Kilbom. 1997. A 33-yr follow-up of peak oxygen uptake and related variables of former physical education students. *Journal of Applied Physiology* 82: 1844–1852.

Borg, G. A. V. 1982. Psychophysical bases of perceived exertion. *Medicine and Science in Sports and Exercise* 14:377–381.

Brooks, G. A., T. D. Fahey, and T. P. White. 1996. *Exercise Physiology: Human Bioenergetics and Its Applications,* 2d ed. Mountain View, Calif.: Mayfield.

Brown, M. D., et al. 1997. Improvement of insulin sensitivity by short-term exercise training in hypertensive African American women. *Hypertension* 30(6): 1549–1553.

Centers for Disease Control and Prevention. 1998. Heat-related mortality—United States, 1997. *Morbidity and Mortality Weekly Report* 47(23):473–476.

Charlton, G. A., and M. H. Crawford. 1997. Physiologic consequences of training. *Cardiology Clinics* 15:345–354.

Chesler, R. M., et al. 1997. Cardiovascular response to sudden strenuous exercise: An exercise echocardiographic study. *Medicine and Science in Sports and Exercise* 29:1299–1303.

Crouse, S. F., et al. 1997. Effects of training and a single session of exercise on lipids and apolipoproteins in hypercholesterolemic men. *Journal of Applied Physiology* 83:2019–2028.

Evans, W. J., and D. Cyr-Campbell. 1997. Nutrition, exercise, and healthy aging. *Journal of the American Dietetics Association* 97:632–638.

Exercise during pregnancy and the postpartum period. ACOG Technical Bulletin Number 189. 1994. *International Journal of Gynaecology and Obstetrics* 45(1): 65–70.

Gibbons, R. J., et al. 1997. ACC/AHA Guidelines for Exercise Testing. A report of the American College of Cardiology/ American Heart Association Task Force on Practice Guidelines (Committee on Exercise Testing). *Journal of the American College of Cardiology* 30:260–311.

Hakim, A. A., et al. 1998. Effects of walking on mortality among nonsmoking retired men. *New England Journal of Medicine* 338(2): 94–99.

Ivy, J. L. 1997. Role of exercise training in the prevention and treatment of insulin resistance and non-insulin-dependent diabetes mellitus. *Sports Medicine* 24:321–336.

Jennings, G. L. 1997. Exercise and blood pressure: Walk, run or swim? *Journal of Hypertension* 15:567–569.

Kelley, G. 1998. Aerobic exercise and lumbar spine bone mineral density in postmenopausal women: A meta-analysis. *Journal of the American Geriatrics Society* 46(2): 143–152.

Mackinnon, L. T., L. Hubinger, and F. Lepre. 1997. Effects of physical activity and diet on lipoprotein(a). *Medicine and Science in Sports and Exercise* 29:1429–1436.

Mengelkoch, L. J., et al. 1997. Effects of age, physical training, and physical fitness on coronary heart disease risk factors in older track athletes at twenty-year follow-up. *Journal of the American Geriatrics Society* 45(12): 1446–1453.

Nicoloff, G., and T. L. Schwenk. 1995. Using exercise to ward off depression. *Physician and Sportsmedicine* 23(9): 44–58.

Radegran, G., and B. Saltin. 1998. Muscle blood flow at onset of dynamic exercise in humans. *American Journal of Physiology* 274(1 Pt 2): H314–H322.

Roitman, J. 1998. *ACSM's Resource Manual for Guidelines for Exercise Testing and Prescription.* 3d ed. Baltimore: Williams and Wilkens.

Sandor, R. P. 1997. Heat illness: On-site diagnosis and cooling. *Physician and Sportsmedicine* 25(6): 35–41.

Shaping Up. 1998. *Consumer Reports,* January.

Shephard, R. J., and P. N. Shek. 1995. Cancer, immune function, and physical activity. *Canadian Journal of Applied Physiology* 20:1–25.

Sipila, S., et al. 1997. Effects of strength and endurance training on muscle fibre characteristics in elderly women. *Clinical Physiology* 17:459–474.

Stamford, B. 1997. Choosing and using exercise equipment. *Physician and Sportsmedicine* 25(1): 107–109.

Tsintzas, K., and C. Williams. 1998. Human muscle glycogen metabolism during exercise. Effect of carbohydrate supplementation. *Sports Medicine* 25(1): 7–23.

Turley, K. R., and J. H. Wilmore. 1997. Cardiovascular responses to treadmill and cycle ergometer exercise in children and adults. *Journal of Applied Physiology* 83:948–957.

Utter, A., et al. 1997. Effect of carbohydrate substrate availability on ratings of perceived exertion during prolonged running. *International Journal of Sports Nutrition* 7(4): 274–285.

Van Boxtel, M. P. J., et al. 1997. Aerobic capacity and cognitive performance in a cross-sectional aging study. *Medicine and Science in Sports and Exercise* 29(10): 1357–1365.

Weltan, S. M., et al. 1998. Preexercise muscle glycogen content affects metabolism during exercise despite maintenance of hyperglycemia. *American Journal of Physiology* 274(1 Pt 1): E83–E88.

LAB 3-1   *Assessing Your Current Level of Cardiorespiratory Endurance*

Before taking any of the cardiorespiratory endurance assessment tests, refer to the fitness prerequisites and cautions given in Table 3-2. For best results, don't exercise strenuously or consume caffeine the day of the test, and don't smoke or eat a heavy meal within about 3 hours of the test.

The 1-Mile Walk Test

Equipment

1.   A track or course that provides a measurement of 1 mile
2.   A stopwatch, clock, or watch with a second hand
3.   A weight scale

Preparation

Measure your body weight (in pounds) before taking the test.

Body weight: _____ lb

Instructions

1.   Warm up before taking the test. Do some walking, easy jogging, or calisthenics and some stretching exercises.
2.   Cover the 1-mile course as quickly as possible. Walk at a pace that is brisk but comfortable. You must raise your heart rate above 120 bpm.
3.   As soon as you complete the distance, note your time and take your pulse for 10 seconds.

     Walking time: _____ min _____ sec

     10-second pulse count: _____ beats

4.   Cool down after the test by walking slowly for several minutes.

Determining Maximal Oxygen Consumption

1.   Convert your 10-second pulse count into a value for exercise heart rate by multiplying it by 6.

     Exercise heart rate: _____ × 6 = _____ bpm
                          _{10-sec pulse count}

2.   Convert your walking time from minutes and seconds to a decimal figure. For example, a time of 14 minutes and 45 seconds would be 14 + (45/60), or 14.75 minutes.

     Walking time: _____ min + (_____ sec ÷ 60 sec/min) = _____ min

3.   Insert values for your age, gender, weight, walking time, and exercise heart rate in the following equation, where

     W = your weight (in pounds)

     A = your age (in years)

     G = your gender (male = 1; female = 0)

     T = your time to complete the 1-mile course (in minutes)

     H = your exercise heart rate (in beats per minute)

     $\dot{V}O_{2max} = 132.853 - (0.0769 \times W) - (0.3877 \times A) + (6.315 \times G) - (3.2649 \times T) - (0.1565 \times H)$

For example, a 20-year-old, 190-pound male with a time of 14.75 minutes and an exercise heart rate of 152 bpm would calculate maximal oxygen consumption as follows:

$$\dot{V}O_{2max} = 132.853 - (0.0769 \times 190) - (0.3877 \times 20) + (6.315 \times 1) - (3.2649 \times 14.75) - (0.1565 \times 152)$$
$$= 45 \ ml/kg/min$$

$$\dot{V}O_{2max} = 132.853 - (0.0769 \times \underline{\hspace{1cm}}) - (0.3877 \times \underline{\hspace{1cm}}) + (6.315 \times \underline{\hspace{1cm}})$$
$$\text{weight (lb)} \qquad\qquad \text{age (years)} \qquad\qquad \text{gender}$$

$$- (3.2649 \times \underline{\hspace{1cm}}) - (0.1565 \times \underline{\hspace{1cm}}) = \underline{\hspace{1cm}} \ \textbf{ml/kg/min}$$
$$\text{walking time (min)} \qquad \text{exercise heart rate (bpm)}$$

4. Copy this value for $\dot{V}O_{2max}$ into the appropriate place in the chart on the final page of this lab.

The 3-Minute Step Test

Equipment

1. A step, bench, or bleacher step that is 16.25 inches from ground level
2. A stopwatch, clock, or watch with a second hand
3. A metronome

Preparation

Practice stepping up and down from the step before you begin the test. Each step has four beats: up-up-down-down. Males should perform the test with the metronome set for a rate of 96 beats per minute, or 24 steps per minute. Females should set the metronome at 88 beats per minute, or 22 steps per minute.

Instructions

1. Warm up before taking the test. Do some walking, easy jogging, and stretching exercises.
2. Set the metronome at the proper rate. Your instructor or a partner can call out starting and stopping times; otherwise, have a clock or watch within easy viewing during the test.
3. Begin the test, and continue to step at the correct pace for 3 minutes.
4. Stop after 3 minutes. Remain standing, and count your pulse for the 15-second period from 5 to 20 seconds into recovery.

    15-second pulse count: _____ beats

5. Cool down after the test by walking slowly for several minutes.

Determining Maximal Oxygen Consumption

1. Convert your 15-second pulse count to a value for recovery heart rate by multiplying by 4.

    Recovery heart rate: _____ × 4 = _____ bpm
    15-sec pulse count

2. Insert your recovery heart rate in the equation below, where

    H = recovery heart rate (in beats per minute)
    Males: $\dot{V}O_{2max} = 111.33 - (0.42 \times H)$
    Females: $\dot{V}O_{2max} = 65.81 - (0.1847 \times H)$

    For example, a man with a recovery heart rate of 162 bpm would calculate maximal oxygen consumption as follows:

    $$\dot{V}O_{2max} = 111.33 - (0.42 \times 162) = 43 \ ml/kg/min$$

    Males: $\dot{V}O_{2max} = 111.33 - (0.42 \times \underline{\hspace{1cm}}) = \underline{\hspace{1cm}} \ \textbf{ml/kg/min}$
    recovery heart rate (bpm)

    Females: $\dot{V}O_{2max} = 65.81 - (0.1847 \times \underline{\hspace{1cm}}) = \underline{\hspace{1cm}} \ \textbf{ml/kg/min}$
    recovery heart rate (bpm)

3. Copy this value for $\dot{V}O_{2max}$ into the appropriate place in the chart on the final page of this lab.

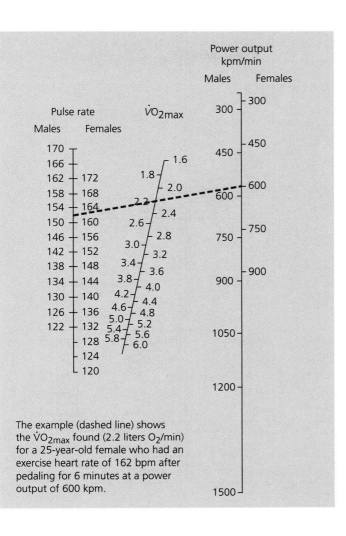

Power output
kpm/min

Males   Females

The example (dashed line) shows
the $\dot{V}O_{2max}$ found (2.2 liters O_2/min)
for a 25-year-old female who had an
exercise heart rate of 162 bpm after
pedaling for 6 minutes at a power
output of 600 kpm.

Nomogram for use with the Åstrand-
Rhyming cycle ergometer test.

c. Divide this number by your weight (in kilograms).

For example, a 135-pound, 25-year-old female whose 10-second count was 27 at a workload
of 600 kpm would calculate maximal oxygen consumption as follows:

1. 27 beats × 6 = 162 bpm

2. Connecting 600 kpm and 162 bpm on the nomogram gives a $\dot{V}O_{2max}$ value of 2.2 l/min

3. The age-adjustment factor for a 25-year-old is 1.00.
    2.2 l/min × 1.00 = 2.2 l/min

4. To convert 135 pounds to kilograms:
    135 lb ÷ 2.2 lb/kg = 61.4 kg

    To convert liters to milliliters:

    2.2 l/min × 1000 ml/l = 2200 ml/min

    To adjust for weight:

    2200 ml/min ÷ 61.4 kg = 35.8 ml/kg/min

Convert body weight to kg: _____ lb ÷ 2.2 lb/kg = _____ kg

Convert from liters to milliliters: _____ l/min × 1000 ml/l = _____ ml/min
                                     age-corrected $\dot{V}O_{2max}$

Adjust for weight:

$\dot{V}O_{2max}$ = _____ ml/min ÷ _____ kg = _____ **ml/kg/min**
        $\dot{V}O_{2max}$ body weight

5. Copy this value for $\dot{V}O_{2max}$ into the appropriate place in the chart below.

Rating Your Cardiovascular Fitness

Record your $\dot{V}O_{2max}$ score(s) and the corresponding fitness rating from the table in the chart below.

Maximal Oxygen Consumption (ml/kg/min)

Women	Very Poor	Poor	Fair	Good	Excellent	Superior
Age: 18–29	Below 30.6	30.6–33.7	33.8–36.6	36.7–40.9	41.0–46.7	Above 46.7
30–39	Below 28.7	28.7–32.2	32.3–34.5	34.6–38.5	38.6–43.8	Above 43.8
40–49	Below 26.5	26.5–29.4	29.5–32.2	32.3–36.2	36.3–40.9	Above 40.9
50–59	Below 24.3	24.3–26.8	26.9–29.3	29.4–32.2	32.3–36.7	Above 36.7
60 and over	Below 22.8	22.8–24.4	24.5–27.1	27.2–31.1	31.2–37.4	Above 37.4
Men						
Age: 18–29	Below 37.1	37.1–40.9	41.0–44.1	44.2–48.1	48.2–53.9	Above 53.9
30–39	Below 35.4	35.4–38.8	38.9–42.3	42.4–46.7	46.8–52.4	Above 52.4
40–49	Below 33.0	33.0–36.7	36.8–39.8	39.9–44.0	44.1–50.3	Above 50.3
50–59	Below 30.2	30.2–33.7	33.8–36.6	36.7–40.9	41.0–47.0	Above 47.0
60 and over	Below 26.5	26.5–30.1	30.2–33.5	33.6–38.0	38.1–45.1	Above 45.1

SOURCE: Based on norms from the Cooper Institute for Aerobics Research, Dallas, Texas; used with permission.

	$\dot{V}O_{2max}$	Cardiovascular Fitness Rating
1-mile walk test		
3-minute step test		
1.5-mile run-walk test	38.76	poor
Åstrand-Rhyming cycle ergometer test		

Is your rating as high as you want it to be? If not, what is your goal for $\dot{V}O_{2max}$? _____

_____

_____

To monitor your progress toward your goal, enter the results of this lab in the Preprogram Assessment column of Appendix D. After several weeks of a cardiorespiratory endurance exercise program, complete this lab again, and enter the results in the Postprogram Assessment column of Appendix D. How do the results compare? (For accuracy, it's best to compare $\dot{V}O_{2max}$ scores for the same test.)

SOURCES: Kline, G. M., et al. 1987. Estimation of $\dot{V}O_{2max}$ from a one-mile track walk, gender, age, and body weight. *Medicine and Science in Sports and Exercise* 19(3): 253–259. McArdle, W. D., F. I. Katch, and V. L. Katch. 1991. *Exercise Physiology: Energy, Nutrition, and Human Performance.* Philadelphia: Lea and Febiger, pp. 225–226. Brooks, G. A., and T. D. Fahey. 1987. *Fundamentals of Human Performance.* New York: Macmillan. Åstrand, P. O., and I. Rhyming. 1954. A nomogram for calculation of aerobic capacity (physical fitness) from pulse rate during submaximal work. *Journal of Applied Physiology* 7:218–221. Used with permission.

LAB 3-2 *Developing an Exercise Program for Cardiorespiratory Endurance*

1. *Goals.* Determine goals for your cardiorespiratory endurance exercise program, and record them below. Goals can be specific or general, short or long term.

_____

_____

_____

_____

2. *Activities.* Refer to the box "Activities and Sports for Developing Cardiorespiratory Endurance" (p. 52) and choose one or more activities for your program. Fill in the activity name and general intensity rating sections on the program plan below.

3. *Duration.* Fill in an appropriate duration for each activity (20–60 minutes).

4. *Intensity.* Determine your exercise intensity, and fill in below.

   a. Calculate your target heart rate range.

   Maximum heart rate: 220 − _____ = _____ bpm

age (years)

   65% training intensity = _____ bpm × 0.65 = _____ bpm

maximum heart rate

   90% training intensity = _____ bpm × 0.90 = _____ bpm

maximum heart rate

   Target heart rate range = _____ to _____ bpm
   (Note: If you are very unfit, use 55% of maximum heart rate as the lower end of your target heart rate range.)

   b. If you prefer, determine an RPE value that corresponds to your target heart rate range (see pp. 52–53 and Figure 3-3).

5. *Frequency.* Fill in how often you plan to participate in each activity.

Program Plan

Activity	General Intensity Rating (L, M, H)	Duration (min)	Intensity (bpm or RPE)	Frequency (check ✓)						
				M	T	W	Th	F	Sa	Su

6. *Monitoring your program.* Complete a log like the one on the next page to monitor your program and track your progress. Fill in the duration of exercise for each workout. To monitor your progress more closely, you can also track another variable, such as distance. For example, if your cardiorespiratory endurance program includes walking and swimming, you can keep track of miles walked and yards swum in addition to the duration of each exercise session.

Activity/Date													
1	Duration												
2	Duration												
3	Duration												
4	Duration												
5	Duration												

Activity/Date													
1	Duration												
2	Duration												
3	Duration												
4	Duration												
5	Duration												

Activity/Date													
1	Duration												
2	Duration												
3	Duration												
4	Duration												
5	Duration												

Muscular Strength and Endurance

LOOKING AHEAD

After reading this chapter, you should be able to answer these questions about muscular strength and endurance:

- What are muscular strength and endurance, and how do they relate to wellness?

- How can muscular strength and endurance be assessed?

- How do weight training exercises affect muscles?

- What type, frequency, and number of weight training exercises make up a successful program?

- What are the most important strategies for avoiding injuries in a weight training program?

- How are common weight training exercises performed using weight machines and free weights?

Exercise experts have long emphasized the importance of cardiovascular fitness. Other physical fitness factors, such as muscle strength and flexibility, were mentioned almost as an afterthought. As more was learned about how the body responds to exercise, however, it became obvious that these other factors are vital to health, wellness, and overall quality of life. Muscles make up over 40% of your body mass. You depend on them for movement, and, because of their mass, they are the site of a large portion of the energy reactions (metabolism) that take place in your body. Strong, well-developed muscles help you perform daily activities with greater ease, protect you from injury, and enhance your well-being in other ways.

This chapter explains the benefits of strength training and describes methods of assessing muscular strength and endurance. It then explains the basics of weight training and provides guidelines for setting up your own weight training program.

BENEFITS OF MUSCULAR STRENGTH AND ENDURANCE

Enhanced muscular strength and endurance can lead to improvements in the areas of performance, injury prevention, body composition, self-image, and lifetime muscle and bone health.

Improved Performance of Physical Activities

A person with a moderate-to-high level of muscular strength and endurance can perform everyday tasks—such as climbing stairs and carrying books or groceries—with ease. Muscular strength and endurance are also important in recreational activities: People with poor muscle strength tire more easily and are less effective in activities like hiking, skiing, and playing tennis. Increased strength can enhance your enjoyment of recreational sports by making it possible to achieve high levels of performance and to handle advanced techniques.

TERMS **tendon** A tough band of fibrous tissue that connects a muscle to a bone or other body part and transmits the force exerted by the muscle.

ligament A tough band of tissue that connects the ends of bones to other bones or supports organs in place.

testosterone The principal male hormone, responsible for the development of secondary sex characteristics and important in the increase of muscle size.

repetition maximum (RM) The maximum amount of resistance that can be moved a specified number of times; 1 RM is the maximum weight that can be lifted once.

repetitions The number of times an exercise is performed during one set.

Injury Prevention

Increased muscle strength provides protection against injury because it helps people maintain good posture and appropriate body mechanics when carrying out everyday activities like walking, lifting, and carrying. Strong muscles in the abdomen, hips, low back, and legs support the back in proper alignment and help prevent low-back pain, which afflicts over 85% of all Americans at some time in their lives. (Prevention of low-back pain is discussed in Chapter 5.) Training for muscular strength also makes the **tendons, ligaments,** and joint surfaces stronger and less susceptible to injury.

Improved Body Composition

As Chapter 2 explained, healthy body composition means that the body has a high proportion of fat-free mass (primarily composed of muscle) and a relatively small proportion of fat. Strength training improves body composition by increasing muscle mass, thereby tipping the body composition ratio toward fat-free mass and away from fat. Building muscle mass through strength training also helps with losing fat because metabolic rate is directly proportional to muscle mass: The more muscle mass, the higher the metabolic rate. A high metabolic rate means that a nutritionally sound diet will not lead to an increase in body fat.

Enhanced Self-Image

Weight training leads to an enhanced self-image by providing stronger, firmer-looking muscles and a toned, healthy-looking body. Men tend to build larger, stronger, more shapely muscles. Women tend to lose inches, increase strength, and develop greater muscle definition. The larger muscles in men combine with high levels of the hormone **testosterone,** the principal androgen, for a strong tissue-building effect; see the box "Gender Differences in Muscular Strength."

Because weight training provides measurable objectives (pounds lifted, repetitions accomplished), a person can easily recognize improved performance, leading to greater self-confidence. It's especially satisfying to work on improving one's personal record.

Improved Muscle and Bone Health with Aging

Research has shown that good muscle strength helps people live healthier lives. A lifelong program of regular strength training prevents muscle and nerve degeneration that can compromise the quality of life and increase the risk of hip fractures and other potentially life-threatening injuries. After age 30, people begin to lose muscle mass. At first they may notice that they can't play sports as well as they could in high school. After more years of inactivity and strength loss, people may have trouble performing even the simple movements of daily life—getting out of a bathtub or automobile, walking up a flight of stairs, or

Men are generally stronger than women because they typically have larger bodies overall and larger muscles. But when strength is expressed per unit of cross-sectional area of muscle tissue, men are only 1–2% stronger than women in the upper body and about equal to women in the lower body. (Men have a larger proportion of muscle tissue in the upper body, so it's easier for them to build upper-body strength than it is for women.) Individual muscle fibers are larger in men, but the metabolism of cells within those fibers is the same in both sexes.

Two factors that help explain these disparities between the sexes are androgen levels and the speed of nervous control of muscle. Androgens are naturally occurring male hormones that are responsible for the development of secondary sex characteristics (facial hair, deep voice, and so forth). Androgens also promote the growth of muscle tissue. Androgen levels are about 6–10 times higher in men than in women, so men tend to have larger muscles. Also, because the male nervous system can activate muscles faster, men tend to have more power.

Some women are concerned that they will develop large muscles from weight training. Most studies show that women do not develop big muscles, but the evidence of top women body builders suggests that they can. Some of these women may have taken drugs to increase their muscle size, but many muscular women have not. Evidence suggests, though, that it is difficult for women to gain a large amount of muscle without training intensely over many years.

The bottom line is that both men and women can increase strength through weight training. Women may not be able to lift as much weight as men, but pound for pound of muscle, they have nearly the same capacity to gain strength as men. The lifetime wellness benefits of strength training are available to everyone.

SOURCE: Fahey, T. D. 1997. *Weight Training for Men and Women*, 3d ed. Mountain View, Calif.: Mayfield.

doing yard work. Poor strength makes it much more likely that a person will be injured during the course of everyday activities.

As a person ages, motor nerves can become disconnected from the portion of muscle they control. Muscle physiologists estimate that by age 70, 15% of the motor nerves in most people are no longer connected to muscle tissue. Aging and inactivity also cause muscles to become slower and therefore less able to perform quick, powerful movements. Strength training helps maintain motor nerve connections and the quickness of muscles.

Osteoporosis is common in people over age 55, particularly postmenopausal women. Osteoporosis leads to fractures that can be life-threatening. Hormonal changes from aging account for much of the bone loss that occurs, but lack of bone stress due to inactivity and a poor diet are contributing factors. Recent research indicates that strength training can lessen bone loss even if it is taken up later in life. Increased muscle strength can also help prevent falls, which are a major cause of injury in people with osteoporosis. (Strategies for preventing osteoporosis are described in Chapter 8.)

ASSESSING MUSCULAR STRENGTH AND ENDURANCE

Muscular strength and muscular endurance are distinct but related components of fitness. Muscular strength, the maximum amount of force a muscle can produce in a single effort, is usually assessed by measuring the maximum amount of weight a person can lift one time. This single maximal movement is referred to as one **repetition maximum (RM)**. You can assess the strength of your major

muscle groups by taking the one-repetition maximum tests for the bench press and the leg press. Refer to Lab 4-1 for guidelines on taking these tests. Instructions for assessing grip strength using a dynamometer are also included in Lab 4-1. For more accurate results, avoid any strenuous weight training for 48 hours beforehand.

Muscular endurance is the ability of a muscle to exert a submaximal force repeatedly or continuously over time. This ability depends on muscular strength because a certain amount of strength is required for any muscle movement. Muscular endurance is usually assessed by counting the maximum number of **repetitions** of a muscular contraction a person can do (such as in push-ups) or the maximum amount of time a person can hold a muscular contraction (such as in the flexed-arm hang). You can test the muscular endurance of major muscle groups in your body by taking the 60-second sit-up test or the curl-up test and the push-up test. Refer to Lab 4-1 for complete instructions on taking these assessment tests.

Record your results and your fitness rating from the assessment tests in Lab 4-1. If the results show that improvement is needed, a weight training program will enable you to make rapid gains in muscular strength and endurance.

FUNDAMENTALS OF WEIGHT TRAINING

Weight training develops muscular strength and endurance in the same way that endurance exercise develops cardiovascular fitness: When the muscles are stressed by a greater load than they are used to, they adapt and improve their function. The type of adaptation that occurs depends on the type of stress applied.

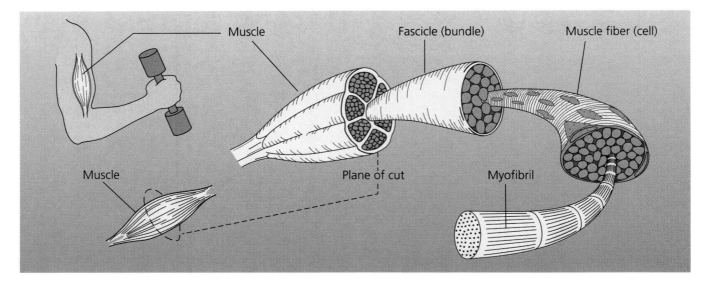

Figure 4-1   Components of skeletal muscle tissue.

Physiological Effects of Weight Training

Muscles move the body and enable it to exert force because they move the skeleton. When a muscle contracts (shortens), it moves a bone by pulling on the tendon that attaches the muscle to the bone. Muscles consist of individual muscle cells, or **muscle fibers,** connected in bundles (Figure 4-1). A single muscle is made up of many bundles of muscle fibers and is covered by layers of connective tissue that hold the fibers together. Muscle fibers, in turn, are made up of smaller units called **myofibrils.** (When your muscles are given the signal to contract, pro-

tein filaments within the myofibrils slide across one another, causing the muscle fiber to shorten.) Weight training causes the size of individual muscle fibers to increase by increasing the number of myofibrils. Larger muscle fibers mean a larger and stronger muscle. The development of large muscle fibers is called **hypertrophy.**

Muscle fibers are classified as fast-twitch or slow-twitch fibers according to their strength, speed of contraction, and energy source. **Slow-twitch fibers** are relatively fatigue-resistant, but they don't contract as rapidly or strongly as fast-twitch fibers. The principal energy system that fuels slow-twitch fibers is aerobic. **Fast-twitch fibers** contract more rapidly and forcefully than slow-twitch fibers but fatigue more quickly. Although oxygen is important in the energy system that fuels fast-twitch fibers, they rely more on anaerobic metabolism than do slow-twitch fibers (see Chapter 3 for a discussion of energy systems).

Most muscles contain a mixture of slow-twitch and fast-twitch fibers. The type of fiber that acts depends on the type of work required. Endurance activities like jogging tend to use slow-twitch fibers, whereas strength and **power** activities like sprinting use fast-twitch fibers. Weight training can increase the size and strength of both fast-twitch and slow-twitch fibers, although fast-twitch fibers are preferentially increased.

To exert force, the body recruits one or more motor units to contract. A **motor unit** is made up of a nerve connected to a number of muscle fibers. When a motor nerve calls upon its fibers to contract, all the fibers contract to their maximum capacity. The number of motor units recruited depends on the amount of strength required: When a person picks up a small weight, he or she uses fewer motor units than when picking up a large weight. Training with weights improves the body's ability to

TERMS   **muscle fiber**   A single muscle cell, usually classified according to strength, speed of contraction, and energy source.

myofibrils   Protein structures that make up muscle fibers.

hypertrophy   An increase in the size of a muscle fiber, usually stimulated by muscular overload.

slow-twitch fibers   Red muscle fibers that are fatigue-resistant but have a slow contraction speed and a lower capacity for tension; usually recruited for endurance activities.

fast-twitch fibers   White muscle fibers that contract rapidly and forcefully but fatigue quickly; usually recruited for actions requiring strength and power.

power   The ability to exert force rapidly.

motor unit   A motor nerve (one that initiates movement) connected to one or more muscle fibers.

isometric   The application of force without movement; also called static.

isotonic   The application of force resulting in movement; also called dynamic.

concentric muscle contraction   An isotonic contraction in which the muscle gets shorter as it contracts.

eccentric muscle contraction   An isotonic contraction in which the muscle lengthens as it contracts.

TABLE 4-1	Physiological Changes and Benefits from Weight Training

Change	Benefits
Increased muscle mass*	Increased muscular strength Improved body composition Higher rate of metabolism Toned, healthy-looking muscles
Increased utilization of motor units during muscle contractions	Increased muscular strength and power
Improved coordination of motor units	Increased muscular strength and power
Increased strength of tendons, ligaments, and bones	Lower risk of injury to these tissues
Increased storage of fuel in muscles	Increased resistance to muscle fatigue
Increased size of fast-twitch muscle fibers (from a high-resistance program)	Increased muscular strength and power
Increased size of slow-twitch muscle fibers (from a high-repetition program)	Increased muscular endurance
Increased blood supply to muscles (from a high-repetition program)	Increased delivery of oxygen and nutrients Increased elimination of wastes

*Due to genetic and hormonal differences, men will build more muscle mass than women.

recruit motor units—a phenomenon called muscle learning—which increases strength even before muscle size increases.

In summary, weight training increases muscle strength because it increases the size of muscle fibers and improves the body's ability to call upon motor units to exert force. The physiological changes and benefits that result from weight training are summarized in Table 4-1.

Types of Weight Training Exercises

Weight training exercises are generally classified as isometric or isotonic. Each involves a different way of using and strengthening muscles.

Isometric Exercise Also called static exercise, **isometric** exercise involves applying force without movement. To perform an isometric exercise, a person can use an immovable object like a wall to provide resistance, or the individual can just tighten a muscle while remaining still (for example, tightening the abdominal muscles while sitting at a desk). In isometrics, the muscle contracts, but there is no movement.

Isometric exercises aren't as widely used as isotonic exercises because they don't develop strength throughout a joint's entire range of motion. However, isometric exercises are useful in strengthening muscles after an injury or surgery, when movement of the affected joint could delay healing. Isometrics are also used to overcome weak points in an individual's range of motion. Isometrically strengthening a muscle at its weakest point will allow more weight to be lifted with that muscle during isotonic exercise. For maximum strength gains, hold the isometric contraction maximally for 6 seconds; do 5–10 repetitions.

This isometric exercise for the arms and upper back involves locking the hands together and attempting to pull them apart. Isometric contractions involve force without movement.

Isotonic Exercise Isotonic (or dynamic) exercise involves applying force with movement. Isotonic exercises are the most popular type of exercises for increasing muscle strength and seem to be most valuable for developing strength that can be transferred to other forms of physical activity. They can be performed with weight machines, free weights, or a person's own body weight (as in sit-ups or push-ups).

There are two kinds of isotonic muscle contractions: concentric and eccentric. A **concentric muscle contraction** occurs when the muscle applies force as it shortens. An **eccentric muscle contraction** occurs when the muscle applies force as it lengthens. For example, in an arm curl, the biceps muscle works concentrically as the weight is raised toward the shoulder and eccentrically as the weight is lowered.

Left: A concentric contraction: The biceps muscle shortens as the arm lifts a weight toward the shoulder. **Right:** An eccentric contraction: The biceps muscle lengthens as the arm lowers a weight toward the thigh.

Two of the most common isotonic exercise techniques are constant resistance exercise and variable resistance exercise. Constant resistance exercise uses a constant load (weight) throughout a joint's entire range of motion. Training with free weights is a form of constant resistance exercise. A problem with this technique is that, because of differences in leverage, there are points in a joint's range of motion where the muscle controlling the movement is stronger and points where it is weaker. The amount of weight a person can lift is limited by the weakest point in the range. In variable resistance exercise, the load is changed to provide maximum load throughout the entire range of motion. This form of exercise uses machines that place more stress on muscles at the end of the range of motion, where a person has better leverage and is capable of exerting more force. The Nautilus pullover machine is an example of a variable resistance exercise machine.

Four other kinds of isotonic techniques, used mainly by athletes for training and rehabilitation, are eccentric loading, plyometrics, speed loading, and isokinetics.

- **Eccentric loading** involves placing a load on a muscle as it lengthens. The muscle contracts eccentrically in order to control the weight. Eccentric loading is practiced during most types of resistance training. For example, you are performing an eccentric movement as you lower the weight to your chest during a bench press in preparation for the active movement.

- **Plyometrics** is the sudden eccentric loading and stretching of muscles followed by a forceful concentric contraction. An example would be jumping from a bench to the ground and then jumping back onto the bench. This type of exercise is used to develop explosive strength.

- **Speed loading** involves moving a weight as rapidly as possible in an attempt to approach the speeds used in movements like throwing a softball or sprinting. In the bench press, for example, speed loading might involve doing 5 repetitions as fast as possible using a weight that is half the maximum load you can lift. You can gauge your progress by timing how fast you can perform the repetitions.

- **Isokinetic** exercise involves exerting force at a constant speed against an equal force exerted by a special strength training machine. The isokinetic machine provides variable resistance at different points in the joint's range of motion, matching the effort applied by the individual, while keeping the speed of the movement constant. In other words, the force exerted by the individual at any point in the range of motion is resisted by an equal force from the isokinetic machine. Isokinetic exercises are excellent for building strength and endurance, but the equipment is expensive and less commonly available than other kinds of weight machines.

TERMS   **eccentric loading**   Loading the muscle while it is lengthening; sometimes called "negatives."

plyometrics   Rapid stretching of a muscle group that is undergoing eccentric stress (the muscle is exerting force while it lengthens), followed by a rapid concentric contraction.

speed loading   Moving a load as rapidly as possible.

isokinetic   The application of force at a constant speed against an equal force.

spotter   A person who assists with a weight training exercise done with free weights.

agonist   A muscle in a state of contraction, opposed by the action of another muscle, its antagonist.

antagonist   A muscle that opposes the action of another muscle, its agonist.

Exercise Machines

Advantages

- Safe
- Convenient
- Don't require spotters
- Don't require lifter to balance bar
- Provide variable resistance
- Require less skill
- Make it easy to move from one exercise to the next
- Allow easy isolation of individual muscle groups
- Support back (on many machines)

Disadvantages

- Limited availability
- Inappropriate for performing dynamic movements
- Allow a limited number of exercises

Free Weights

Advantages

- Allow dynamic movements
- Allow the user to develop control of the weights
- Allow a greater variety of exercises
- Widely available
- Truer to real-life situations; strength transfers to daily activities

Disadvantages

- Not as safe
- Require spotters
- Require more skill
- Cause more blisters and calluses

Comparing the Different Types of Exercise   Isometric exercises require no equipment, so they can be done virtually anywhere. They build strength rapidly and are useful for rehabilitating injured joints. On the other hand, they have to be performed at several different angles for each joint to improve strength throughout the joint's entire range of motion. Isotonic exercises can be performed without equipment (calisthenics) or with equipment (weight lifting). They are excellent for building strength and endurance, and they tend to build strength through a joint's full range of motion.

Most people develop muscular strength and endurance using isotonic exercises. Ultimately, the type of exercise a person chooses depends on individual goals, preferences, and access to equipment.

CREATING A SUCCESSFUL WEIGHT TRAINING PROGRAM

To get the most out of your weight training program, you must design it to achieve maximum fitness benefits with a low risk of injury. Before you begin, seriously consider the type and amount of training that's right for you.

Choosing Equipment: Weight Machines Versus Free Weights

Your muscles will get stronger if you make them work against a resistance. Resistance can be provided by free weights, by your own body weight, or by sophisticated exercise machines. Weight machines are preferred by many people because they are safe, convenient, and easy to use. You just set the resistance (usually by placing a pin in the weight stack), sit down at the machine, and start working. Machines make it easy to isolate and work specific muscles. You don't need a **spotter,** someone who stands by to assist when free weights are used, and you don't have to worry about dropping a weight on yourself.

Free weights require more care, balance, and coordination to use, but they strengthen your body in ways that are more adaptable to real life. Free weights are more popular with athletes for developing explosive strength for sports.

Unless you are training seriously for a sport that requires a great deal of strength, training on machines is probably safer, more convenient, and just as effective as training with free weights. However, you can increase strength either way; which to use is a matter of personal preference. The box "Exercise Machines Versus Free Weights" can help you make a decision.

Selecting Exercises

A complete weight training program works all the major muscle groups. It usually takes about 8–10 different exercises to get a complete workout. For overall fitness, you need to include exercises for your neck, upper back, shoulders, arms, chest, abdomen, lower back, thighs, buttocks, and calves. If you are also training for a particular sport, include exercises to strengthen the muscles important for optimal performance *and* the muscles most likely to be injured. A program of weight training exercises for general fitness is presented later in this chapter.

It is important to balance exercises between **agonist** and **antagonist** muscle groups. (When a muscle contracts, it is known as the agonist; the opposing muscle, which must relax and stretch to allow contraction by the agonist, is known as the antagonist.) If you do an exercise that moves a joint in one direction, also select an exercise that works the joint in the opposite direction. For example, if you do knee extensions to develop the muscles on the front of your thighs, also do leg curls to develop the antagonistic muscles on the back of your thighs.

The order of exercises can also be important. Do exercises for large muscle groups or for more than one joint before you do exercises that use small muscle groups or single joints. This allows for more effective overload of the larger, more powerful muscle groups. Small muscle groups fatigue more easily than larger ones, and small muscle fatigue limits your capacity to overload larger muscle groups. For example, lateral raises, which work the shoulder muscles, should be performed after bench presses, which work the chest and arms in addition to the shoulders. If you fatigue your shoulder muscles by doing lateral raises first, you won't be able to lift as much weight and effectively fatigue all the key muscle groups used during the bench press.

Resistance

The amount of weight (resistance) you lift in weight training exercises is equivalent to intensity in cardiorespiratory endurance training. It determines the way your body will adapt to weight training and how quickly these adaptations will occur. Choose weights based on your current level of muscular fitness and your fitness goals. To build strength rapidly, you should lift weights as heavy as 80% of your maximum capacity (1 RM). If you're more interested in building endurance, choose a lighter weight, perhaps 40–60% of 1 RM. For example, if your maximum capacity for the leg press is 160 pounds, you might lift 130 pounds to build strength and 80 pounds to build endurance. For a general fitness program to develop both strength and endurance, choose a weight in the middle of this range, perhaps 70% of 1 RM.

Because it can be tedious and time-consuming to continually reassess your maximum capacity for each exercise, you might find it easier to choose a weight based on the number of repetitions of an exercise you can perform with a given resistance.

Repetitions and Sets

In order to improve fitness, you must do enough repetitions of each exercise to fatigue your muscles. The number of repetitions needed to cause fatigue depends on the amount of resistance: the heavier the weight, the fewer repetitions to reach fatigue. In general, a heavy

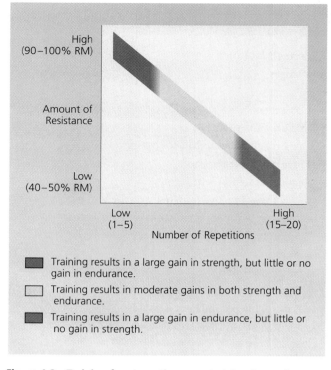

Figure 4-2   Training for strength versus training for endurance.

weight and a low number of repetitions (1–5) build strength, whereas a light weight and a high number of repetitions (15–20) build endurance (Figure 4-2). For a general fitness program to build both strength and endurance, try to do about 8–12 repetitions of each exercise; a few exercises, such as abdominal crunches and calf raises, may require more. Choose a weight heavy enough to fatigue your muscles but light enough for you to complete the repetitions with good form. Due to an increased risk of injury, it is recommended that older and more frail people (approximately 50–60 years of age and above) perform more repetitions (10–15) using a lighter weight.

In weight training, a **set** refers to a group of repetitions of an exercise followed by a rest period. Surprisingly, exercise scientists have not identified the optimal number of sets for increasing strength. For developing strength and endurance for general fitness, a single set of each exercise is sufficient, provided you use enough resistance to fatigue your muscles. (You should just barely be able to complete the 8–12 repetitions for each exercise.) Doing more than 1 set of each exercise may increase strength development, and most serious weight trainers do at least 3 sets of each exercise (see below for additional guidelines for more advanced programs).

If you perform more than 1 set of an exercise, you need to rest long enough between sets to allow your muscles to work at a high enough intensity to increase fitness. The length of the rest interval depends on the amount of resistance. In a program to develop a combination of strength

TERMS   set   A group of repetitions followed by a rest period.

Guidelines

Type of activity: 8–10 weight training exercises that focus on major muscle groups

Frequency: 2–3 days per week

Resistance: Weights heavy enough to cause muscle fatigue when performed for the selected number of repetitions

Repetitions: 8–12 of each exercise (10–15 with a lower weight for people over age 50–60)

Sets: 1 (Doing more than 1 set per exercise may result in faster and greater strength gains.)

Sample Program

1. Warm-up (5–10 minutes)
2. Weight training exercises (see table at right)
3. Cool-down (5–10 minutes)

Exercise	Resistance (lb)	Repetitions	Sets
Bench press	60	10	1
Overhead press	40	10	1
Lat pulls	40	10	1
Lateral raises	5	10	1
Biceps curls	25	10	1
Squats	30	10	1
Toe raises	25	15	1
Abdominal curls	—	30	1
Spine extensions	—	10	1
Neck flexion	—	10	1

and endurance for wellness, a rest period of 1–3 minutes between sets is appropriate; if you are lifting heavier loads to build maximum strength, rest 3–5 minutes between sets. You can save time in your workouts if you alternate sets of different exercises. Each muscle group can rest between sets while you work on other muscles.

The Warm-Up and Cool-Down

As with cardiorespiratory endurance exercise, you should warm up before every weight training session and cool down afterward. You should do both a general warm-up—several minutes of walking or easy jogging—and a warm-up for the weight training exercises you plan to perform. For example, if you plan to do 1 or more sets of 10 repetitions of bench presses with 125 pounds, you might do 1 set of 10 repetitions with 50 pounds as a warm-up. Do similar warm-up exercises for each exercise in your program.

To cool down after weight training, relax for 5–10 minutes after your workout. Including a period of post-exercise stretching may help prevent muscle soreness; warmed-up muscles and joints make this a particularly good time to work on flexibility.

Frequency of Exercise

For general fitness, the American College of Sports Medicine recommends a frequency of 2–3 days per week for weight training. Allow your muscles at least 1 day of rest between workouts; if you train too often, your muscles won't be able to work at a high enough intensity to improve their fitness, and soreness and injury are more likely to result. If you enjoy weight training and would

like to train more often, try working different muscle groups on alternate days. For example, work your arms and upper body one day, work your lower body the next day, and then return to upper-body exercises on the third day. Refer to the box "A Sample Weight Training Program for General Fitness" for suggestions on beginning a program.

Making Progress

The first few weeks of weight training should be devoted to learning the exercises. You need to learn the movements, and your nervous system needs to practice communicating with your muscles so you can develop strength effectively. To start, choose a weight that you can move easily through 8–12 repetitions, and do only 1 set of each exercise. Gradually add weight and (if you want) sets to your program over the first few weeks until you are doing 1–3 sets of 8–12 repetitions of each exercise.

As you progress, add weight when you can do more than 12 repetitions of an exercise. If adding weight means you can do only 7 or 8 repetitions, stay with that weight until you can again complete 12 repetitions per set. If you can do only 4–6 repetitions after adding weight, you've added too much and should take some off.

You can expect to improve rapidly during the first 6–10 weeks of training: a 10–30% increase in the amount of weight lifted. Gains will then come more slowly. Your rate of improvement will depend on how hard you work and how your body responds to resistance training. There will be individual differences in the rate of improvement. Factors such as age, motivation, and heredity will affect your progress.

Your ultimate goal depends on you. After you have achieved the level of strength and muscularity that you

Exercise/Date		9/14	9/16	9/18	9/21	9/23	9/25	9/28	9/30	10/2	10/5	10/7	10/9	10/12	10/14	10/16							
Bench press	Wt.	70	70	70	75	75	75	80	80	80	90	90	95	105	105	105							
	Sets	1	1	1	1	1	1	1	1	1	1	1	1	1	1	1							
	Reps.	10	10	12	10	12	12	10	9	12	12	12	12	8	7	8							
Overhead press	Wt.	40	40	40	55	55	60	60	60	70	70	75	75	75	80	85							
	Sets	1	1	1	1	1	1	1	1	1	1	1	1	1	1	1							
	Reps.	10	10	12	10	12	10	10	12	10	12	8	11	12	12	8							
Lat pulls	Wt.	50	50	50	60	60	60	60	60	60	70	70	70	80	80	80							
	Sets	1	1	1	1	1	1	1	1	1	1	1	1	1	1	1							
	Reps.	10	10	12	8	8	10	8	11	12	10	10	12	8	8	8							
Lateral raises	Wt.	5	5	5	7.5	7.5	7.5	7.5	7.5	7.5	7.5	7.5	7.5	10	10	10							
	Sets	1	1	1	1	1	1	1	1	1	1	1	1	1	1	1							
	Reps.	10	10	10	7	8	7	10	8	8	11	12	12	7	7	8							
Biceps curls	Wt.	35	35	35	40	40	40	45	45	45	50	50	50	50	50	50							
	Sets	1	1	1	1	1	1	1	1	1	1	1	1	1	1	1							
	Reps.	10	10	10	10	12	12	10	12	12	10	8	8	10	10	10							
Squats	Wt.	—	—	—	45	45	85	85	105	115	125	135	135	145	145	145							
	Sets	1	1	1	1	1	1	1	1	1	1	1	1	1	1	1							
	Reps.	10	10	10	12	15	10	12	12	15	12	10	12	9	8	9							
Toe raises	Wt.	—	—	—	45	45	85	85	105	115	125	135	135	145	145	145							
	Sets	1	1	1	1	1	1	1	1	1	1	1	1	1	1	1							
	Reps.	15	15	15	15	15	15	15	15	15	15	15	15	15	15	15							
Abdominal curls	Wt.	—	—	—	—	—	—	—	—	—	—	—	—	—	—	—							
	Sets	1	1	1	1	1	1	1	1	1	1	1	1	1	1	1							
	Reps.	20	20	20	20	20	20	25	25	25	30	30	30	30	30	30							
Spine extensions	Wt.	—	—	—	—	—	—	—	—	—	—	—	—	—	—	—							
	Sets	1	1	1	1	1	1	1	1	1	1	1	1	1	1	1							
	Reps.	5	5	5	8	8	8	10	10	10	10	10	10	10	10	10							
Neck flexion	Wt.	—	—	—	—	—	—	—	—	—	—	—	—	—	—	—							
	Sets	1	1	1	1	1	1	1	1	1	1	1	1	1	1	1							
	Reps.	5	5	5	10	10	10	10	10	10	10	10	10	10	10	10							

Figure 4-3   A sample workout card.

want, you can maintain your gains by training 2–3 days per week. You can monitor the progress of your program by recording the amount of resistance and the number of repetitions and sets you perform on a workout card like the one shown in Figure 4-3.

More Advanced Strength Training Programs

The weight training program described in this section—1 set of 8–12 repetitions of 8–10 exercises, performed 2–3 days per week—is sufficient to develop and maintain muscular strength and endurance for general fitness. If you have a different goal, you may need to adjust your program accordingly. As described above, performing more sets of a smaller number of repetitions with a heavier load will cause greater increases in strength. A program designed to build strength might include 3–5 sets of 4–6 repetitions each; the load used should be heavy enough to cause fatigue with the smaller number of repetitions. Be sure to rest long enough after a set to allow your muscles to recover and to work intensely during the next set.

Experienced weight trainers often engage in some form of cycle training, in which the exercises, number of sets and repetitions, and intensity are varied within a workout and/or between workouts. For example, you might do a particular exercise more intensely during some sets or on some days than others; you might also vary the exercises you perform for particular muscle groups. For information on these more advanced training techniques, consult your instructor, your coach, or the trainer at your school's weight room or the local gym; several of the books listed in the For More Information section at the end of the chapter also provide information on program design. If you decide to adopt a more advanced training regimen, start off slowly to give your body a chance to adjust and to minimize the risk of injury.

Weight Training Safety

Injuries do happen in weight training. Maximum physical effort, elaborate machinery, rapid movements, and heavy weights can combine to make the weight room a dangerous place if proper precautions aren't taken. To help ensure that your workouts are safe and productive, follow the guidelines in the box "Safe Weight Training" and the suggestions given below.

Use Proper Lifting Technique   Every exercise has a proper technique that is important for obtaining maximum benefits and preventing injury. Your instructor or weight room attendant can help explain the specific tech-

- Lift weights from a stabilized body position.
- Be aware of what's going on around you. Stay away from other people when they're doing exercises. If you bump into someone, you could cause an injury.
- Don't use defective equipment. Report any equipment malfunctions immediately.
- Protect your back by maintaining control of your spine (protect your spine from dangerous positions). Observe proper lifting techniques, and use a weight-lifting belt when doing heavy lifts.
- Don't hold your breath while doing weight training exercises.
- Always warm up before training, and cool down afterward.
- Don't exercise if you're ill, injured, or overtrained.

(a)

(b)

Spotters should be present when a person trains with free weights. **(a)** If two spotters are used, one spotter should stand at each end of the barbell. **(b)** If one spotter is present, he or she should stand behind the lifter.

niques for performing different exercises and using different weight machines. Perform exercises smoothly and with good form. Lift or push the weight forcefully during the active phase of the lift and then lower it slowly with control. Perform all lifts through the full range of motion.

Use Spotters and Collars with Free Weights   Spotters are necessary when an exercise has potential for danger: A weight that is out of control or falls can cause a serious injury. A spotter can assist you if you cannot complete a lift or if the weight tilts. A spotter can also help you move a weight into position before a lift and provide help or additional resistance during a lift. Spotting requires practice and coordination between the lifter and spotter(s).

Collars are devices that secure weights to a barbell or dumbbell. Although people lift weights without collars, doing so is dangerous. It is easy to lose your balance or to raise one side of the weight faster than the other. Without collars, the weights on one side of the bar will slip off, and the weights on the opposite side will crash to the floor.

Proper lifting technique for free weights also includes the following:

- Keep weights as close to your body as possible.
- Do most of your lifting with your legs. Keep your hips and buttocks tucked in.
- When you pick a weight up from the ground, keep your back straight and your head level or up. Don't bend at the waist with straight legs.
- Don't twist your body while lifting.

- Lift weights smoothly and slowly; don't jerk them. Control the weight through the entire range of motion.
- Don't bounce weights against your body during an exercise.
- Never hold your breath when you lift. Exhale when exerting the greatest force, and inhale when moving the weight into position for the active phase of the lift. (Holding your breath causes a decrease in blood returning to the heart and can make you become dizzy and faint.)
- Rest between sets if you perform more than one set of each exercise. Fatigue hampers your ability to obtain maximum benefits from your program and is a prime cause of injury.
- When lifting barbells and dumbbells, wrap your thumbs around the bar when gripping it. You can easily drop the weight when using a "thumbless" grip.
- Gloves are not mandatory but may prevent calluses on your hands.
- When doing standing lifts, maintain a good posture so that you protect your back.
- Don't lift beyond the limits of your strength.

Use Common Sense When Exercising on Weight Machines   Although notable for their safety, weight

Temporalis

Masseter

Sternocleidomastoid
[Scalenus]

Deltoid

[Pectoralis minor]

Pectoralis major

Biceps

Brachialis

Brachioradialis

Quadriceps { Rectus femoris
[Vastus intermedius]
Vastus lateralis
Vastus medialis

Tibialis anterior

Soleus

Trapezius

Biceps

Triceps

External oblique

Rectus abdominis

Adductor longus

Sartorius

Patella

Gastrocnemius
(calf)

Anterior view

Figure 4-4 The muscular system. The muscle names enclosed in brackets refer to deep muscles.

machines are not completely danger-free. The following strategies can help prevent injuries.

- Keep away from moving weight stacks. Pay attention when you're changing weights. Someone may jump on the machine ahead of you and begin an exercise while your fingers are close to the weight stack.

- Stay away from moving parts of the machine that could pinch your skin.

- Adjust each machine for your body so that you don't have to work in an awkward position. Lock everything in place before you begin.

- Beware of broken bolts, frayed cables, broken chains, or loose cushions that can give way and cause serious injury. If you notice a broken or frayed part, tell an instructor immediately.

- Make sure the machines are clean. Dirty vinyl is a breeding ground for germs that can cause skin diseases. Carry a towel around with you and place it on the machine where you will sit or lie down.

- Be aware of what's happening around you. Talking between exercises is a great way to relax and have fun, but inattention can lead to injury.

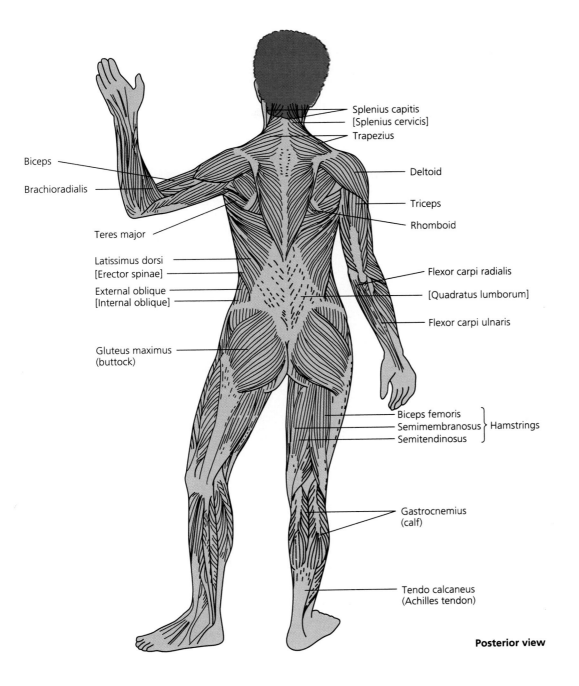

Splenius capitis
[Splenius cervicis]
Trapezius
Deltoid
Triceps
Rhomboid
Flexor carpi radialis
[Quadratus lumborum]
Flexor carpi ulnaris
Biceps femoris
Semimembranosus ⎫ Hamstrings
Semitendinosus ⎭
Gastrocnemius
(calf)
Tendo calcaneus
(Achilles tendon)

Biceps
Brachioradialis
Teres major
Latissimus dorsi
[Erector spinae]
External oblique
[Internal oblique]
Gluteus maximus
(buttock)

Posterior view

Be Alert for Injuries Report any obvious muscle or joint injuries to your instructor or physician, and stop exercising the affected area. Training with an injured joint or muscle can lead to a more serious injury. Make sure you get the necessary first aid. Even minor injuries heal faster if you use the R-I-C-E principle of treating injuries described in Chapter 3.

Consult a physician if you're having any unusual symptoms during exercise or if you're uncertain whether weight training is a proper activity for you. Conditions such as heart disease and high blood pressure can be aggravated during weight training. Symptoms such as headaches, dizziness, labored breathing, numbness, vision disturbances, and chest, neck, or arm pains should be reported immediately.

Weight Training Exercises

A general book on fitness and wellness cannot include a detailed description of all weight training exercises. Here we present a basic program for developing muscular strength and endurance for general fitness using free weights and Nautilus weight machines. Instructions for each exercise are accompanied by photographs and a listing of the muscles being trained. (Figure 4-4 is a diagram

Body Part	Nautilus	Universal Gym	Free Weights
Neck	4-way neck	Neck conditioning station	Neck harness Manual exercises
Trapezius ("Traps")	Overhead press Lateral raise Reverse pullover Compound row Shoulder shrug Rowing back	Shoulder press Shoulder shrug Upright row Bent-over row Rip-up Front raise Pull-up	Overhead press Lateral raise Shoulder shrug Power clean Upright row
Deltoids	Lateral raise Overhead press Reverse pullover Double chest 10° chest 50° chest Seated dip Bench press Compound row Rotary shoulder	Bench press Shoulder shrug Shoulder press Upright row Rip-up Front raise Pull-up	Raise Bench press Shoulder press Upright row Pull-up
Biceps	Biceps curl Lat pull	Biceps curl Lat pull	Biceps curl Lat pull Pull-up
Triceps	Triceps extension Seated dip Triceps exten. (lat machine) Bench press Overhead press	French curl Dip Triceps exten. (lat machine) Bench press Seated press	French curl Dip Triceps exten. (lat machine) Bench press Military press
Latissimus dorsi ("Lats")	Pullover Behind neck Torso arm Lat pull Seated dip Compound row	Pull-up Lat pull Bent-over row Pull-over Dip	Pull-up Pull-over Dip Bent-over row Lat pull
Abdominals	Abdominal Rotary torso	Hip flexor Leg raise Crunch Sit-up Side-bend	Hip flexor Leg raise Crunch Sit-up Side-bend Isometric tightener
Lower back	Lower back	Back extension Back leg raise	Back extension Good-morning
Thigh and buttocks	Leg press Leg extension Leg curl Hip adductor Hip abductor	Leg press Leg curl Leg extension Adductor kick Abductor kick Back hip extension	Squat Leg press Leg extension Leg curl Power clean Snatch Dead lift
Calf	Seated calf Heel raise: multiexercise	Calf press	Heel raise

TABLE 4-2 *Weight Training Exercises for Machines and Free Weights*

TABLE 4-3 — Weight Training for Sports and Activities

Emphasize these muscle groups when training for the following sports and activities. Although it is important to condition all major muscle groups, specific activities require extra conditioning in specific muscles.

Activity or Sport	Neck	Shoulders	Chest	Arms	Forearms	Upper Back	Lower Back	Abdominals	Thighs	Hamstrings	Calves
Badminton		✔	✔	✔	✔	✔			✔	✔	✔
Basketball		✔	✔	✔		✔	✔	✔	✔	✔	✔
Billiards		✔		✔	✔	✔	✔				
Canoeing		✔	✔	✔	✔	✔	✔	✔			
Cycling		✔		✔	✔	✔	✔	✔	✔	✔	✔
Dancing							✔	✔	✔	✔	✔
Field hockey		✔	✔	✔	✔	✔	✔	✔	✔	✔	✔
Fishing				✔	✔				✔	✔	✔
Football	✔	✔	✔	✔	✔	✔	✔	✔	✔	✔	✔
Golf		✔		✔	✔	✔	✔	✔	✔	✔	✔
Gymnastics	✔	✔	✔	✔	✔	✔	✔	✔	✔	✔	✔
Jogging		✔		✔		✔	✔	✔	✔	✔	✔
Rock climbing		✔	✔	✔	✔	✔	✔	✔	✔	✔	✔
Scuba diving				✔		✔	✔	✔	✔	✔	
Skating, in-line		✔				✔	✔	✔	✔	✔	✔
Skiing, cross-country		✔		✔	✔	✔	✔	✔	✔	✔	✔
Skiing, downhill		✔		✔		✔	✔	✔	✔	✔	✔
Squash		✔	✔	✔	✔	✔	✔	✔	✔	✔	✔
Swimming		✔	✔	✔	✔	✔	✔	✔	✔	✔	
Table tennis		✔		✔	✔	✔			✔	✔	✔
Tennis		✔	✔	✔	✔	✔	✔	✔	✔	✔	✔
Triathlon		✔	✔	✔	✔	✔	✔	✔	✔	✔	✔
Volleyball		✔	✔	✔	✔	✔	✔	✔	✔	✔	✔
Water skiing	✔	✔		✔	✔	✔	✔	✔	✔	✔	✔
Wrestling	✔	✔	✔	✔	✔	✔	✔	✔	✔	✔	✔

of the muscular system.) Table 4-2 lists alternative and additional exercises that can be performed on Nautilus or Universal machines or with free weights. If you are interested in learning how to do these exercises, ask your instructor or coach for assistance.

If you want to develop strength for a particular activity, your program should contain exercises for general fitness, exercises for the muscle groups most important for the activity, and exercises for muscle groups most often injured.

To create a weight training program for your favorite sport or activity, choose from among the exercises listed in Table 4-3, as well as from those listed in Table 4-2. Regardless of the goals of your program or the type of equipment you use, your program should be structured so that you obtain maximum results without risking injury. You should train at least 2 days per week, and each exercise session should contain a warm-up, 1 or more sets of 8–12 repetitions of 8–10 exercises, and a period of rest.

WEIGHT TRAINING EXERCISES
Free Weights

EXERCISE 1

BENCH PRESS

Muscles developed: Pectoralis major, triceps, deltoids

Instruction: (a) Lying on a bench on your back with your feet on the floor, grasp the bar with palms upward and hands shoulder-width apart. **(b)** Lower the bar to your chest. Then return it to the starting position. The bar should follow an elliptical path, during which the weight moves from a low point at the chest to a high point over the chin. If your back arches too much, try doing this exercise with your feet on the bench.

 (a)

 (b)

EXERCISE 2

SHOULDER PRESS (Overhead or Military Press)

Muscles developed: Deltoids, triceps, trapezius

Instructions: This exercise can be done standing or seated, with dumbbells or barbells. The shoulder press begins with the weight at your chest, preferably on a rack. **(a)** Grasp the weight with your palms facing away from you. **(b)** Push the weight overhead until your arms are extended. Then return to the starting position (weight at chest). Be careful not to arch your back excessively.

If you are a more advanced weight trainer, you can "clean" the weight to your chest (lift it from the floor to your chest). The clean should be attempted only after instruction from a knowledgeable coach; otherwise, it can lead to injury.

 (a)

 (b)

Although a spotter does not appear in these demonstration photographs, spotters should be used for most exercises with free weights.

LAT PULL

Muscles developed: Latissimus dorsi, biceps

Instructions: Begin in a seated or kneeling position, depending on the type of lat machine and the manufacturer's instructions. **(a)** Grasp the bar of the machine with arms fully extended. **(b)** Slowly pull the weight down until it reaches the back of your neck. Slowly return to the starting position.

(a)   (b)

LATERAL RAISE

Muscles developed: Deltoids

Instructions: **(a)** Stand with feet shoulder-width apart and a dumbbell in each hand. Hold the dumbbells parallel to each other. **(b)** With elbows slightly bent, slowly lift both weights until they reach shoulder level. Keep your wrists in a neutral position, in line with your forearms. Return to the starting position.

(a)   (b)

BICEPS CURL

Muscles developed: Biceps, brachialis

Instructions: (a) From a standing position, grasp the bar with your palms upward and your hands shoulder-width apart. **(b)** Keeping your upper body rigid, flex (bend) your elbows until the bar reaches a level slightly below the collarbone. Return the bar to the starting position.

(a)　　　　　　　　　　　　　　　(b)

SQUAT

Muscles developed: Quadriceps, gluteus maximus, hamstrings, gastrocnemius

Instructions: Stand with feet shoulder-width apart and toes pointed slightly outward. **(a)** Rest the bar on the back of your shoulders, holding it there with hands facing forward. **(b)** Keeping your head up and lower back straight, squat down until your thighs are almost parallel with the floor. Drive upward toward the starting position, keeping your back in a fixed position throughout the exercise.

(a)　　　　　　　　　　　　　　　(b)

Although a spotter does not appear in these demonstration photographs, spotters should be used for most exercises with free weights.

TOE RAISE

Muscles developed: Gastrocnemius, soleus

Instructions: Stand with feet shoulder-width apart and toes pointed straight ahead. **(a)** Rest the bar on the back of your shoulders, holding it there with hands facing forward. **(b)** Press down with your toes while lifting your heels. Return to the starting position.

(a)   (b)

CURL-UP OR CRUNCH

Muscles developed: Rectus abdominis, obliques

Instructions: (a) Lie on your back on the floor with your arms folded across your chest and your feet on the floor or on a bench. **(b)** Curl your trunk up and forward by raising your head and shoulders from the ground. Lower to the starting position.

(a)   (b)

SPINE EXTENSIONS (Isometric Exercises)

Muscles developed: Erector spinae, gluteus maximus, hamstrings, deltoids

Instructions: Begin on all fours with your knees below your hips and your hands below your shoulders.

Unilateral spine extension: (a) Extend your right leg to the rear, and reach forward with your right arm. Keep your neck neutral and your raised arm and leg in line with your torso. Don't arch your back or let your hip or shoulder sag. Hold this position for 10–30 seconds. Repeat with your left leg and left arm.

Bilateral spine extension: (b) Extend your left leg to the rear, and reach forward with your right arm. Keep your neck neutral and your raised leg in line with your torso. Don't arch your back or let your hip or shoulder sag. Hold this position for 10–30 seconds. Repeat with your right leg and left arm.

You can make this exercise more difficult by attaching weights to your ankles and wrists.

(a)

(b)

NECK FLEXION AND LATERAL FLEXION (Isometric Exercises)

Muscles developed: Sternocleidomastoids, scaleni

Instructions:

Neck Flexion: (a) Place your hand on your forehead with fingertips pointed up. Using the muscles at the back of your neck, press your head forward and resist the pressure with the palm of your hand.

Lateral flexion: (b) Place your hand on the right side of your face, fingertips pointed up. Using the muscles on the left side of your neck, press your head to the right and resist the pressure with the palm of your hand. Repeat on the left side.

(a)

(b)

Nautilus Weight Machines

EXERCISE 1

BENCH PRESS

Muscles developed: Pectoralis major, anterior deltoids, triceps

Instructions: Lie on the bench so the tops of the handles are aligned with the tops of your armpits. Place your feet flat on the floor; if they don't reach, place them on the bench. (a) Grasp the handles with your palms facing away from you. (b) Push the bars until your arms are fully extended. Return to the starting position.

(a)

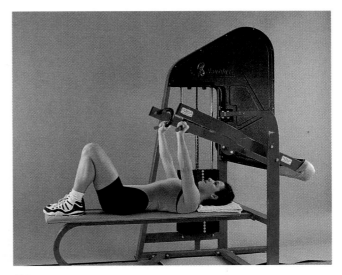

(b)

EXERCISE 2

OVERHEAD PRESS (Shoulder Press)

Muscles developed: Deltoids, trapezius, triceps

Instructions: Adjust the seat so the two bars are slightly above your shoulders. (a) Sit down, facing away from the machine, and grasp the bars with your palms facing inward. (b) Press the weight upward until your arms are extended. Return to the starting position.

(a)

(b)

PULLOVER

Muscles developed: Latissimus dorsi, pectoralis major and minor, triceps, abdominals

Instructions: Adjust the seat so your shoulders are aligned with the cams. Push down on the foot pads with your feet to bring the bar forward until you can place your elbows on the pads. Rest your hands lightly on the bar. If possible, place your feet flat on the floor. **(a)** To get into the starting position, let your arms go backward as far as possible. **(b)** Pull your elbows forward until the bar almost touches your abdomen. Return to the starting position.

(a)   (b)

LATERAL RAISE

Muscles developed: Deltoids, trapezius

Instructions: **(a)** Adjust the seat so the pads rest just above your elbows when your upper arms are at your sides, your elbows are bent, and your forearms are parallel to the floor. **(b)** Lightly grasp the handles and push outward and up with your arms until the pads are shoulder height. Lead with your elbows rather than trying to lift the bars with your hands. Return to the starting position.

(a)   (b)

MULTITRICEPS

Muscles developed: Triceps

Instructions: Adjust the seat so your elbows are slightly lower than your shoulders when you sit down. (**a**) Place your elbows on the support cushions and your forearms on the bar pads. (**b**) Extend your elbows as much as possible. Return to the starting position.

(a)

(b)

LEG PRESS

Muscles developed: Gluteus maximus, quadriceps, hamstrings

Instructions: (**a**) Adjust the seat so your knees are bent at a 90-degree angle. (**b**) Sit with your hands on the side handles, your feet on the pedals, and your legs fully extended. (**c**) From this position, bend your right leg 90 degrees, and then forcefully extend it. Repeat with your left leg. Alternate between right and left legs.

(a)

(b)

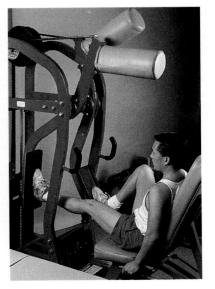

(c)

LEG EXTENSION (Knee Extension)

Muscles developed: Quadriceps

Instructions: (a) Sit on the seat with your shins under the knee-extension pads. **(b)** Extend your knees until they are straight. Return to the starting position.

Knee extensions cause kneecap pain in some people. If you have kneecap pain during this exercise, check with an orthopedic specialist before repeating it.

(a)

(b)

PRONE LEG CURL (Knee Flexion)

Muscles developed: Hamstrings

Instructions: (a) Lie on your stomach, resting the pads of the machine just below your calf muscles and with your knees just off the edge of the bench. **(b)** Flex your knees until they approach your buttocks. Return to the starting position.

(a)

(b)

TOE RAISE

Muscles developed: Gastrocnemius, soleus

Instructions: **(a)** Stand with your head between the pads and one pad on each shoulder. **(b)** Press down with your toes while lifting your heels. Return to the starting position. Changing the direction your feet are pointing (straight ahead, inward, and outward) will work different portions of your calf muscles.

(a)   (b)

ABDOMINAL CURL

Muscles developed: Rectus abdominis, internal and external obliques

Instructions: **(a)** Adjust the seat so the machine rotates at the level of your navel, the pad rests on your upper chest, and your feet can rest comfortably on the floor. **(b)** Move your trunk forward as far as possible. Return to the starting position.

(a)   (b)

LOW-BACK MACHINE (Back Extensions)

Muscles developed: Erector spinae, quadratus lumborum

Instructions: (a) Sit on the seat with your upper legs under the thigh-support pads, your back on the back roller pad, and your feet on the platform. **(b)** Extend backward until your back is straight. Return to the starting position. Try to keep your spine rigid during the exercise.

(a) (b)

FOUR-WAY NECK MACHINE

Muscles developed: Sternocleidomastoids, scaleni (flexion and lateral flexion); splenius capitis, splenius cervicis, trapezius (extension)

Instructions:

Flexion: (a) Adjust the seat so the front of your forehead rests in the center of the two pads. Bend your head forward as far as possible, using your neck muscles, and then return to the starting position.

Lateral flexion: (b) Adjust the seat so the side of your head rests in the center of the two pads. Bend your head sideways toward your shoulder as far as possible, and then return to the starting position. Perform the exercise for both the right and left sides of your head.

Extension: (c) Adjust the seat so the back of your head rests in the center of the two pads. Bend your head backward as far as possible, and then return to the starting position.

(a) (b) (c)

How long must I weight train before I begin to see changes in my body? You will increase strength very rapidly during the early stages of a weight training program, primarily the result of muscle learning (the increased ability of the nervous system to recruit muscle fibers to exert force). Actual changes in muscle size usually begin after about 6–8 weeks of training.

I am concerned about my body composition. Will I gain weight if I do resistance exercises? Your weight probably will not change significantly as a result of a recreational-type weight training program: 1 set of 8–12 repetitions of 8–10 exercises. You will tend to increase muscle mass and lose body fat, so your weight will stay about the same. (Men will tend to build larger muscles than women because of the tissue-building effects of male hormones.) Increased muscle mass will help you control body fat. Muscle increases your metabolism, which means you burn up more calories every day. If you combine resistance exercises with endurance exercises, you will be on your way to developing a healthier body composition. Concentrate on fat loss rather than weight loss.

Do I need more protein in my diet when I train with weights? No. While there is some evidence that power athletes involved in heavy training have a higher-than-normal protein requirement, there is no reason for most people to consume extra protein. Most Americans take in more protein than they need, so even if there is an increased protein need during heavy training, it is probably supplied by the average diet. (See Chapter 8 for more on dietary needs of athletes.)

Are there any supplements or drugs that will help me make larger and more rapid increases in strength and endurance? No nutritional supplement or drug will change a weak, un-trained person into a strong, fit person. Those changes require regular training that stresses the muscles, heart, lungs, and metabolism and causes the body to adapt. Supplements or drugs that are promoted as instant or quick "cures" usually don't work and are either dangerous or expensive, or both. **Anabolic steroids**—the drugs most often taken in an effort to build strength and power—have dangerous side effects, described in Table 4-4. You are better off staying with proven principles of nutrition and a steady, progressive fitness program.

What causes muscle soreness the day or two following a weight training workout? The muscle pain you feel a day or two after a heavy weight training workout is caused by injury to the muscle fibers and surrounding connective tissue. Contrary to popular belief, delayed-onset muscle soreness is not caused by lactic acid buildup. Scientists believe that injury to muscle fibers causes the release of excess calcium into muscles. The calcium causes the release of substances called **proteases**, which break down part of the muscle tissue and

cause pain. After a bout of intense exercise that causes muscle injury and delayed-onset muscle soreness, the muscles produce protective proteins that prevent soreness during future workouts. If you don't work out regularly, you lose these protective proteins and become susceptible to muscle soreness again.

Will strength training improve my sports performance? Strength developed in the weight room does not automatically increase your power in sports such as skiing, tennis, or cycling. Hitting a forehand in tennis or making a turn on skis is highly specific and requires precise coordination between your nervous system and muscles. In skilled people, movements become reflex—you don't think about them when you do them. Increasing strength can disturb this coordination. Only by simultaneously practicing a sport and improving fitness can you expect to become more powerful in the skill. Practice helps you integrate your new strength with your skills, which makes you more powerful. Consequently, you can hit the ball harder in tennis or make more graceful turns on the ski slopes. (Refer to Chapter 2 for more on the concept of specificity of physical training.)

Will I improve faster if I train every day? No. Your muscles need time to recover between training sessions. Doing resistance exercises every day will cause you to become over-trained, which will increase your chance of injury and impede your progress. If you find that your strength training program has reached a plateau, try one of these strategies:

- Train less frequently. If you are currently training the same muscle groups three or more times per week, you may not be allowing your muscles to fully recover from intense workouts.

- Change exercises. Using different exercises for a particular muscle group may stimulate further strength development.

- Vary the load and number of repetitions. Try increasing or decreasing the loads you are using and changing the number of repetitions accordingly.

- Vary the number of sets. If you have been performing 1 set of each exercise, add sets.

- If you are training alone, find a motivated training partner. A partner can encourage you and assist you with difficult lifts, forcing you to work harder.

If I stop weight training, will my muscles turn to fat? No. Fat and muscle are two different kinds of tissue, and one cannot turn into the other. Muscles that aren't used become smaller (atrophy), and body fat may increase if caloric intake exceeds calories burned. Although the result of inactivity may be smaller muscles and more fat, the change is caused by two separate processes.

anabolic steroids Synthetic male hormones taken to enhance athletic performance and body composition.

proteases Enzymes that break down proteins.

TERMS

TABLE 4-4	Performance Aids Marketed to Weight Trainers		
Substance	Supposed Effects	Actual Effects	Selected Potential Side Effects
Adrenal steroids: DHEA, androstenedione	Increased testosterone, muscle mass, and strength; decreased body fat	Increased testosterone, strength, and fat-free mass and decreased fat in older subjects (more studies needed in younger people)	Gonadal suppression, prostate hypertrophy, breast development in males, masculinization in women and children. Long-term effects unknown
Amino acids	Increased muscle mass	No effects if dietary protein intake is adequate	Minimal side effects; unbalanced amino acid intake can cause problems with protein metabolism
Anabolic steroids	Increased muscle mass, strength, power, psychological aggressiveness, and endurance	Increased strength, power, fat-free mass, and aggression; no effects on endurance	Minor to severe: gonadal suppression, liver disease, acne, breast development in males, masculinization in women and children, heart disease, cancer. Steroids are controlled substances[a]
Chromium picolinate	Increased muscle mass; decreased body fat	Well-controlled studies show no significant effect on fat-free mass or body fat	Moderate doses (50–200 μg) appear safe; higher doses may cause DNA damage and other serious effects. Long-term effects unknown
Creatine monohydrate	Increased muscle creatine phosphate, muscle mass, and capacity for high-intensity exercise	Increased muscle mass and performance in some types of high-intensity exercise	Minimal side effects; some reports of muscle cramping. Long-term effects unknown
Ephedrine	Decreased body fat; increased training intensity due to stimulant effect	Decreased appetite, particularly when taken with caffeine; no evidence for increased training intensity	Abnormal heart rhythms, nervousness, headache, and gastrointestinal distress. Not recommended
Ginseng	Decreased effects of physical and emotional stress; increased oxygen consumption	Most well-controlled studies show no effect on performance	No serious side effects; high doses can cause high blood pressure, nervousness, and insomnia
Growth hormone	Increased muscle mass, strength, and power; decreased body fat	Increased muscle mass and strength	Diabetes, acromegaly (disease characterized by increased growth of bones in hands and face), enlarged heart and other organs. An extremely expensive controlled substance[a]
HMB (beta-hydroxy-beta-methylbutyrate)	Increased strength and muscle mass; decreased body fat	Some studies show increased fat-free mass and decreased fat; more research needed	No reported side effects. Long-term effects unknown
"Metabolic optimizer" meals for athletes	Increased muscle mass; energy supply; decreased body fat	No proven effects beyond that of balanced meals	No reported side effects; extremely expensive
Plant sterols	Increased muscle mass and strength; enhanced release of growth hormone and testosterone	No evidence of beneficial effects on body composition or performance	No known side effects; can cause allergic reactions in some people
Protein	Increased muscle mass	No effects if dietary protein intake is adequate	Can be dangerous for people with liver or kidney disease

[a]Possession of a controlled substance is illegal without a prescription, and physicians are not allowed to prescribe them for the improvement of athletic performance. In addition, the use of anabolic steroids, growth hormone, or any of several other substances listed on this table is banned for athletic competition.

SOURCES: Williams, M. H. 1998. *The Ergogenics Edge: Pushing the Limits of Sports Performance.* Champaign, Ill.: Human Kinetics. Armsey, T. D., and G. A. Green. 1997. Nutrition supplements: Science vs. hype. *The Physician and Sportsmedicine* 25(4). Brooks, G. A., T. D. Fahey, and T. P. White. 1996. *Exercise Physiology: Human Bioenergetics and Its Applications,* 2d ed. Mountain View, Calif.: Mayfield.

SUMMARY

- Improvements in muscular strength and endurance lead to enhanced physical performance, protection against injury, improved body composition, better self-image, and improved muscle and bone health with aging.

- Muscular strength can be assessed by determining the amount of weight that can be lifted in one repetition of an exercise; muscular endurance can be assessed by determining the number of repetitions of a particular exercise that can be performed.

- Hypertrophy, increased muscle fiber size, occurs when weight training causes the number of myofibrils to increase; total muscle size thereby increases. Strength also increases through muscle learning.

- Isometric exercises (contraction without movement) are most useful when a person is recovering from an injury or surgery or needs to overcome weak points in a range of motion.

- Isotonic exercises involve contraction that results in movement. The two most common types are constant resistance (free weights) and variable resistance (weight machines).

- Free weights and weight machines are basically equally effective in producing fitness, although machines tend to be safer.

- Lifting heavy weights for only a few repetitions helps develop strength. Lifting lighter weights for more repetitions helps develop muscular endurance.

- A weight training program for general fitness includes at least 1 set of 8–12 repetitions (enough to cause fatigue) of 8–10 exercises, along with warm-up and cool-down periods; the program should be carried out 2–3 times a week.

- Safety guidelines for weight training include using proper technique, using spotters and collars when necessary, using common sense and remaining alert, and taking care of injuries.

FOR MORE INFORMATION

Information on and programs in weight training are available through physical education and athletics departments, private health clubs, and weight-lifting clubs.

Books

Fahey, T. D. 1997. *Basic Weight Training for Men and Women,* 3d ed. Mountain View, Calif.: Mayfield. *A practical guide to developing training programs using free weights tailored to individual needs.*

Fleck, S. J., and W. J. Kraemer. 1997. *Designing Resistance Training Programs.* Champaign, Ill.: Human Kinetics. *A book aimed at personal trainers or serious weight trainers who want a thorough discussion of program design methods for weight training.*

Ward, P. E., and R. D. Ward. 1997. *The Encyclopedia of Weight Training.* Los Angeles: Q P T Publishing. *An authoritative guide to weight training for athletes and body builders written by two of America's top strength coaches.*

Westcott, W. 1996. *Building Strength and Stamina: New Nautilus Training for Total Fitness.* Champaign, Ill.: Human Kinetics. *An updated guide to training using Nautilus machines.*

Williams, M. H. 1998. *The Ergogenics Edge: Pushing the Limits of Sports Performance.* Champaign, Ill.: Human Kinetics. *Written by one of the top sports nutrition researchers in the world, this is an excellent book on the scientific basis of substances and techniques used to improve athletic performance.*

Organizations and Web Sites

Biomechanics World Wide. A resource site with links to many other sites relating to biomechanics; topics include muscle mechanics and sports techniques.

　http://www.per.ualberta.ca/biomechanics

Human Anatomy On-line. Provides text, illustrations, and animation about the muscular system, nerve-muscle connections, muscular contraction, and other topics.

　http://www.innerbody.com/indexbody.html

National Strength and Conditioning Association. Provides education and certification for professionals in strength and conditioning.

　402-476-6669

　http://www.nsca-cc.org

Nicholas Institute of Sports Medicine and Athletic Trauma. Includes information on exercise physiology, physical therapy, sports medicine, and training.

　http://www.nismat.org

University of California, San Diego/Muscle Physiology Home Page. Provides an introduction to muscle physiology, including information about types of muscle fibers and energy cycles.

　http://muscle.ucsd.edu

University of Michigan/Muscles in Action. Interactive descriptions of muscle movements.

　http://www.med.umich.edu/lrc/Hypermuscle/Hyper.html

See also the listings in Chapter 2.

SELECTED BIBLIOGRAPHY

American College of Sports Medicine. 1995. *Guidelines for Exercise Testing and Prescription,* 5th ed. Baltimore: Williams & Wilkins.

American College of Sports Medicine. 1998. Position Stand: The Recommended Quantity and Quality of Exercise for Developing and Maintaining Cardiorespiratory and Muscular Fitness, and Flexibility in Healthy Adults. *Medicine and Science in Sports and Exercise* 30(6): 975–991.

Ashe, J. 1997. Force and the motor cortex. *Behavioral Brain Research* 86:1–15.

Bohannon, R. W. 1997. Hand-held dynamometry: Factors influencing reliability and validity. *Clinical Rehabilitation* 11:263–264.

Brooks, G. A., T. D. Fahey, and T. P. White. 1996. *Exercise Physiology: Human Bioenergetics and Its Applications,* 2d ed.

Mountain View, Calif.: Mayfield.

Burr, D. B. 1997. Muscle strength, bone mass, and age-related bone loss. *Journal of Bone Mineral Research* 12:1547–1551.

Chandler, J. M., et al. 1998. Is lower extremity strength gain associated with improvement in physical performance and disability in frail, community-dwelling elders? *Archives of Physical Medicine and Rehabilitation* 79(1): 24–30.

Chilibeck, P. D., et al. 1998. A comparison of strength and muscle mass increases during resistance training in young women. *European Journal of Applied Physiology* 77(1–2): 170–175.

Delecluse, C. 1997. Influence of strength training on sprint running performance. Current findings and implications for training. *Sports Medicine* 24:147–156.

Feigenbaum, M. S., and M. L. Pollock. 1997. Strength training: Rationale for current guidelines for adult fitness programs. *The Physician and Sportsmedicine* 25(2): 44–49.

Geliebter, A., et al. 1997. Effects of strength or aerobic training on body composition, resting metabolic rate, and peak oxygen consumption in obese dieting subjects. *American Journal of Clinical Nutrition* 66:557–563.

Harris, T. 1997. Muscle mass and strength: Relation to function in population studies. *Journal of Nutrition* 127:1004S–1006S.

Klinge, K., et al. 1997. The effect of strength and flexibility training on skeletal muscle electromyographic activity, stiffness, and viscoelastic stress relaxation response. *American Journal of Sports Medicine* 25:710–716.

Lindle, R. S., et al. 1997. Age and gender comparisons of muscle strength in 654 women and men aged 20–93 yr. *Journal of Applied Physiology* 83:1581–1587.

Longhurst, J. C., and C. L. Stebbins. 1997. The power athlete. *Cardiology Clinics* 15:413–429.

Mayhew, J. L., et al. 1997. Changes in upper body power following heavy-resistance strength training in college men. *International Journal of Sports Medicine* 18:516–520.

Pincivero, D. M., S. M. Lephart, and R. G. Karunakara. 1997. Effects of rest interval on isokinetic strength and functional performance after short-term high intensity training. *British Journal of Sports Medicine* 31:229–234.

Ploutz-Snyder, L. L., P. A. Tesch, and G. A. Dudley. 1998. Increased vulnerability to eccentric exercise-induced dysfunction and muscle injury after concentric training. *Archives of Physical Medicine and Rehabilitation* 79(1): 58–61.

Pollock, M. L., et al. 1997. Twenty-year follow-up of aerobic power and body composition of older track athletes. *Journal of Applied Physiology* 82:1508–1516.

Stanford, B. 1998. Weight training basics: Part 1: Choosing the best options. *The Physician and Sportsmedicine* 26(2).

Thompson, H. S., et al. 1997. The effects of oral contraceptives on delayed onset muscle soreness following exercise. *Contraception* 56:59–65.

Toji, J., K. Suei, and M. Kaneko. 1997. Effects of combined training loads on relations among force, velocity, and power development. *Canadian Journal of Applied Physiology* 22: 328–336.

Vandenberghe, K., et al. 1997. Long-term creatine intake is beneficial to muscle performance during resistance training. *Journal of Applied Physiology* 83:2055–2063.

Van Etten, L. M., et al. 1997. Effect of an 18-wk weight-training program on energy expenditure and physical activity. *Journal of Applied Physiology* 82:298–304.

Vincent, H. K., and K. R. Vincent. 1997. The effect of training status on the serum creatine kinase response, soreness and muscle function following resistance exercise. *International Journal of Sports Medicine* 18:431–437.

Wiemann, K., and K. Hahn. 1997. Influences of strength, stretching and circulatory exercises on flexibility parameters of the human hamstrings. *International Journal of Sports Medicine* 18:340–346.

Wu, F. C. 1997. Endocrine aspects of anabolic steroids. *Clinical Chemistry* 43:1289–1292.

Name _____ **Section** _____ **Date** _____

LAB 4-1 *Assessing Your Current Level of Muscular Strength*

For best results, don't do any strenuous weight training within 48 hours of any test.

The Maximum Bench Press Test

Equipment

1. Universal Gym Dynamic Variable Resistance machine
2. Weight scale

Maximum bench press test.

The ratings for this test were developed using the Universal Gym Dynamic Variable Resistance machine; results will be somewhat less accurate if the test is performed on another type of machine or with free weights.

If free weights are used, the following equipment is needed:

1. Flat bench (with or without racks)
2. Barbell
3. Assorted weight plates
4. Collars to hold weight plates in place
5. One or two spotters
6. Weight scale

Preparation

Try a few bench presses with a small amount of weight so you can practice your technique, warm up your muscles, and, if you use free weights, coordinate your movements with those of your spotters. Weigh yourself, and record the results.

Body weight: _____ lb

Instructions

1. Set the machine (or place weights on the barbell) for a weight that is lower than the amount you believe you can lift.
2. Lie on the bench with your feet firmly on the floor. If you are using a weight machine, grasp the handles with palms away from you; the tops of the handles should be aligned with the tops of your armpits.

    If you are using free weights, grasp the bar at shoulder width with your palms away from you. If you have one spotter, she or he should stand directly behind the bench; if you have two spotters, they should stand to the side, one at each end of the barbell. Lower the bar to your chest in preparation for the lift.
3. Push the bars or barbell until your arms are fully extended. Exhale as you lift. If you are using free weights, the bar should follow an elliptical path, during which the weight moves from a low point at the chest to a high point over the chin. Keep your feet firmly on the floor, don't arch your back, and push the weight evenly with your right and left arms. Don't bounce the weight on your chest.
4. Rest for several minutes, then repeat the lift with a heavier weight. It will probably take several attempts to determine the maximum amount of weight you can lift (1 RM).

    1 RM: _____ lb

Rating Your Bench Press Result

1. Divide your 1 RM value by your body weight.

    1 RM _____ lb ÷ body weight _____ lb = _____

2. Find this ratio in the table below to determine your bench press strength rating. Record the result here and in the chart at the end of this lab.

Bench press strength rating: _____

Strength Ratings for the Maximum Bench Press Test

	Pounds Lifted/Body Weight (lb)					
Men	*Very Poor*	*Poor*	*Fair*	*Good*	*Excellent*	*Superior*
Age: Under 20	Below 0.89	0.89–1.05	1.06–1.18	1.19–1.33	1.34–1.75	Above 1.75
20–29	Below 0.88	0.88–0.98	0.99–1.13	1.14–1.31	1.32–1.62	Above 1.62
30–39	Below 0.78	0.78–0.87	0.88–0.97	0.98–1.11	1.12–1.34	Above 1.34
40–49	Below 0.72	0.72–0.79	0.80–0.87	0.88–0.99	1.00–1.19	Above 1.19
50–59	Below 0.63	0.63–0.70	0.71–0.78	0.79–0.89	0.90–1.04	Above 1.04
60 and over	Below 0.57	0.57–0.65	0.66–0.71	0.72–0.81	0.82–0.93	Above 0.93
Women						
Age: Under 20	Below 0.53	0.53–0.57	0.58–0.64	0.65–0.76	0.77–0.87	Above 0.87
20–29	Below 0.51	0.51–0.58	0.59–0.69	0.70–0.79	0.80–1.00	Above 1.00
30–39	Below 0.47	0.47–0.52	0.53–0.59	0.60–0.69	0.70–0.81	Above 0.81
40–49	Below 0.43	0.43–0.49	0.50–0.53	0.54–0.61	0.62–0.76	Above 0.76
50–59	Below 0.39	0.39–0.43	0.44–0.47	0.48–0.54	0.55–0.67	Above 0.67
60 and over	Below 0.38	0.38–0.42	0.43–0.46	0.47–0.53	0.54–0.71	Above 0.71

SOURCE: Based on norms from the Cooper Institute for Aerobics Research, Dallas, Texas; used with permission.

The Maximum Leg Press Test

Equipment

1. Universal Gym Dynamic Variable Resistance leg press machine (If you're using a Universal Gym leg press with two sets of pedals, use the lower pedals.)
2. Weight scale

The ratings for this test were developed using the Universal Gym Dynamic Variable Resistance machine; results will be somewhat less accurate if the test is performed on another type of machine.

Maximum leg press test.

Preparation

Try a few leg presses with the machine set for a small amount of weight so you can practice your technique and warm up your muscles. Weigh yourself, and record the results.

Body weight: _____ lb

Instructions

1. Set the machine for a weight that is lower than the amount you believe you can press.
2. Adjust the seat so that your knees are bent at a 70-degree angle to start.
3. Grasp the side handlebars, and push with your legs until your knees are fully extended.
4. Rest for several minutes, then repeat the press with a higher weight setting. It will probably take several attempts to determine the maximum amount of weight you can press.

1 RM: _____ lb

Rating Your Leg Press Result

1. Divide your 1 RM value by your body weight.

    1 RM _____ lb ÷ body weight _____ lb = _____

2. Find this ratio in the table below to determine your leg press strength rating. Record the result below and in the chart at the end of this lab.

    Leg press strength rating: _____

Strength Ratings for the Maximum Leg Press Test

			Pounds Lifted/Body Weight (lb)			
Men	*Very Poor*	*Poor*	*Fair*	*Good*	*Excellent*	*Superior*
Age: Under 20	Below 1.70	1.70–1.89	1.90–2.03	2.04–2.27	2.28–2.81	Above 2.81
20–29	Below 1.63	1.63–1.82	1.83–1.96	1.97–2.12	2.13–2.39	Above 2.39
30–39	Below 1.52	1.52–1.64	1.65–1.76	1.77–1.92	1.93–2.19	Above 2.19
40–49	Below 1.44	1.44–1.56	1.57–1.67	1.68–1.81	1.82–2.01	Above 2.01
50–59	Below 1.32	1.32–1.45	1.46–1.57	1.58–1.70	1.71–1.89	Above 1.89
60 and over	Below 1.25	1.25–1.37	1.38–1.48	1.49–1.61	1.62–1.79	Above 1.79
Women						
Age: Under 20	Below 1.22	1.22–1.37	1.38–1.58	1.59–1.70	1.71–1.87	Above 1.87
20–29	Below 1.22	1.22–1.36	1.37–1.49	1.50–1.67	1.68–1.97	Above 1.97
30–39	Below 1.09	1.09–1.20	1.21–1.32	1.33–1.46	1.47–1.67	Above 1.67
40–49	Below 1.02	1.02–1.12	1.13–1.22	1.23–1.36	1.37–1.56	Above 1.56
50–59	Below 0.88	0.88–0.98	0.99–1.09	1.10–1.24	1.25–1.42	Above 1.42
60 and over	Below 0.85	0.85–0.92	0.93–1.03	1.04–1.17	1.18–1.42	Above 1.42

SOURCE: Based on norms from the Cooper Institute for Aerobics Research, Dallas, Texas; used with permission.

Hand Grip Strength Test

Equipment

Grip strength dynamometer

Preparation

If necessary, adjust the hand grip size on the dynamometer into a position that is comfortable for you; then lock the grip in place. The second joint of your fingers should fit snugly under the handle of the dynamometer.

Instructions

Hand grip strength test.

1. Stand with the hand to be tested first at your side, away from your body. The dynamometer should be in line with your forearm and held at the level of your thigh. Squeeze the dynamometer as hard as possible without moving your arm; exhale as you squeeze. During the test, don't let the dynamometer touch your body or any other object.

2. Perform two trials with each hand. Rest for about a minute between trials. Record the scores for each hand to the nearest kilogram.

    Right hand: Trial 1: _____ kg   Trial 2: _____ kg

    Left hand: Trial 1: _____ kg   Trial 2: _____ kg

(Scores on the dynamometer should be given in kilograms. If the dynamometer you are using gives scores in pounds, convert pounds to kilograms by dividing your score by 2.2.)

Rating Your Hand Grip Strength

Your total score is the sum of the best trial for each hand.

Right hand best trial   _____ kg

Left hand best trial   _____ kg

Total score   _____ kg

Refer to the table below for a rating of your grip strength. Record the result below and in the chart at the end of this lab.

Rating for hand grip strength: _____

Grip Strength* (kg)

Men	Needs Improvement	Fair	Good	Very Good	Excellent
Age: 15–19	Below 84	84–94	95–102	103–112	Above 112
20–29	Below 97	97–105	106–112	113–123	Above 123
30–39	Below 97	97–104	105–112	113–122	Above 122
40–49	Below 94	94–101	102–109	110–118	Above 118
50–59	Below 87	87–95	96–101	102–109	Above 109
60–69	Below 79	79–85	86–92	93–101	Above 101
Women					
Age: 15–19	Below 54	54–58	59–63	64–70	Above 70
20–29	Below 55	55–60	61–64	65–70	Above 70
30–39	Below 56	56–60	61–65	66–72	Above 72
40–49	Below 55	55–58	59–64	65–72	Above 72
50–59	Below 51	51–54	55–58	59–64	Above 64
60–69	Below 48	48–50	51–53	54–59	Above 59

*Combined right and left hand grip strength.

Source: *The Canadian Physical Activity, Fitness and Lifestyle Appraisal: CSEP's Plan for Healthy Active Living, 1996.* Reprinted by permission from the Canadian Society for Exercise Physiology.

Summary of Results

Maximum bench press test

Weight pressed: _____ lb   Rating: _____

Maximum leg press test

Weight pressed: _____ lb   Rating: _____

Hand grip strength test

Total score: _____ kg   Rating: _____

Remember that muscular strength is specific: Your ratings may vary considerably for different parts of your body. You can use these results to guide you in planning a weight training program.

To monitor your progress toward your goal, enter the results of this lab in the Preprogram Assessment column of Appendix D. After several weeks of a weight training program, do this lab again, and enter the results in the Postprogram Assessment column of Appendix D. How do the results compare?

Name _____ Section _____ Date _____

LAB 4-3 *Designing and Monitoring a Weight Training Program*

1. *Set goals.* List the goals of your weight training program. Goals can be general, such as developing greater muscle definition, or specific, such as increasing the power in a golf swing. If your goals involve the development of a specific muscle group, note that also.

    1. _____

    2. _____

    3. _____

    4. _____

2. *Choose exercises.* Based on your goals, choose 8–10 exercises to perform during each weight training session. If your goal is general training for wellness, use the sample program in the box "A Sample Weight Training Program for General Fitness" on p. 77. If your goals relate to a specific sport, use Table 4-3 to put together a program to develop the important muscle groups. List your exercises and the muscles they develop in the space provided in the program plan below.

3. *Choose starting weights.* Experiment with different amounts of weight until you settle on a good starting weight, one that you can lift easily for 10–12 repetitions. As you progress in your program, you can add more weight. Fill in the starting weight for each exercise on the program plan.

4. *Choose a starting number of sets and repetitions.* Include at least 1 set of 8–12 repetitions of each exercise. (As you add weight, you may have to decrease the number of repetitions slightly until your muscles adapt to the heavier load.) If your program is focusing on strength alone, your sets can contain fewer repetitions using a heavier load. If you are over approximately 50–60 years of age, your sets should contain more repetitions (10–15) using a lighter load. Fill in the starting number of sets and repetitions of each exercise on the program plan.

5. *Choose the number of training sessions per week.* Work out at least 2 days per week. Indicate the days you will train on your program plan; be sure to include days of rest to allow your body to recover.

6. *Monitor your progress.* Use the workout card on the next page to monitor program progress and keep track of exercises, weights, sets, and repetitions. (A more extensive series of weight training logs is included in the Daily Fitness Log booklet.)

Program Plan for Weight Training

Exercise	Muscle(s) Developed	Weight (lb)	Repetitions	Sets	Frequency (check ✓)						
					M	T	W	Th	F	Sa	Su

WORKOUT CARD FOR _____

Exercise/Date	Wt	Sets	Reps	Wt	Sets	Reps	Wt	Sets	Reps	Wt	Sets	Reps	Wt	Sets	Reps	Wt	Sets	Reps	Wt	Sets	Reps	Wt	Sets	Reps	Wt	Sets	Reps	Wt	Sets	Reps	Wt	Sets	Reps	Wt	Sets	Reps

Flexibility

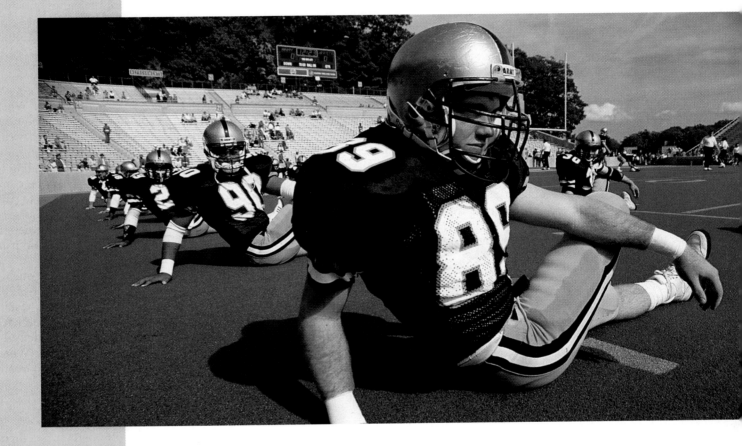

LOOKING AHEAD

After reading this chapter, you should be able to answer these questions about flexibility and stretching exercises:

• What are the potential benefits of flexibility and stretching exercises?

• What determines the amount of flexibility in each joint?

• What are the different types of stretching exercises, and how do they affect muscles?

• What type, intensity, duration, and frequency of stretching exercises will develop the greatest amount of flexibility with the lowest risk of injury?

• What are some common stretching exercises for major joints?

• How can low-back pain be prevented and managed?

Flexibility—the ability of a joint to move through its full **range of motion**—is extremely important for general fitness and wellness. The smooth and easy performance of everyday and recreational activities is impossible if flexibility is poor. Flexibility is a highly adaptable physical fitness component. It increases in response to a regular program of stretching exercises and decreases with inactivity. Flexibility is also specific: Good flexibility in one joint doesn't necessarily mean good flexibility in another. Flexibility can be increased through stretching exercises for all major joints.

There are two basic types of flexibility: static and dynamic. Static flexibility refers to the ability to assume and maintain an extended position at one end or point in a joint's range of motion; it is what most people mean by the term *flexibility*. Dynamic flexibility, unlike static flexibility, involves movement; it is the ability to move a joint quickly through its range of motion with little resistance. For example, static shoulder flexibility would determine how far you could extend your arm across the front of your body or out to the side. Dynamic shoulder flexibility would affect your ability to pitch a softball, swing a golf club, or swim the crawl stroke. For a gymnast to perform a split on the balance beam, she must have good static flexibility in her legs and hips; in order to perform a split leap, she must have good dynamic flexibility.

Static flexibility depends on many factors, including the structure of a joint and the tightness of muscles, tendons, and ligaments that are attached to it. Dynamic flexibility is dependent on static flexibility, but it also involves such factors as strength, coordination, and resistance to movement. Dynamic flexibility can be important for both daily activities and sports. However, because static flexibility is easier to measure and better researched, most assessment tests and stretching programs—including those presented in this chapter—target static flexibility.

This chapter describes the factors that affect flexibility and the benefits of maintaining good flexibility. It provides guidelines for assessing your current level of flexibility and putting together a successful stretching program. It also examines the common problem of low-back pain.

BENEFITS OF FLEXIBILITY AND STRETCHING EXERCISES

Good flexibility provides benefits for the entire muscular and skeletal system; it may also prevent injuries and soreness and improve performance in sports and other activities.

Joint Health

Good flexibility is essential to good joint health. When the muscles and other tissues that support a joint are tight, the joint is subject to abnormal stresses that can cause joint deterioration. For example, tight thigh muscles cause excessive pressure on the kneecap, leading to pain in the knee joint. Tight shoulder muscles can compress sensitive soft tissues in the shoulder, leading to pain and disability in the joint. Poor joint flexibility can also cause abnormalities in joint lubrication, leading to deterioration of the sensitive cartilage cells lining the joint; pain and further joint injury can result.

Improved flexibility can greatly improve your quality of life, particularly as you get older. Aging decreases the natural elasticity of muscles, tendons, and joints, resulting in stiffness. The problem is compounded if you have arthritis. Flexibility exercises improve the elasticity in your tissues, making it easier to move your body. When you're flexible, everything from tying your shoes to reaching for a jar on an upper shelf becomes easier.

Low-Back Pain and Injuries

Low-back pain is sometimes related to poor spinal alignment, which puts pressure on the nerves leading out from the spinal column. Good strength and flexibility in the back, pelvis, and thighs may help prevent this type of back pain. Unfortunately, research studies have not yet clearly defined the relationship between back pain and lack of flexibility.

Poor flexibility does increase one's risk for injury. A general stretching program has been shown to be effective in reducing the frequency of injuries as well as their severity. When injuries do occur, flexibility exercises can be used in treatment: They reduce symptoms and help restore normal range of motion in affected joints.

Overstretching—stretching muscles to extreme ranges of motion—may actually decrease the stability of a joint. While some activities, such as gymnastics and ballet, re-

TERMS **range of motion** The full motion possible in a joint.

delayed-onset muscle soreness Soreness that occurs 1–2 days after exercising, probably caused by tissue damage that stimulates the release of calcium and enzymes that break down muscle fibers.

joint capsules Semielastic structures, composed primarily of connective tissue, that surround major joints.

soft tissues Tissues of the human body that include skin, fat, linings of internal organs and blood vessels, connective tissues, tendons, ligaments, muscles, and nerves.

collagen White fibers that provide structure and support in connective tissue.

elastin Yellow fibers that make connective tissue flexible.

titin A filament in muscle that helps align proteins that cause muscle contraction; titin has elastic properties and also plays a role in flexibility.

quire extreme joint movements, such flexibility is not recommended for the average person. In fact, extreme flexibility may increase risk of injury in activities such as skiing, basketball, and volleyball. Again, as with other types of exercise, moderation is the key to safe training.

Additional Potential Benefits

- *Reduction of postexercise muscle soreness.* **Delayed-onset muscle soreness,** occurring 1–2 days after exercise, is thought to be caused by damage to the muscle fibers and supporting connective tissue. Some studies (though not others) have shown that stretching after exercise decreases the degree of muscle soreness.

- *Relief of aches and pains.* Flexibility exercises help relieve pain that develops from stress or prolonged sitting. Studying or working in one place for a long time can cause your muscles to become tense. Stretching helps relieve tension, so you can go back to work refreshed and effective.

- *Improved body position and strength for sports (and life).* Good flexibility lets a person assume more efficient body positions and exert force through a greater range of motion. For example, swimmers with more flexible shoulders have stronger strokes because they can pull their arms through the water in the optimal position. Flexible joints and muscles let you move more fluidly without constraint. Some studies also suggest that flexibility training enhances strength development.

- *Maintenance of good posture.* Good flexibility also contributes to body symmetry and good posture. Bad postural habits can gradually change your body structures. Sitting in a slumped position, for example, can lead to tightness in the muscles in the front of your chest and overstretching and looseness in the upper spine, causing a rounding of the upper back. This condition, called kyphosis, is common in older people. It may be prevented by doing stretching exercises regularly.

- *Relaxation.* Flexibility exercises are a great way to relax. Studies have shown that doing flexibility exercises reduces mental tension, slows your breathing rate, and reduces blood pressure.

Flexibility and Lifetime Wellness

Part of wellness is being able to move without pain or hindrance. Flexibility exercises are an important part of this process. Sedentary people often effectively lose their mobility at an early age. Even relatively young people are often handicapped by back, shoulder, knee, and ankle pain. As they age, the pain can become debilitating, leading to injuries and a lower quality of life. Good flexibility helps keep your joints and muscles moving without pain so that you can do all the things you enjoy.

The flexibility of a joint is affected by its structure, by muscle elasticity and length, and by nervous system activity. Some factors—joint structure, for example—can't be changed. Other factors, such as the length of resting muscle fibers, can be changed through exercise; these factors should be the focus of a program to develop flexibility.

Joint Structure

The amount of flexibility in a joint is determined in part by the nature and structure of the joint. Hinge joints such as those in your fingers and knees allow only limited forward and backward movement; they lock when fully extended. Ball-and-socket joints like the hip enable movement in many different directions and have a greater range of motion. Major joints are surrounded by **joint capsules,** semielastic structures that give joints strength and stability but limit movement. Heredity also plays a part in joint structure and flexibility; for example, although everyone has a broad range of motion in the ball-and-socket hip joint, not everyone can do a split.

Muscle Elasticity and Length

Soft tissues, including skin, muscles, tendons, and ligaments, also limit the flexibility of a joint. Muscle tissue is the key to developing flexibility because it can be lengthened if it is regularly stretched. As described in Chapter 4, muscles contain proteins that create movement by causing muscles to contract. These contractile proteins can also stretch, and they are involved in the development of flexibility. However, the most important component of muscle tissue related to flexibility is the connective tissue that surrounds and envelops every part of muscle tissue, from individual muscle fibers to entire muscles. Connective tissue provides structure, elasticity, and bulk and makes up about 30% of muscle mass. Two principal types of connective tissue are **collagen,** white fibers that provide structure and support, and **elastin,** yellow fibers that are elastic and flexible. Muscles contain both collagen and elastin, closely intertwined, so muscle tissue exhibits the properties of both types of fibers. A recently discovered structural protein in muscles called **titin** also has elastic properties and contributes to flexibility.

When a muscle is stretched, the wavelike elastin fibers straighten; when the stretch is relieved, they rapidly snap back to their resting position. If gently and regularly stretched, connective tissues will lengthen and flexibility will improve (Figure 5-1). Without regular stretching, the process reverses: these tissues shorten, resulting in decreased flexibility. Regular stretching also contributes to flexibility by lengthening muscle fibers through the addition of contractile units called sarcomeres.

The stretch characteristics of connective tissue in

Relaxed: In the resting state, the fibers have a wavelike structure.

Stretching 1: The wavelike structure of the fibers straightens.

Stretching 2: The fibers lengthen.

Figure 5-1 Relaxed versus stretched connective tissue in muscle.

muscle are important considerations for a stretching program. The amount of stretch a muscle will tolerate is limited, and as the limits of its flexibility are reached, connective tissue becomes more brittle and may rupture if overstretched (Figure 5-2). A safe and effective program stretches muscles enough to slightly elongate the tissues but not so much that they are damaged. Research has shown that flexibility is improved best by stretching when muscles are warm (following exercise or the application of heat) and the stretch is applied gradually and conservatively. Sudden, high-stress stretching is less effective and can lead to muscle damage.

Nervous System Activity

Muscles contain **stretch receptors** that control their length. If a muscle is stretched suddenly, stretch receptors send signals to the spinal cord, which then sends a signal back to the same muscle, causing it to contract. These reflexes occur frequently in active muscles. They help the body know what the muscles are doing and allow for fine control of muscle length.

Small movements that only slightly stimulate these receptors cause small reflex actions. Rapid, powerful, and sudden movements that strongly stimulate the receptors cause large, powerful reflex muscle contractions. Stretches that involve rapid, bouncy movements are considered dangerous because they may stimulate a reflex muscle contraction during a stretch. A muscle that contracts at the same time it's being stretched can be easily injured, so slow, gradual stretches are always safest.

Strong muscle contractions produce a reflex of the opposite type—one that causes muscles to relax and keeps them from contracting too hard. This inverse stretch reflex has recently been introduced as an aid to improving flexibility: Contracting a muscle prior to stretching it causes it to relax, allowing it to stretch farther. The contraction-stretch technique for developing flexibility is called **proprioceptive neuromuscular facilitation (PNF)**. More research needs to be done, however, to determine precisely the degree to which PNF techniques cause muscle relaxation and help develop flexibility.

Doing each stretching exercise several times in a row can "reset" the sensitivity of muscle stretch receptors. Stretching a muscle, relaxing, and then stretching it again cause

the stretch receptors to become slightly less sensitive, thereby enabling the muscle to stretch farther. It is not known if stretch receptor sensitivity continues to change following prolonged flexibility training, but it's likely that neural changes do occur to help increase flexibility.

ASSESSING FLEXIBILITY

Because flexibility is specific to each joint, there are no tests of general flexibility. The most commonly used flexibility test is the sit-and-reach test. This test rates the flexibility of the muscles in the lower back and hamstrings; flexibility in these muscles may be important in preventing low-back pain. To assess your flexibility and identify inflexible joints, complete Lab 5-1.

CREATING A SUCCESSFUL PROGRAM TO DEVELOP FLEXIBILITY

A successful program for developing flexibility contains safe exercises executed with the most effective techniques.

Types of Stretching Techniques

Stretching techniques vary from simply stretching the muscles during the course of normal activities to sophisticated methods based on patterns of muscle reflexes. Improper stretching techniques can do more harm than good, so it's important to understand the different types of stretching exercises and how they affect the muscles. Three common techniques are static stretches, ballistic stretches, and PNF.

Static Stretching In **static stretching**, each muscle is gradually stretched, and the stretch is held for 10–30 seconds. (Holding the stretch longer than 30 seconds will not further improve flexibility, while stretching for less than 10 seconds will provide little benefit.) A slow stretch prompts less reaction from stretch receptors, and the muscles can safely stretch farther than usual. Static stretching is the type most often recommended by fitness

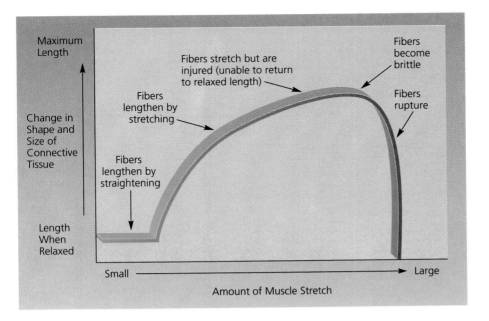

Figure 5-2   The effect of stretch on connective tissue.

In the figure:
- Maximum Length
- Change in Shape and Size of Connective Tissue
- Length When Relaxed
- Fibers lengthen by straightening
- Fibers lengthen by stretching
- Fibers stretch but are injured (unable to return to relaxed length)
- Fibers become brittle
- Fibers rupture
- Small ———→ Large
- Amount of Muscle Stretch

experts because it's safe and effective. The key to this technique is to stretch the muscles and joints to the point where a pull is felt, but not to the point of pain.

Ballistic Stretching   The technique of **ballistic stretching** involves dynamic muscle action whereby the muscles are stretched suddenly in a bouncing movement. For example, touching the toes repeatedly in rapid succession is a ballistic stretch for the hamstrings. The problem with this technique is that the heightened activity of stretch receptors caused by the rapid stretches can continue for some time, possibly causing injuries during any physical activities that follow. For this reason, ballistic stretching is not recommended.

Proprioceptive Neuromuscular Facilitation   As mentioned earlier, PNF techniques use reflexes initiated by muscle and joint receptors to cause greater training effects. The most popular PNF stretching technique is the contract-relax stretching method, in which a muscle is contracted before it is stretched. For example, in a seated stretch of calf muscles, the first step in PNF is to contract the calf muscles: A partner can provide resistance for an isometric contraction. Following a brief period of relaxation, the next step is to stretch the calf muscles by pulling the tops of the feet toward the body. A duration of 6 seconds for the contraction and 10–30 seconds for the stretch is recommended. PNF appears to allow for more effective stretching, but it tends to cause more muscle stiffness and soreness than static stretching; furthermore, it usually requires a partner and takes more time.

Passive and Active Stretching

Stretches can be done either passively or actively.

Passive Stretching   In **passive stretching**, an outside force or resistance provided by yourself, a partner, gravity, or a weight helps your joints move through their range of motion. For example, a seated stretch of the hamstring and back muscles can be done by reaching the hands toward the feet until a "pull" is felt in those muscles. You can achieve a greater range of motion (a more intense stretch) using passive stretching. However, because the stretch is not controlled by the muscles themselves, there is a greater risk of injury. Communication between partners in passive stretching is very important so joints aren't forced outside their normal functional range of motion.

Active Stretching   In **active stretching**, a muscle is stretched by a contraction of the opposing muscle (the muscle on the opposite side of the limb). For example, an

TERMS

stretch receptors   Sense organs in skeletal muscles that initiate a nerve signal to the spinal cord in response to a stretch; a contraction follows.

proprioceptive neuromuscular facilitation (PNF)   A technique in which the inverse stretch reflex induces relaxation in a muscle prior to its being stretched, allowing for more stretch and more rapid development of joint flexibility.

static stretching   A technique in which a muscle is slowly and gently stretched and then held in the stretched position.

ballistic stretching   A technique in which muscles are stretched by the force generated as a body part is repeatedly bounced, swung, or jerked.

passive stretching   A technique in which muscles are stretched by force applied by an outside source.

active stretching   A technique in which muscles are stretched by the contraction of the opposing muscles.

TACTICS AND TIPS | *Safe Stretching*

- Do stretching exercises statically. Stretch to the point of mild discomfort, and hold the position for 10–30 seconds, rest for 30–60 seconds, and repeat, trying to stretch a bit farther.

- Do not stretch until the point of pain.

- Relax and breathe easily as you stretch. Try to relax the muscles being stretched.

- Perform all exercises on both sides of your body.

- Increase intensity and duration gradually over time. Improved flexibility takes many months to develop.

- Stretch when your muscles are warm. Do gentle warm-up exercises such as easy jogging or calisthenics before doing a pre-exercise stretching routine.

- There are large individual differences in joint flexibility. Don't feel you have to compete with others during stretching workouts.

In passive stretching (left), an outside force—such as pressure exerted by another person—helps move the joint and stretch the muscles. In active stretching (right), the force to move the joint and stretch the muscles is provided by a contraction of the opposing muscles.

active seated stretch of the calf muscles occurs when a person actively contracts the muscles on the top of the shin. The contraction of this opposing muscle produces a reflex that relaxes the muscles to be stretched. The muscle can be stretched farther with a low risk of injury.

The only disadvantage of active stretching is that a person may not be able to produce enough stress (enough stretch) to increase flexibility using only the contraction of opposing muscle groups. The safest and most convenient technique is active static stretching, with an occasional passive assist. For example, you might stretch your calves both by contracting the muscles on the top of your shin and by pulling your feet toward you. This way you combine the advantages of active stretching—safety and the relaxation reflex—with those of passive stretching—greater range of motion.

Intensity and Duration

For each exercise, slowly apply stretch to your muscles to the point of slight tension or mild discomfort. Hold the stretch for 10–30 seconds. As you hold the stretch, the feeling of slight tension should slowly subside; at that point, try to stretch a bit farther. Throughout the stretch, try to relax and breathe easily. Rest for about 30–60 seconds between each stretch, and do at least 4 repetitions of each stretch. A complete flexibility workout usually takes about 20–30 minutes.

Frequency

The American College of Sports Medicine recommends that stretching exercises be performed a minimum of 2–3 days per week. Many people do flexibility training more often—3–5 days per week—for even greater benefits. It's best to stretch when your muscles are warm, so try incorporating stretching into your cool-down after cardiorespiratory endurance exercise or weight training. Stretching can also be a part of your warm-up, but it's best to increase the temperature of your muscles first by doing the active part of the warm-up (for example, walking or slow jogging).

Refer to the box "Safe Stretching" for additional tips on creating a safe and successful stretching program, and complete Lab 5-2 when you're ready to start your own program.

Exercises to Improve Flexibility

There are hundreds of exercises that can improve flexibility. Your program should include exercises that work all the major joints of the body by stretching their associated muscles. The exercises illustrated here are simple to do and pose a minimum risk of injury. Use these exercises, or substitute your favorite stretches, to create a well-rounded program for developing flexibility. Be sure to perform each stretch using the proper technique. Hold each position for 10–30 seconds, and perform at least 4 repetitions of each exercise.

FLEXIBILITY EXERCISES

EXERCISE 1

HEAD TURNS AND TILTS

Areas stretched: Neck, upper back

Instructions:

Head turns: Turn your head to the right and hold the stretch. Repeat to the left.

Head tilts: Tilt your head to the left and hold the stretch. Repeat to the right.

Variation: Place your right palm on your right cheek; try to turn your head to the right as you resist with your hand. Repeat on the left side.

EXERCISE 2

TOWEL STRETCH

Areas stretched: Triceps, shoulders, chest

Instructions: Roll up a towel and grasp it with both hands, palms down. With your arms straight, slowly lift it back over your head as far as possible. The closer together your hands are, the greater the stretch.

Variation: Repeat the stretch with your arms down and the towel behind your back. Grasp the towel with your palms forward and thumbs pointing out. Gently raise your arms behind your back.

EXERCISE 3

ACROSS-THE-BODY STRETCH

Areas stretched: Shoulders, upper back

Instructions: Keeping your back straight, cross your left arm in front of your body and grasp it with your right hand. Stretch your arm, shoulders, and back by gently pulling your arm as close to your body as possible. Repeat the stretch with your right arm.

Variation: Bend your right arm over and behind your head. Grasp your right hand with your left, and gently pull your arm until you feel the stretch. Repeat for your left arm.

EXERCISE 4

UPPER-BACK STRETCH

Areas stretched: Upper back

Instructions: Stand with your feet shoulder-width apart, knees slightly bent, and pelvis tucked under. Clasp your hands in front of your body, and press your palms forward.

Variation: In the same position, wrap your arms around your body as if you were giving yourself a hug.

EXERCISE 5

LATERAL STRETCH

Areas Stretched: Trunk muscles

Instructions: Stand with your feet shoulder-width apart, knees slightly bent, and pelvis tucked under. Raise one arm over your head and bend sideways from the waist. Support your trunk by placing the hand or forearm of your other arm on your thigh or hip for support. Be sure you bend directly sideways, and don't move your body below the waist. Repeat on the other side.

Variation: Perform the same exercise in a seated position.

EXERCISE 6

STEP STRETCH

Areas stretched: Hip, front of thigh (quadriceps)

Instructions: Step forward and flex your forward knee, keeping your knee directly above your ankle. Stretch your other leg back so that it is parallel to the floor. Press your hips forward and down to stretch. Your arms can be at your sides, on top of your knee, or on the ground for balance. Repeat on the other side.

SIDE LUNGE

Areas stretched: Inner thigh, hip, calf

Instructions: Stand in a wide straddle with your legs turned out from your hip joints and your hands on your thighs. Lunge to one side by bending one knee and keeping the other leg straight. Keep your knee directly over your ankle; do not bend it more than 90 degrees. Repeat on the other side.

Variation: In the same position, lift the heel of the bent knee to provide additional stretch. The exercise may also be performed with your hands on the floor for balance.

SOLE STRETCH

Areas stretched: Inner thigh, hip

Instructions: Sit with the soles of your feet together. Push your knees toward the floor using your hands or forearms.

Variation: When you first begin to push your knees toward the floor, use your legs to resist the movement. Then relax and press your knees down as far as they will go.

TRUNK ROTATION

Areas stretched: Trunk, outer thigh and hip, lower back

Instructions: Sit with your right leg straight, left leg bent and crossed over the right knee, and left hand on the floor next to your left hip. Turn your trunk as far as possible to the left by pushing against your left leg with your right forearm or elbow. Keep your left foot on the floor. Repeat on the other side.

ALTERNATE LEG STRETCHER

Areas stretched: Back of the thigh (hamstring), hip, knee, ankle, buttocks

Instructions: Lie flat on your back with both legs straight. **(a)** Grasp your left leg behind the thigh, and pull in to your chest. **(b)** Hold this position, and then extend your left leg toward the ceiling. **(c)** Hold this position, and then bring your left knee back to your chest and pull your toes toward your shin with your left hand. Stretch the back of the leg by attempting to straighten your knee. Repeat for the other leg.

Variation: Perform the stretch on both legs at the same time.

(a)

(b)

(c)

MODIFIED HURDLER STRETCH
(Seated Single-Toe Touch)

Areas stretched: Back of the thigh (hamstring), lower back

Instructions: Sit with your right leg straight and your left leg tucked close to your body. Reach toward your right foot as far as possible. Repeat for the other leg.

Variation: As you stretch forward, alternately flex and point the foot of your extended leg.

LOWER LEG STRETCH

Areas stretched: Back of the lower leg (calf, soleus, Achilles tendon)

Instructions: Stand with one foot about 1–2 feet in front of the other, with both feet pointing forward. **(a)** Keeping your back leg straight, lunge forward by bending your front knee and pushing your rear heel backward. Hold this position. **(b)** Then pull your back foot in slightly, and bend your back knee. Shift your weight to your back leg. Hold. Repeat on the other side.

Variation: Place your hands on a wall and extend one foot back, pressing your heel down to stretch; or stand with the balls of your feet on a step or bench and allow your heels to drop below the level of your toes.

(a) (b)

Over 85% of Americans will experience back pain at some time in their lives. Low-back pain is the second most common ailment in the United States—headache tops the list—and the second most common reason for absences from work. Low-back pain is estimated to cost as much as $50 billion per year in lost productivity, medical and legal fees, and disability insurance and compensation.

Back pain can result from sudden traumatic injuries, but it is more often the long-term result of weak and inflexible muscles, poor posture, or poor body mechanics during activities like lifting and carrying. Any abnormal strain on the back can result in pain. Most cases of low-back pain clear up on their own within a few weeks, but some people have recurrences or suffer from chronic pain.

Function and Structure of the Spine

The spinal column performs many important functions in the body.

- It provides structural support for the body, especially the thorax (upper-body cavity).
- It surrounds and protects the spinal cord.
- It supports much of the body's weight and transmits it to the lower body.
- It serves as an attachment site for a large number of muscles, tendons, and ligaments.
- It allows movement of the neck and back in all directions.

The spinal column is made up of bones called **vertebrae** (Figure 5-3). The spine consists of 7 cervical vertebrae in the neck, 12 thoracic vertebrae in the upper back, and 5 lumbar vertebrae in the lower back. The 9 vertebrae at the base of the spine are fused into two sections and form the sacrum and the coccyx (tailbone). The spine has four curves: the cervical, thoracic, lumbar, and sacral curves. These curves help bring the body weight supported by the spine in line with the axis of the body.

Although the structure of vertebrae depends on their location on the spine, the different types of vertebrae do share common characteristics. Each consists of a body, an arch, and several bony processes (Figure 5-4). The vertebral body is cylindrical, with flattened surfaces where **intervertebral disks** are attached. The vertebral body is designed to carry the stress of body weight and physical activity. The vertebral arch surrounds and protects the spinal cord. The bony processes serve as joints for adjacent vertebrae and attachment sites for muscles and ligaments. **Nerve roots** from the spinal cord pass through notches in the vertebral arch.

Intervertebral disks, which absorb and disperse the stresses placed on the spine, separate vertebrae from each other. Disks are made up of a gel- and water-filled nucleus surrounded by a series of fibrous rings. The liquid

vertebrae Bony segments composing the spinal column that **TERMS** provide structural support for the body and protect the spinal cord.

intervertebral disk A tough, elastic disk located between adjoining vertebrae consisting of a gel- and water-filled nucleus surrounded by fibrous rings; it serves as a shock absorber for the spinal column.

nerve root The base of one of the 31 pairs of spinal nerves that branch off the spinal cord through spaces between vertebrae.

Spinal curves   **Vertebrae**

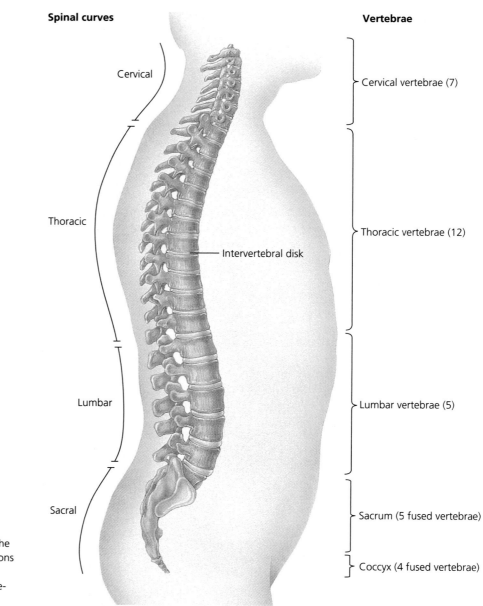

Cervical

Thoracic

Intervertebral disk

Cervical vertebrae (7)

Thoracic vertebrae (12)

Lumbar

Lumbar vertebrae (5)

Sacral

Sacrum (5 fused vertebrae)

Coccyx (4 fused vertebrae)

Figure 5-3   The spinal column.   The spine is made up of five separate regions and has four distinct curves. An intervertebral disk is located between verte-brae.

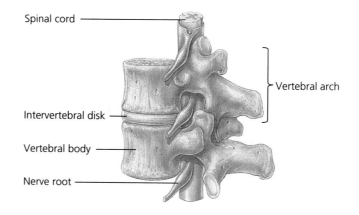

Spinal cord

Vertebral arch

Intervertebral disk

Vertebral body

Nerve root

Figure 5-4   Vertebrae and an intervertebral disk.

Risk Factors for Low-Back Pain

- Age greater than 34 years
- Degenerative disease (e.g., osteoporosis, arthritis)
- Family history of back pain
- History of back trauma
- Lack of physical activity
- Low job satisfaction
- Low muscular strength relative to body weight
- Low socioeconomic status
- Male sex (in some studies)
- Obesity

- Occupations or activities requiring frequent lifting, twisting, bending, or standing up
- Occupations with high concentration demands (e.g., computer programming)
- Physically hard work
- Poor posture
- Psychological depression
- Repetitive strain in forced positions over long time periods
- Smoking (linked to increased disk degeneration)
- Vibration affecting the whole body (such as experienced by truck drivers)

nucleus can change shape when it is compressed, allowing the disk to absorb shock. The intervertebral disks also help maintain the spaces between vertebrae where the spinal nerve roots are located.

Causes of Back Pain

Back pain can occur at any point along your spine; the lumbar area, because it bears the majority of your weight, is the most common site. Any movement that causes excessive stress on the spinal column can cause injury and pain. The spine is well equipped to bear body weight and the force or stress of body movements along its long axis. However, it is less capable of bearing loads at an angle to its long axis. You do not have to carry a heavy load or participate in a vigorous contact sport to injure your back. Picking a pencil up from the floor using poor body mechanics—reaching too far out in front of you or bending over with your knees straight, for example—can also result in back pain (see the box "Risk Factors for Low-Back Pain").

Underlying causes of back pain include weak or inflexible muscles in the back, hips, abdomen, and legs; excess body weight; poor posture when standing, sitting, or sleeping; and poor body mechanics when performing actions like lifting and carrying, or sports movements. Abnormal spinal loading resulting from any of these causes can have short-term or long-term direct and indirect effects on the spine. Strained muscles, tendons, or ligaments can cause pain and can, over time, lead to injuries to vertebrae or the intervertebral disks.

Stress can cause disks to break down and lose some of their ability to absorb shock. A damaged disk may bulge out between vertebrae and put pressure on a nerve root, a condition commonly referred to as a slipped disk. Painful pressure on nerves can also occur if damage to a disk narrows the space between two vertebrae. With age, you lose fluid from the disks, making them more likely to bulge and put pressure on nerve roots. Depending on the amount of pressure on a nerve, symptoms may include numbness in the back, hip, leg, or foot; radiating pain; loss of muscle function; depressed reflexes; and muscle spasm. If the pressure is severe enough, loss of function can be permanent.

Preventing Low-Back Pain

Incorrect posture when standing, sitting, lying, and lifting is responsible for many back injuries. In general, think about moving your spine as a unit, with the force directed through its long axis. Strategies for maintaining good posture during daily activities are presented in the box "Avoiding Low-Back Pain." Follow the same guidelines for posture and movement when you engage in sports or recreational activities. Maintain control over your body movements, and warm up thoroughly before you exercise. Take special care when lifting weights as part of a strength training program. (Refer to Chapter 4 for more information on proper weight-lifting technique.)

The role of exercise in preventing and treating back pain is still being investigated. However, many experts do recommend exercise, especially for people who have already experienced an episode of low-back pain. Lifestyle physical activity such as walking is often recommended for the prevention of back pain. When walking, stand up straight, keep your head centered over your body, and swing your arms freely. Movement helps lubricate your spinal disks and increases muscle fitness in your trunk and legs. To help maintain a healthy back, you should also regularly perform exercises that stretch and strengthen the major muscle groups that affect your back. The following exercises focus on the key areas: the abdominal muscles, the muscles along your spine and sides, and the muscles of your hips and thighs. If you have back problems, check with your physician before beginning any exercise program. Perform the exercises slowly, and progress very gradually. Stop and consult your physician if any exercise causes back pain.

Changes in everyday behavior can help prevent and alleviate low-back pain.

- *Lying down.* When resting or sleeping, lie on your side with your knees and hips bent. If you lie on your back, place a pillow under your knees. Don't lie on your stomach. If your mattress isn't firm, place a plywood board under it.

- *Sitting.* Sit with your lower back slightly rounded, knees bent, and feet flat on the floor. Alternate crossing your legs, or use a foot rest to keep your knees higher than your hips. If this position is uncomfortable or if your back flattens when you sit, try using a lumbar roll pillow behind your lower back.

- *Lifting.* If you need to lower yourself to grasp an object, bend at the knees and hips rather than at the waist. Your feet should be about shoulder-width apart. Lift gradually, keeping your arms straight, by standing up or by pushing with your leg muscles. Keep the object close to your body. Don't twist; if you have to turn with the object, change the position of your feet.

- *Standing.* When you are standing, a straight line should run from the top of your ear through the center of your shoulder, the center of your hip, the back of your kneecap, and the front of your ankle bone. Support your weight mainly on your heels, with one or both knees slightly bent. Try to keep your lower back flat by placing one foot on a stool. Don't let your pelvis tip forward or your back arch. Shift your weight back and forth from foot to foot. Avoid prolonged standing. (To check your posture, stand in a normal way with your back to a wall. Your upper back and buttocks should touch the wall; your heels may be a few inches away. Slide one hand into the space between your lower back and the wall. It should slide in easily but should almost touch both your back and the wall. Adjust your posture as needed, and try to hold this position as you walk away from the wall.)

- *Walking.* Walk with your toes pointed straight ahead. Keep your back flat, head up, and chin in. Don't wear high-heeled shoes.

LOW-BACK EXERCISES

EXERCISE 1

WALL STRETCH

Areas stretched: Back of thigh (hamstring), calf

Instructions: Sit on the floor with one leg extended and your foot flat against a wall or other immovable object. Bend the other leg and place your foot flat on the floor next to the knee of the straight leg. Clasp your hands behind your back or rest them loosely on the floor behind you. Bend forward from your hips, keeping your lower back flat and straight. Your bent knee can be moved slightly to the side to make room for your upper body as you lean forward. Repeat with the other leg.

EXERCISE 2

STEP STRETCH (see Exercise 6 in the flexibility program)

EXERCISE 3

ALTERNATE LEG STRETCHER (see Exercise 10 in the flexibility program)

EXERCISE 4

DOUBLE KNEE-TO-CHEST

Areas stretched: Lower back, hips

Instructions: Lie on your back with both knees bent and feet flat on the floor. **(a)** With one hand on the back of each thigh, slowly pull both knees to your chest; hold the stretch. **(b)** Then straighten your knees so that both legs are extended toward the ceiling. Return to the starting position by drawing your legs back to your chest and then placing your feet on the floor.

(a)

(b)

TRUNK TWIST

Area stretched: Lower back, sides

Instructions: Lie on your side with top knee bent, lower leg straight, lower arm extended out in front of you on the floor, and upper arm at your side. Push down with your upper knee while you twist your trunk backward. Try to get your shoulders and upper body flat on the floor, turning your head as well. Return to the starting position, and then repeat on the other side.

BACK BRIDGE

Areas strengthened: Hips, buttocks

Instructions: Lie on your back with knees bent and arms extended to the side. Tuck your pelvis under, and then lift your tailbone, buttocks, and lower back from the floor. Hold this position for 5–10 seconds with your weight resting on your feet, arms, and shoulders, and then return to the starting position. Work up to 10 repetitions of the exercise.

PELVIC TILT

Areas strengthened: Abdomen, buttocks

Instructions: Lie on your back with knees bent and arms extended to the side. Tilt your pelvis under, and try to flatten your lower back against the floor. Tighten your buttock and abdominal muscles while you hold this position for 5–10 seconds. Don't hold your breath. Work up to 10 repetitions of the exercise. Pelvic tilts can also be done standing or leaning against a wall.

MODIFIED SIT-UP

Areas strengthened: Abdomen

Instructions: Lie on your back with knees bent and arms crossed on your chest. Tilt your pelvis under, flattening your back. Tuck your chin in and slowly curl up, one vertebra at a time as you lift your head first and then your shoulders. Stop when you can see your heels, and hold for 5–10 seconds before returning to the starting position. Do 10 repetitions.

Variation: Add a twist to develop other abdominal muscles. When you have curled up so that your shoulder blades are off the floor, twist your upper body so that one shoulder is higher than the other; reach past your knee with your upper arm. Hold, and then return to the starting position. Repeat on the opposite side.

PRESS-UP

Areas stretched: Lower back, abdomen

Instructions: Lie face down with your hands under your face. Slowly push yourself up until your upper body is resting on your forearms. Relax and hold for 5–10 seconds. Gradually progress to straightening your elbows while keeping your pubic bone on the floor. (Stop if this exercise produces any pain.)

WALL SQUAT (Phantom Chair)

Areas strengthened: Lower back, thighs, abdomen

Instructions: Lean against a wall and bend your knees as though you are sitting in a chair. Support your weight with your legs. Begin by holding the position for 5–10 seconds. Build up to 1 minute or more.

SPINE EXTENSIONS (see Exercise 9 in the free weights program in Chapter 4, p. 88)

COMMON QUESTIONS ANSWERED

Are there any stretching exercises I shouldn't do? Yes. Avoid exercises that put excessive pressure on your joints, particularly your spine and knees. Previous injuries and poor flexibility may make certain exercises dangerous for some people. Exercises that may cause problems are described in the box "Stretches to Avoid."

Is stretching the same as warming up? People often confuse stretching and pre-exercise warm-up. While they are complementary, they're two distinct activities. A warm-up involves light exercise that increases body temperature so that your metabolism works better when you're exercising at high intensity. Stretching increases the movement capability of your joints, so you can move more easily, with less risk of injury.

Whenever you stretch, you should ideally first spend 5–10 minutes engaged in some form of low-intensity exercise, such as walking, jogging, or low-intensity calisthenics. When your muscles are warmed, begin your stretching routine. Warmed muscles stretch better than cold ones and are less prone to injury.

How much flexibility do I need? This question is not always easy to answer. If you're involved in a sport such as gymnastics, figure skating, or ballet, you are often required to reach extreme joint motions to achieve success. However, nonathletes do not need to reach these extreme joint positions. In fact, too much flexibility may, in some cases, increase your risk of injury. As with other types of fitness, moderation is the key. You should regularly stretch your major joints and muscle groups but not aspire to reach extreme flexibility.

Can I stretch too far? Yes. As muscle tissue is progressively stretched, it reaches a point where it becomes damaged and may rupture. The greatest danger occurs during passive stretching when a partner is doing the stretching for you. It is critical that your stretching partner not force your joint outside its normal functional range of motion.

Does weight training limit flexibility? Weight training, or any physical activity, will decrease flexibility if the exercises are not performed through a full range of motion. When done properly, weight training increases flexibility.

Does jogging impair flexibility? Because of the limited range of motion used during the running stride, jogging tends to compromise flexibility. It is very important for runners to practice flexibility exercises for the hamstrings and quadriceps regularly.

SUMMARY

- Flexibility, the ability of joints to move through their full range of motion, is highly adaptable and specific to each joint.
- The benefits of flexibility include preventing abnormal stresses that lead to joint deterioration and possibly reducing the risk of injuries and low-back pain.
- Range of motion can be limited by joint structure, by limited muscle elasticity, and by stretch receptor activity.
- Developing flexibility depends on stretching the elastic tissues within muscles regularly and gently until they lengthen. Overstretching can make connective tissue brittle and lead to rupture.
- Signals sent between stretch receptors and the spinal cord can enhance flexibility because contracting a muscle stimulates a relaxation response, thereby allowing a longer muscle stretch, and because stretch receptors become less sensitive after repeated stretches, initiating fewer contractions.
- The sit-and-reach test is most often used to assess flexibility; comparisons can also be made to a chart showing normal range of motion for major joints.
- Static stretching is done slowly and held to the point of mild tension; ballistic stretching consists of bouncing stretches and can lead to injury. Proprioceptive neuromuscular facilitation uses muscle receptors in contracting and relaxing a muscle.
- Passive stretching, using an outside force in moving muscles and joints, achieves a greater range of motion (and has a higher injury risk) than active stretching, which uses opposing muscles to initiate a stretch.
- Stretches should be held for 10–30 seconds; perform at least 4 repetitions. Flexibility training should be done 2 or more days a week, preferably following activity when muscles are warm.

The safe alternatives listed here are described and illustrated on pages 115–119 as part of the complete program of safe flexibility exercises presented in this chapter.

Standing Toe Touch

Problem: Puts excessive strain on the spine

Alternatives: Alternate leg stretcher (Exercise 10), modified hurdler stretch (Exercise 11), and lower leg stretch (Exercise 12)

Full Squat

Problem: Puts excessive strain on the ankles, knees, and spine

Alternatives: Alternate leg stretcher (Exercise 10) and lower leg stretch (Exercise 12)

Standing Ankle-to-Buttocks Quadriceps Stretch

Problem: Puts excessive strain on the ligaments of the knee

Alternative: Step stretch (Exercise 6)

Prone Arch

Problem: Puts excessive strain on the spine, knees, and shoulders

Alternatives: Towel stretch (Exercise 2) and step stretch (Exercise 6)

Standing Hamstring Stretch

Problem: Puts excessive strain on the knee and lower back

Alternatives: Alternate leg stretcher (Exercise 10) and modified hurdler stretch (Exercise 11)

Yoga Plow

Problem: Puts excessive strain on the neck, shoulders, and back

Alternatives: Head turns and tilts (Exercise 1), across-the-body stretch (Exercise 3), and upper-back stretch (Exercise 4)

Hurdler Stretch

Problem: Turning out the bent leg can put excessive strain on the ligaments of the knee

Alternative: Modified hurdler stretch (Exercise 11)

- The spinal column consists of vertebrae separated by intervertebral disks. It provides structure and support for the body and protects the spinal cord.
- In addition to good posture, proper body mechanics, and regular physical activity, a program for preventing low-back pain includes exercises that stretch and strengthen major muscle groups that affect the lower back.

FOR MORE INFORMATION

Books

Alter, M. J. 1996. *Science of Flexibility,* 2d ed. Champaign, Ill.: Human Kinetics. *An extremely well researched book that discusses the scientific basis of stretching exercises and flexibility.*

Anderson, B., and J. Anderson. 1997. *Stretching at Your Computer or Desk.* Bolinas, Calif.: Shelter Publications. *Stretching routines for workplace and school settings.*

Maharam, L. 1998. *A Healthy Back: A Sports Medicine Doctor's Back-Care Program for Everybody.* New York: Henry Holt. *Lifestyle advice for preventing and eliminating back pain.*

Martins, P. 1997. *The New York City Ballet Workout: Fifty Stretches and Exercises Anyone Can Do for a Strong, Graceful, and Sculpted Body.* New York: William Morrow. *Stretching exercises with a dance orientation.*

Smith, B. 1997. *Flexibility for Sport.* Wiltshire, Eng.: Crowood Press. *Stretching workouts for people interested in various sports.*

St. George, F. 1997. *Stretching for Flexibility and Health.* Freedom, Calif.: Crossing Press. *A good basic book on stretching exercises.*

Web Sites

Back Pain Prevention. Tips for use at home, at work, and during exercise.
http://cst.lanl.gov/CST/backpain/mainback.html

FitnessLink/Stretching Exercises. Information on a safe, effective stretching program.
http://www.fitnesslink.com/exercise/stretch.htm

NIH Back Pain Fact Sheet. Provides basic information on the prevention and treatment of back pain.
http://www.ninds.nih.gov/HEALINFO/DISORDER/back%20pain/backpain.htm

Southern California Orthopedic Institute. Provides information about a variety of orthopedic problems, including back injuries; also has illustrations of spinal anatomy.
http://www.scoi.com

Stretching and Flexibility. Provides information about the physiology of stretching and different types of stretching exercises.
http://www.cs.huji.ac.il/papers/rma/stretching_toc.html

See also the listings for Chapters 2 and 4.

SELECTED BIBLIOGRAPHY

Agency for Health Care Policy and Research. 1994. *Clinical Practice Guidelines. Acute Low Back Problems in Adults.* Silver Spring, Md.: Publications Clearinghouse.

Alter, M. J. 1996. *The Science of Flexibility,* 2d ed. Champaign, Ill.: Human Kinetics.

American College of Sports Medicine. 1998. ACSM Position Stand: The Recommended Quantity and Quality of Exercises for Developing and Maintaining Cardiorespiratory and Muscular Fitness, and Flexibility in Healthy Adults. *Medicine and Science in Sports and Exercise* 30(6): 975–991.

American Medical Association. 1995. *The AMA Pocket Guide to Back Pain.* New York: Random House.

Andersson, G. B. 1997. Low back pain. *Journal of Rehabilitation Research and Development* 34:IX–X.

Bandy, W. D., J. M. Irion, and M. Briggler. 1997. The effect of time and frequency of static stretching on flexibility of the hamstring muscles. *Physical Therapy* 77:1090–1096.

Burton, A. K., and E. Erg. 1997. Back injury and work loss. Biomechanical and psychosocial influences. *Spine* 22: 2575–2580.

Callaghan, J. P., J. L. Gunning, and S. M. McGill. 1998. The relationship between lumbar spine load and muscle activity during extensor exercises. *Physical Therapy* 78(1): 8–18.

Craib, M. W., et al. 1996. The association between flexibility and running economy in sub-elite male distance runners. *Medicine and Science in Sports and Exercise* 28:737–743.

Daltroy, L. H., et al. 1997. A controlled trial of an educational program to prevent low back injuries. *New England Journal of Medicine* 337:322–328.

Dempsey, P. G., A. Burdorf, and B. S. Webster. 1997. The influence of personal variables on work-related low-back disorders and implications for future research. *Journal of Occupational and Environmental Medicine* 39:748–759.

Hurwitz, E. L., and H. Morgenstern. 1997. Correlates of back problems and back-related disability in the United States. *Journal of Clinical Epidemiology* 50:669–681.

Jackson, A. W., et al. 1998. Relations of sit-up and sit-and-reach tests to low back pain in adults. *Journal of Orthopaedic and Sports Physical Therapy* 27(1): 22–26.

Leboeuf-Yde, C., J. M. Lauritsen, and T. Lauritzen. 1997. Why has the search for causes of low back pain largely been non-conclusive? *Spine* 22:877–881.

Nieman, D. C. 1999. *Exercise Testing and Prescription: A Health-Related Approach,* 4th ed. Mountain View, Calif.: Mayfield.

Schwartz, E., R. E. Yodaiken, and R. Sokas. 1997. An educational program to prevent disabling low back pain. *New England Journal of Medicine* 337:1923–1924.

Shiple, D. O. 1997. Relieving low-back pain with exercise. *The Physician and Sportsmedicine* 25(8): 67–68.

Wiemann, K., and K. Hahn. 1997. Influences of strength, stretching and circulatory exercises on flexibility parameters of the human hamstrings. *International Journal of Sports Medicine* 18:340–346.

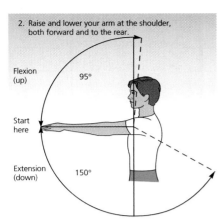

2. Raise and lower your arm at the shoulder, both forward and to the rear.

Flexion (up)

95°

Start here

Extension (down)

150°

A. Comparison Method (✓)

Flexion: Average or above _____ Needs improvement _____

Extension: Average or above _____ Needs improvement _____

B. Measurement Method

Flexion: _____ °   Rating: _____

Extension: _____ °   Rating: _____

Ratings

	Flexion	Extension
Below average	<92°	<145°
Average	92°–95°	145°–150°
Above average	96°–99°	151°–156°
Excellent	>99°	>156°

---

3. Bend and straighten your elbow.

Flexion (up) 55°

Start here

Extension (down) 89°

A. Comparison Method (✓)

Flexion: Average or above _____ Needs improvement _____

Extension: Average or above _____ Needs improvement _____

B. Measurement Method

Flexion: _____ °   Rating: _____

Extension: _____ °   Rating: _____

Ratings

	Flexion	Extension
Below average	<51°	<88°
Average	51°–55°	88°–89°
Above average	56°–60°	90°–91°
Excellent	>60°	>91°

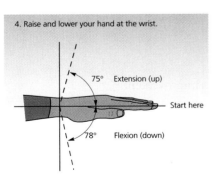

4. Raise and lower your hand at the wrist.

75° Extension (up)

Start here

78° Flexion (down)

A. Comparison Method (✓)

Extension: Average or above _____ Needs improvement _____

Flexion: Average or above _____ Needs improvement _____

B. Measurement Method

Extension: _____ °   Rating: _____

Flexion: _____ °   Rating: _____

Ratings

	Extension	Flexion
Below average	<70°	<73°
Average	70°–75°	73°–78°
Above average	76°–81°	79°–84°
Excellent	>81°	>84°

5. Bend directly sideways at your waist. (To prevent injury, keep your knees slightly bent, and support your trunk by placing your hand or forearm on your thigh.)

Start here

40°   40°

A. Comparison Method (✓)

Right lateral flexion: Average or above _____ Needs improvement _____

Left lateral flexion: Average or above _____ Needs improvement _____

B. Measurement Method:

Right lateral flexion: _____ ° Rating: _____

Left lateral flexion: _____ ° Rating: _____

Ratings

	Right or Left Lateral Flexion
Below average	<36°
Average	36°–40°
Above average	41°–45°
Excellent	>45

6. Raise leg to the side at the hip.

45°   26°
Abduction   Adduction
(out)   (in)

Start here

A. Comparison Method (✓)

Abduction: Average or above _____ Needs improvement _____

Adduction: Average or above _____ Needs improvement _____

B. Measurement Method

Abduction: _____ ° Rating: _____

Adduction: _____ ° Rating: _____

Ratings

	Abduction	*Adduction*
Below average	<40°	<23°
Average	40°–45°	23°–26°
Above average	46°–51°	27°–30°
Excellent	>51°	>30°

7. Raise and lower your leg forward at the hip.

125°   Flexion

Start here

A. Comparison Method (✓)

Average or above _____ Needs improvement _____

B. Measurement Method

Flexion: _____ ° Rating: _____

Ratings

	Flexion
Below average	<121°
Average	121°–125°
Above average	126°–130°
Excellent	>130°

8. Bend and straighten your knee.

140°

Flexion

Start here

A. Comparison Method (✓)

    Average or above _____ Needs improvement _____

B. Measurement Method

    Flexion: _____ °   Rating: _____

Ratings

	Flexion
Below average	<136°
Average	136°–140°
Above average	141°–145°
Excellent	>145°

9. Raise and lower your foot at the ankle.

Start here

Dorsiflexion (pull toes toward shin) 13° 55° Plantar flexion (point toes)

A. Comparison Method (✓)

    Dorsiflexion: Average or above _____ Needs improvement _____

    Plantar flexion: Average or above _____ Needs improvement _____

B. Measurement Method

    Dorsiflexion: _____ °   Rating: _____

    Plantar flexion: _____ °   Rating: _____

Ratings

	Dorsiflexion	*Plantar flexion*
Below average	<9°	<50°
Average	9°–13°	50°–55°
Above average	14°–17°	56°–60°
Excellent	>17°	>60°

10. With knees extended and one leg flat on the floor, raise and lower your leg at the hip.

Flexion

81°

0°

Start here

A. Comparison Method (✓)

    Average or above _____ Needs improvement _____

B. Measurement Method

    Flexion: _____ °   Rating: _____

Ratings

	Flexion
Below average	<79°
Average	79°–81°
Above average	82°–84°
Excellent	>84°

Rating Your Flexibility

Sit-and-Reach Test

     Score: _____ in.   Rating: _____

Range of Motion Assessment

Joint		Average ROM	Comparison Method (✓)		Measurement Method	
			Average or above	Needs improvement	Current range of motion (°)	Rating
Shoulder (side-to-side)	Abduction	95°				
	Adduction	127°				
Shoulder (front-to-back)	Flexion	95°				
	Extension	150°				
Elbow (up-and-down)	Flexion	55°				
	Extension	89°				
Wrist (up-and-down)	Extension	75°				
	Flexion	78°				
Low back (side-to-side)	Right flexion	40°				
	Left flexion	40°				
Hip (side-to-side)	Abduction	45°				
	Adduction	26°				
Hip (bent knee)	Flexion	125°				
Knee	Flexion	140°				
Ankle	Dorsiflexion	13°				
	Plantar flexion	55°				
Hip (straight knee)	Flexion	81°				

To monitor your progress toward your goal, enter the results of this lab in the Preprogram Assessment column of Appendix D. After following the stretching program for several weeks, do this lab again, and enter the results in the Postprogram Assessment column of Appendix D. How do the results compare?

Name _____   Section _____   Date _____

LAB 5-2   *Creating a Personalized Program for Developing Flexibility*

Complete the program plan below, and start on your flexibility program.

Exercises: The exercises contained in the program plan below are those from the general stretching program presented in Chapter 5. You can add or delete exercises depending on your needs, goals, and preferences. For any exercises you add, fill in the areas of the body affected.

Frequency: A minimum frequency of 2–3 days per week is recommended. You may want to do your stretching exercises the same days you plan to do cardiorespiratory endurance exercise or weight training, because muscles stretch better following exercise, when they are warm.

Intensity: All stretches should be done to the point of mild discomfort, not pain.

Duration: All stretches should be held for 10–30 seconds. (PNF techniques should include a 6-second contraction followed by a 10–30-second assisted stretch.)

Repetitions: All stretches should be performed at least 4 times.

Program Plan for Flexibility

Exercise	Areas Stretched	Frequency (check ✔)						
		M	T	W	Th	F	Sa	Su
Head turns and tilts	Neck, upper back							
Towel stretch	Triceps, shoulders, chest							
Across-the-body stretch	Shoulders, upper back							
Upper-back stretch	Upper back							
Lateral stretch	Trunk muscles							
Step stretch	Hip, front of thigh (quadriceps)							
Side lunge	Inner thigh, hip, calf							
Sole stretch	Inner thigh, hip							
Trunk rotation	Trunk, outer thigh and hip, lower back							
Alternate leg stretcher	Backs of the thigh (hamstring), hip, knee, ankle, buttocks							
Modified hurdler stretch	Back of the thigh (hamstring), lower back							
Lower leg stretch	Back of the lower leg (calf, soleus, Achilles tendon)							

You can monitor your program using a chart like the one on the next page.

Flexibility Program Chart

Fill in the dates you perform each stretch, the number of seconds you hold each stretch (should be 10–30), and the number of repetitions of each (should be at least 4). For an easy check on the duration of your stretches, count "one thousand one, one thousand two," and so on. You will probably find that over time you'll be able to hold each stretch longer (in addition to being able to stretch farther).

Exercise/Date																			
	Duration																		
	Reps																		
	Duration																		
	Reps																		
	Duration																		
	Reps																		
	Duration																		
	Reps																		
	Duration																		
	Reps																		
	Duration																		
	Reps																		
	Duration																		
	Reps																		
	Duration																		
	Reps																		
	Duration																		
	Reps																		
	Duration																		
	Reps																		
	Duration																		
	Reps																		
	Duration																		
	Reps																		
	Duration																		
	Reps																		
	Duration																		
	Reps																		
	Duration																		
	Reps																		
	Duration																		
	Reps																		
	Duration																		
	Reps																		

Body Composition

6

LOOKING AHEAD

After reading this chapter, you should be able to answer these questions about body composition:

- What are fat-free mass, essential fat, and nonessential fat, and what are their functions in the body?

- How does body composition affect wellness?

- How are body composition and body fat distribution measured?

- What is recommended body weight, and how is it determined?

Body composition, the body's relative amount of fat and fat-free mass, is an important component of fitness for wellness. People whose body composition is optimal tend to be healthier, to move more efficiently, and to feel better about themselves. To reach wellness, you must determine what body composition is right for you and then work to achieve and maintain it.

Although people pay lip service to the idea of exercising for health, a more immediate goal for many is to look fit and healthy. Unfortunately, many people don't succeed in their efforts to obtain a fit and healthy body because they emphasize short-term weight loss rather than the permanent changes in lifestyle that lead to fat loss and a healthy body composition. Successful management of body composition requires the coordination of many aspects of a wellness program, including proper nutrition, adequate exercise, and stress management.

This chapter focuses on defining and measuring body composition and determining recommended body weight; Chapter 9 provides specific strategies for changing your lifestyle to reach your body composition goal.

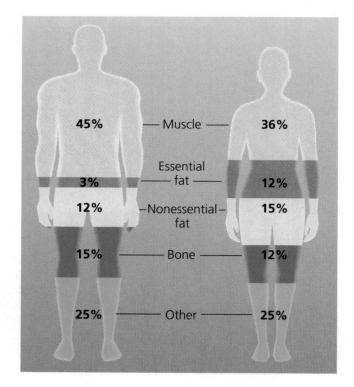

Figure 6-1 **Body composition of a typical man and woman, 20–24 years old.** SOURCE: Adapted from Brooks, G. A., T. D. Fahey, and T. P. White. 1996. *Exercise Physiology: Human Bioenergetics and Its Applications,* 2d ed. Mountain View, Calif.: Mayfield.

WHAT IS BODY COMPOSITION, AND WHY IS IT IMPORTANT?

The human body can be divided into fat-free mass and body fat. Fat-free mass is composed of all the body's non-fat tissues: bone, water, muscle, connective tissue, organ tissues, and teeth. Body fat includes both essential and nonessential body fats (Figure 6-1). **Essential fat** includes lipids incorporated into the nerves, brain, heart, lungs, liver, and mammary glands. These fat deposits, crucial for normal body functioning, make up approximately 3% of total body weight in men and 12% in women. (The larger percentage in women is due to fat deposits in the breasts, uterus, and other sites specific to females.) **Nonessential (storage) fat** exists primarily within fat cells, or **adipose tissue**, often located just below the skin and around major organs. The amount of storage fat varies from individual to individual based on many factors, including gender, age, heredity, metabolism, diet, and activity level. Excess storage fat is usually the result of consuming more energy (as food) than is expended (in metabolism and physical activity).

How much body fat is too much? In the past, many people relied on height-weight tables based on insurance company mortality statistics to answer this question. Unfortunately, these tables can be highly inaccurate for some people; at best, they provide only an indirect measure of fatness. Because, as explained in Chapter 4, muscle tissue is denser and heavier than fat, a fit person can easily weigh more and an unfit person weigh less than recommended weights on a height-weight table.

The most important consideration when a person is looking at body composition is the proportion of the body's total weight that is fat—the **percent body fat.** For example, two women may both be 5 feet, 5 inches tall and weigh 130 pounds. But one woman, a runner, may have only 15% of her body mass as fat, whereas the second, sedentary woman could have 33% body fat. While neither woman is overweight by most standards, the second woman is overfat. Too much body fat (not total weight) has a negative effect on health and well-being.

Some of the most commonly used methods to assess and classify body composition are described later in the chapter. Although less accurate than standards based on body fat, some methods are based on total body weight because it is easier to measure. **Overweight** is usually defined as total body weight above the recommended range for good health (as determined by large-scale population surveys). **Obesity** is defined as a more serious degree of overweight; the cutoff point for obesity may be set in terms of percent body fat, as in Table 6-1, or in terms of some measure of total body weight.

By any measure, Americans are getting fatter. Since 1960, the number of Americans having a body composition categorized as obese has nearly doubled (from 13% to 22%), and more than 50% of American adults are now overweight. The reason for increased body fat in the pop-

Negative Health Consequences of Obesity

An obese person is at increased risk for the following:

Early death

Death from CVD, including sudden death

Hypertension

Diabetes

Gallbladder disease

Cancer of the colon, prostate, esophagus, gallbladder, ovary, endometrium, breast, and cervix

Arthritis and gout

Back pain

Complications during pregnancy

Menstrual abnormalities

Shortness of breath

Sleep apnea (intermittent cessation of breathing while sleeping)

Obesity is also associated with the following:

Increased LDL and triglyceride concentrations

Decreased HDL concentration

Impaired heart function (ventricles)

Impaired immune function

---

ulation is not totally clear, but it is related to decreased physical activity and increased caloric consumption. As discussed in Chapter 2, more than half of all Americans do not meet the minimum recommendation of 30 minutes per day of moderate physical activity. More people are working in white-collar and service professions than in jobs involving physical activity. And increased access to items such as home computers and cable television has also contributed to more sedentary lifestyles. In addition to exercising less, Americans are eating more. The Centers for Disease Control and Prevention has estimated that caloric intake has increased by 100–300 calories per day during the past decade. (For more on the causes of obesity, see Chapter 9.)

Though not as prevalent a problem, having too little body fat is also dangerous (see Table 6-1). Too much or too little body fat can have negative effects on health, performance, and self-image.

Health

Obesity is associated with a wide variety of health problems, many of which are listed in the box "Negative Health Consequences of Obesity." Obese people have an overall mortality rate almost twice that of nonobese people. They are more than five times as likely to develop diabetes (see the box "Diabetes"). In 1998, the American Heart Association classified obesity as one of the five major risk factors for heart disease. It is estimated that if all Americans had a healthy body composition, the incidence of coronary heart disease would drop by 25%.

The distribution of fat is also an important indicator of future health. People who tend to gain weight in the abdominal area ("apples") have a risk of coronary heart disease, high blood pressure, diabetes, and stroke twice as high as that of people who tend to gain weight in the hip area ("pears"). The reason for this increased risk is not

TABLE 6-1 Percent Body Fat Classifications

Percent Body Fat

Males	Females	Classification
Less than 5%	Less than 8%	Excessively lean
5–11%	8–19%	Lean
12–20%	20–30%	Acceptable
21–25%	31–33%	Borderline obese
More than 25%	More than 33%	Obese

These represent approximate standards for body composition; the healthy range varies, depending on health status and risk factors for disease. For example, a man with high blood pressure and high cholesterol levels might want to reduce his percentage of body fat, even if it is within the acceptable range for the general population.

TERMS

essential fat   The fat in the body necessary for normal body functioning.

nonessential (storage) fat   Extra fat or fat reserves stored in the body.

adipose tissue   Connective tissue in which fat is stored.

percent body fat   The percentage of total body weight that is composed of fat.

overweight   Characterized by a body weight above a recommended range for good health; ranges are set through large-scale population surveys.

obese   Severely overweight, characterized by an excessive accumulation of body fat: more than 25% of body weight as fat in men, and more than 33% as fat in women. Obesity may also be defined in terms of some measure of total body weight.

Diabetes mellitus is a disease that causes a disruption of normal metabolism. The pancreas, a long, thin organ located behind the stomach, normally secretes the hormone insulin, which stimulates cells to take up glucose to produce energy. In a person with diabetes, this process is disrupted, causing a buildup of glucose in the bloodstream. Over the long term, diabetes is associated with kidney failure, nerve damage, circulation problems, retinal damage and blindness, and increased rates of heart attack, stroke, and hypertension. The rate of diabetes has increased steadily over the past 40 years, and it is currently the seventh leading cause of death in the United States.

Types of Diabetes

Approximately 16 million Americans—nearly 6% of the population—have one of two major forms of diabetes. About 5–10% of people with diabetes have the more serious form, known as Type 1 diabetes. In this type of diabetes, the pancreas produces little or no insulin, so daily doses of insulin are required. (Without insulin, a person with Type 1 can lapse into a coma.) Type 1 diabetes usually strikes before age 20.

The remaining 15 million Americans with diabetes have Type 2 diabetes. This condition can develop slowly, and about half of affected individuals are unaware of their condition. In Type 2 diabetes, the pancreas doesn't produce enough insulin, the cells don't respond to the hormone, or both. This condition is usually diagnosed in people over age 40. About one-third of people with Type 2 diabetes must inject insulin; others may take medications that increase insulin production or stimulate cells to take up glucose.

A third type of diabetes occurs in some women during pregnancy. So-called *gestational diabetes* usually disappears after pregnancy, but more than half of women who experience it eventually develop Type 2 diabetes.

The major factors involved in the development of diabetes are age, obesity, physical inactivity, a family history of diabetes, and lifestyle. Excess body fat reduces cell sensitivity to insulin, and it is a major risk factor for Type 2 diabetes. Ethnic background also plays a role. African Americans and people of Hispanic background are 55% more likely than non-Hispanic whites to develop Type 2 diabetes. Native Americans also have a higher-than-average incidence of diabetes.

Treatment

There is no cure for diabetes, but it can be successfully managed. Treatment involves keeping blood sugar levels within safe limits through diet, exercise, and, if necessary, medication. Blood sugar levels can be monitored using a home test. Recent research indicates that close monitoring and control of glucose levels can significantly reduce the rate of serious complications among people with diabetes. Nearly 90% of people with Type 2 diabetes are overweight when diagnosed, and an important step in treatment is to lose weight. Even a small amount of weight loss can be beneficial. People with diabetes should eat regular meals with an emphasis on complex carbohydrates and ample

dietary fiber; a physician or dietitian can help design a healthy eating plan. Regular exercise and a healthy diet are often sufficient to control Type 2 diabetes.

Prevention

Recent studies have shown that exercise can help prevent the development of Type 2 diabetes, a benefit especially important in individuals with one or more risk factors for the disease. Exercise burns excess sugar and makes cells more sensitive to insulin. Exercise also helps keep body fat at healthy levels.

Eating a moderate diet to help control body fat is perhaps the most important dietary recommendation for the prevention of diabetes. However, there is some evidence that the composition of the diet may also be important. In a long-term study of over 65,000 nurses, a diet low in fiber and high in sugar and refined carbohydrates was found to increase risk for Type 2 diabetes. The foods most closely linked to higher diabetes risk were regular (non-diet) cola beverages, white bread, white rice, french fries, and potatoes; consumption of cereal fibers such as those found in cold breakfast cereals was associated with lower risk. (Chapter 8 includes more information on different types of carbohydrates as well as specific strategies for increasing fiber intake.)

Warning Signs and Testing

A wellness lifestyle that includes a healthy diet and regular exercise is the best strategy for preventing diabetes. If you do develop diabetes, the best way to avoid complications is to recognize the symptoms and get early diagnosis and treatment. Be alert for the following warning signs:

- Frequent urination
- Extreme hunger or thirst
- Unexplained weight loss
- Extreme fatigue
- Blurred vision
- Frequent infections, especially of the bladder, gums, skin, or vagina
- Cuts and bruises that are slow to heal
- Tingling or numbness in the hands and feet
- Generalized itching, with no rash

Type 2 diabetes is often asymptomatic in the early stages, and major health organizations now recommend routine screening for people over age 45 and anyone younger who is at high risk. (The Web site for the American Diabetes Association, listed in the For More Information section at the end of the chapter, includes an interactive diabetes risk assessment.) Screening involves a blood test to check glucose levels after either a period of fasting or the administration of a set dose of glucose. If you are concerned about your risk for diabetes, talk with your physician about being tested.

If you gaze into the mirror and wish you could change the way your body looks, consider getting some exercise—not to re-shape your contours but to firm up your self-image. According to a recent study from University College London, women who worked out on a regular basis rated their bodies as more attractive and healthy than women who didn't get much physical activity. Of course, the exercisers may have had particularly attractive bodies, but it should be noted that they were more satisfied than the sedentary women, even though they weighed an average of 11–12 pounds more, suggesting that active women are more comfortable bucking the model-thin look that has become our cultural ideal.

One reason for the findings may be that women who exercise regularly often gain a sense of mastery and competence that enhances their self-esteem and body image. In addition, exercise contributes to a more toned look, which some women prefer. Then, too, participating in sports where size and height are advantageous, like volleyball or basketball, may help tall, relatively large women appreciate their body size and shape enough to see beyond cultural stereotypes. Finally, regular exercise and a positive family environment go hand in hand; family support

provides the security to accept "sporty" body shapes even if they aren't picture-perfect by society's standards.

None of this is to say that whether a woman exercises regularly is the only factor that influences the way her body looks to her. Even the sport she prefers or engages in plays a role. In the British study, female body builders, not surprisingly, rated muscular physiques more favorably than women who chose rowing as their sport. In another study in which women were randomly assigned to weight training or brisk walking, body image improved for both groups, but more so for the weight lifters. Despite these other factors, though, the research suggests that as a group, physically active women are more comfortable with their bodies than sedentary women and are particularly tolerant of shapes that deviate from the model-thin icons.

SOURCES: Adapted from "Shape Up Your Body Image." 1995. *Tufts University Diet and Nutrition Letter*, May, p. 8. Tucker, L. A., and R. Mortell. 1993. Comparison of the effects of walking and weight training programs on body image in middle-aged women: An experimental study. *American Journal of Health Promotion* 8(1): 34–42.

---

entirely clear, but it appears that fat in the abdomen is more easily mobilized and sent into the bloodstream, increasing disease-related blood fat levels. In general, men tend to gain weight in the abdominal area and women in the hip area, but women who exhibit the male pattern of fat distribution face the increased health risks associated with it. Researchers have also found ethnic differences in the relative significance of increased abdominal fat, but more studies are needed to clarify the relationship among fat distribution, ethnicity, and disease.

Body fat distribution is usually assessed by calculating the waist-to-hip ratio (the relative circumference of the waist and hips) or by simply measuring the waist. A person doesn't have to be technically overfat to have fat distribution be a risk factor, nor do all overfat people face this increased risk. However, individuals in the obese range should not be complacent about their body composition regardless of their fat distribution—all obesity has serious health consequences.

Is it possible to be too lean? Health experts have generally viewed too little body fat—less than 8% for women and 5% for men—as a threat to health and well-being. Extreme leanness has been linked with reproductive, circulatory, and immune system disorders. Extremely lean people may experience muscle wasting and fatigue; they are also more likely to suffer from a dangerous eating disorder. For women, an extremely low percentage of body fat is associated with **amenorrhea** and loss of bone mass. However, a recent study from Harvard Medical School found that among nonsmoking women who did not suffer from eating disorders, the leanest lived longer than

women of "normal" weight. The authors of this study concluded that even mild to moderate overweight is associated with a substantial increase in the risk of premature death. Additional research is needed to determine all the effects of extremely low body fat levels on health.

Performance of Physical Activities

Too much body fat makes all types of physical activity more difficult because just moving the body through everyday activities means working harder and using more energy. In general, overfat people are less fit than others and don't have the muscular strength, endurance, and flexibility that make normal activity easy. Because exercise is more difficult, they do less of it, depriving themselves of an effective way to improve body composition.

Self-Image

The "fashionable" body image has changed dramatically during the past 50 years, varying from slightly plump to an almost unhealthy thinness. Today a fit and healthy-looking body, developed through a healthy lifestyle, is the goal for most people (see the box "Exercise and Body Image"). And the key to this "look" is a balance of proper nutrition and exercise—in short, a lifestyle that emphasizes wellness.

amenorrhea   Absent or infrequent menstruation, sometimes   **TERMS**
related to low levels of body fat and excessive quantity or
intensity of exercise.

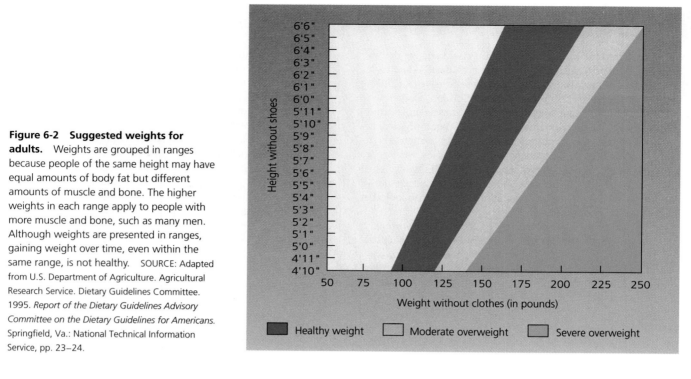

Figure 6-2 Suggested weights for adults. Weights are grouped in ranges because people of the same height may have equal amounts of body fat but different amounts of muscle and bone. The higher weights in each range apply to people with more muscle and bone, such as many men. Although weights are presented in ranges, gaining weight over time, even within the same range, is not healthy. SOURCE: Adapted from U.S. Department of Agriculture. Agricultural Research Service. Dietary Guidelines Committee. 1995. *Report of the Dietary Guidelines Advisory Committee on the Dietary Guidelines for Americans.* Springfield, Va.: National Technical Information Service, pp. 23–24.

Goals for body composition should be realistic, however; a person's ability to change body composition through diet and exercise depends not only on a wellness program, but also on heredity. Unrealistic expectations about body composition can have a negative impact on self-image and can lead to the development of eating disorders. (For more information on eating disorders, see Chapter 9.)

For most people, body fat percentage falls somewhere between ideal and a level that is significantly unhealthy. If they consistently maintain a wellness lifestyle that includes a healthy diet and regular exercise, the right body composition will naturally develop.

Wellness for Life

A healthy body composition is vital for wellness throughout life. Strong scientific evidence suggests that controlling your weight will increase your life span; reduce the risk of heart disease, cancer, diabetes, and back pain; increase your energy level; and improve your self-esteem.

ASSESSING BODY COMPOSITION

The morning weighing ritual on the bathroom scale can't reveal whether a fluctuation in weight is due to a change in muscle, body water, or fat and can't differentiate between overweight and overfat. A 260-pound football player may be overweight according to population height-weight standards yet actually have much less body fat than average. Likewise, a 40-year-old woman may weigh the same as she did 20 years earlier yet have a considerably different body composition. Despite these limitations, the U.S. Food and Drug Administration (FDA) and the Department of Health and Human Services have published new height and weight recommendations, shown in Figure 6-2.

There are a number of simple, inexpensive ways to estimate body composition that are superior to the bathroom scale. These methods include body mass index and skinfold measurements.

Body Mass Index

Body mass index (BMI) is a rough measure of body composition that is useful if you don't have access to sophisticated equipment. Though more accurate than height-weight tables, body mass index is also based on the concept that a person's weight should be proportional to height. The measurement is fairly accurate for people who do not have an unusual amount of muscle mass and

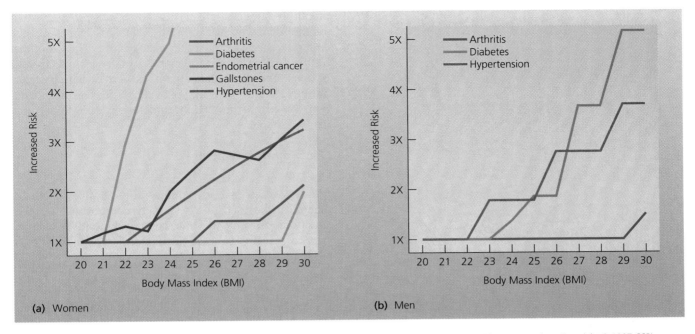

Figure 6-3 BMI and risk of health problems. SOURCE: How's your weight? 1997. *Nutrition Action Healthletter,* December. Copyright © 1997 CSPI. Adapted from Nutrition Action Health Letter (1875 Connecticut Avenue, N. W., Suite 300, Washington D. C. 20009-5728. $24.00 for 10 issues.)

TABLE 6-2	*Classification of Overweight and Obesity by BMI*				
				Disease risk relative to normal weight and waist circumference[a]	
Classification	**BMI (kg/m^2)**	**Obesity class**		**Men ≤ 40 in. (102 cm) Women ≤ 35 in. (88 cm)**	**> 40 in. (102 cm) > 35 in. (88 cm)**
Underweight[b]	less than 18.5			—	—
Normal[c]	18.5–24.9			—	—
Overweight	25.0–29.9			Increased	High
Obesity	30.0–34.9	I		High	Very high
	35.0–39.9	II		Very high	Very high
Extreme obesity	40.0 and higher	III		Extremely high	Extremely high

[a]Disease risk for type 2 diabetes, hypertension, and CVD. The waist circumference cutoff points for increased risk are 40 inches (102 cm) for men and 35 inches (88 cm) for women.

[b]Research suggests that a low BMI can be healthy in some cases, as long as it is not the result of smoking, an eating disorder, or an underlying disease process.

[c]Increased waist circumference can also be a marker for increased risk even in persons of normal weight.

SOURCE: Adapted from National Heart, Lung, and Blood Institute. 1998. *Clinical Guidelines on the Identification, Evaluation, and Treatment of Overweight and Obesity in Adults: The Evidence Report.* Bethesda, Md.: National Institutes of Health.

who are not very short. BMI is calculated by dividing your body weight (expressed in kilograms) by the square of your height (expressed in meters). For example, a person who weighs 130 pounds (59 kilograms) and is 5 feet, 3 inches tall (1.6 meters) would have a BMI of 59 kg ÷ (1.6 m)^2, or 23 kg/m^2. (Refer to Lab 6-1 for instructions on how to calculate your BMI.)

The relative risk for several health problems associated with different values of BMI is shown in Figure 6-3. At high values of BMI, the risk of arthritis, diabetes, hypertension, endometrial cancer, and other disorders increases substantially. The increased risk of diabetes at even fairly low values of BMI especially among women is of particular concern.

Proper technique is important in skinfold measurement. It's best to take several measurements at each site to ensure accuracy.

In June 1998, new federal guidelines for classifying overweight and obesity on the basis of BMI were released by the National Heart, Lung, and Blood Institute (NHLBI), a division of the National Institutes of Health. Under these guidelines, a person is classified as overweight if he or she has a BMI of 25 or above and obese if he or she has a BMI of 30 or above (Table 6-2). Previously, the cutoff point for defining overweight was higher; the new guidelines reflect standards used in other countries as well as by the World Health Organization. Nearly 55% of American adults have a BMI of 25 or above.

In classifying the health risks associated with overweight and obesity, the new NHLBI guidelines consider body fat distribution and other disease risk factors in addition to BMI. As described earlier, excess fat in the abdomen is of greater concern than excess fat in other areas. Methods of assessing body fat distribution are discussed later in the chapter; the NHLBI guidelines use measurement of waist circumference (see Table 6-2). At a given level of overweight, people with a large waist circumference and/or additional disease risk factors are at greater risk for health problems. For example, a man with a BMI of 27, a waist circumference above 40 inches, and high

blood pressure is at greater risk for health problems than another man who has a BMI of 27 but has a smaller waist circumference and no other risk factors. Thus, optimal BMI for good health depends on many factors; if your BMI is 25 or above, consult a physician for help in determining a healthy BMI for you. (Weight loss recommendations based on the NHLBI guidelines are discussed further in Chapter 9.)

Skinfold Measurements

Skinfold measurement is a simple, inexpensive, and practical way to assess body composition. Skinfold measurements can be used to assess body composition because equations can link the thickness of skinfolds at various sites to percent body fat calculations from more precise laboratory techniques.

Skinfolds are measured with a device called a **caliper**, which consists of a pair of spring-loaded, calibrated jaws. High-quality calipers are made of metal and have parallel jaw surfaces and constant spring tension. Inexpensive plastic calipers are also available; to ensure accuracy, plastic calipers should be spring-loaded and have metal jaws.

Refer to Lab 6-1 for the procedure for taking skinfold measurements. Taking accurate measurements with calipers requires patience, experience, and considerable practice. It's best to take several measurements at each site (or have several different people take each measurement) to help ensure accuracy. Be sure to take the measurements in the exact location called for in the procedure. Because the amount of water in your body changes during the day, skinfold measurements taken in the morning and evening often differ. If you repeat the measurements in the future to track changes in your body composition, measure skinfolds at approximately the same time of day.

Other Methods of Measuring Body Composition

Most of the many other methods for determining body composition are very sophisticated and require expensive equipment. Two methods available in many health clubs and sports medicine clinics are underwater weighing and bioelectrical impedance analysis.

Underwater Weighing Hydrostatic (underwater) weighing is considered the most accurate indirect way to measure body composition. It is the standard used for other techniques, including skinfold measurements. For this method, an individual is submerged and weighed under water. The percentages of fat and fat-free weight are calculated from body density. Muscle has a higher density and fat a lower density than water (1.1 grams per cubic centimeter for fat-free mass, 0.91 gram per cubic centimeter for fat, and 1 gram per cubic centimeter for water). Therefore, fat people tend to float and weigh less under water, and lean people tend to sink and weigh more under water.

TERMS **caliper** A pressure-sensitive measuring instrument with two jaws that can be adjusted to determine thickness.

This man is having his body composition assessed in an underwater weighing tank. Muscle has a higher density than water, so people with more lean body mass weigh more under water.

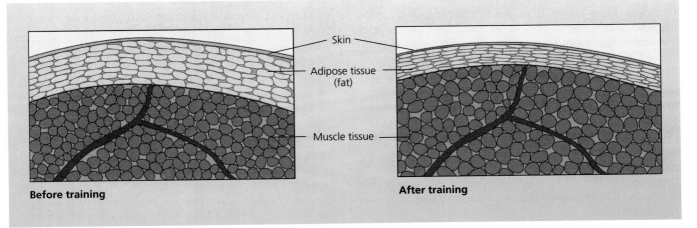

Before training **After training**

Skin
Adipose tissue (fat)
Muscle tissue

Figure 6-4 Effects of exercise on body composition. Endurance exercise and strength training reduce body fat and increase muscle mass.

Although somewhat cumbersome and expensive, this method is not beyond limited budgets. A harness and a spring-loaded scale can be connected to a diving board, and the school pool can be used as the underwater weighing tank. Most university exercise physiology departments or sports medicine laboratories will have an underwater weighing facility. If you want an accurate assessment of your body composition, find a place that does underwater weighing.

Bioelectrical Impedance Analysis (BIA) The technique works by sending a small electrical current through the body and measuring the body's resistance to it. Fat-free tissues, where most body water is located, are good conductors of electrical current, while fat is not. Thus, the amount of resistance to electrical current is related to the amount of fat-free tissue in the body can be used to estimate percent body fat. Bioelectrical impedance analysis is fairly accurate for most people (about the same as skinfold measurements). To avoid error, it is important to follow the manufacturer's instructions carefully and to avoid overhydration or underhydration (more or less body water than normal). Because measurement varies with the type of BIA analyzer, use the same instrument to compare measurements over time.

Assessing Body Fat Distribution

Researchers have studied many different methods for determining the risk associated with body fat distribution. Two of the simplest to perform are waist circumference measurement and waist-to-hip ratio calculation. In the first method, you measure your waist circumference; in the second, you divide your waist circumference by your hip circumference. More research is needed to determine the precise degree of risk associated with specific values for these two assessments of body fat distribution. However, a total waist measurement over 40 inches (102 cm) for men and 35 inches (88 cm) for women and a waist-to-hip ratio above 0.95 for men and 0.86 for women are associated with a significantly increased risk of disease. Follow the instructions in Lab 6-1 to measure and rate your body fat distribution.

DETERMINING RECOMMENDED BODY WEIGHT

If the assessment tests indicate that fat loss would be beneficial for you, your first step is to establish a goal. Use the ratings in Table 6-1 or Table 6-2 to choose a target value for percent body fat or BMI (depending on which type of assessment you completed). Select a goal for percent body fat or BMI that is realistic for you and will ensure good health. Make sure your goal is realistic. Genetics may limit your capacity to change your body composition. Few people can expect to develop the body of a fashion model or competitive body builder. However, you can improve your body composition through a regular program of exercise and a healthy diet. If you have known risk factors for disease, such as high blood pressure or high levels of blood cholesterol, consult your physician to determine the ideal body composition for your individual risk profile.

Once you've established your goal, you can calculate a target body weight. (Though body weight is not an accurate means of assessing body composition, it's a useful method for tracking progress in a program to change body composition. If you're losing a small or moderate amount of weight and exercising, you're probably losing fat while building muscle mass.) Follow the instructions in Lab 6-2 to put the results of all the assessment tests together, get an overview of your body composition, and determine a range for recommended body weight.

Using percent body fat or BMI will generate a fairly accurate target body weight for most people. However, it's best not to stick rigidly to a recommended body weight calculated from any formula; individual genetic, cultural, and lifestyle factors are also important. Decide whether the body weight that the formulas generate for you is realistic, meets all your goals, is healthy, *and* is reasonable for you to maintain.

After selecting your overall goal, set realistic intermediate goals. For example, if you want to lose a total of 10 pounds, you might set short-term goals of losing 2 pounds during the first month of your program and 2 more pounds during the second month. To help ensure success, reevaluate your program and your goals frequently.

Track your progress toward your target body composition by checking your body weight periodically. To get a more accurate idea of your progress, especially when weight loss is large, you should directly reassess your body composition occasionally during your program: Body composition changes as weight changes. Losing a lot of weight usually includes losing some muscle mass no matter how hard a person exercises, partly because carrying less weight requires the muscular system to bear a smaller burden. (Conversely, a large gain in weight without exercise still causes some gain in muscle mass because muscles are working harder to carry the extra weight.)

See Chapter 9 for specific strategies for losing or gaining weight and improving body composition.

COMMON QUESTIONS ANSWERED

Is spot reducing effective?   No. Spot reducing refers to attempts to lose body fat in specific parts of the body by doing exercises for those parts. For example, a person might try to spot reduce in the legs by doing leg lifts. Spot-reducing exercises contribute to fat loss only to the extent that they burn calories. The only way you can reduce fat in any specific area is to create an overall negative energy balance: Take in less energy (food) than you use up through exercise and metabolism.

How does exercise affect body composition?   Cardiorespiratory endurance exercise burns calories, thereby helping create a negative energy balance. Weight training does not use many calories and therefore is of little use in creating a negative

energy balance. However, weight training increases muscle mass, which maintains a high metabolic rate (the body's energy level) and helps improve body composition. To minimize body fat and increase muscle mass, thereby improving body composition, combine cardiorespiratory endurance exercise and weight training (Figure 6-4).

How do I develop a toned, healthy-looking body?   The development of a healthy-looking body requires regular exercise, proper diet, and other good health habits. However, it helps to have heredity on your side. Some people put on or take off fat more easily than others just as some people are taller than

(continued)

others. Be realistic in your goals, and be satisfied with the improvements in body composition you can make by observing the principles of a wellness lifestyle.

Are people who have a desirable body composition physically fit? Having a healthy body composition is not necessarily associated with overall fitness. For example, many body builders have very little body fat but have poor cardiorespiratory capacity and flexibility. To be fit, you must rate high on all the components of fitness.

What is liposuction, and will it help me lose body fat? Suction lipectomy, popularly known as liposuction, has become the most popular type of elective surgery in the United States. The procedure involves removing limited amounts of fat from specific areas. Typically, no more than 2.5 kg (5.5 lb) of adipose tissue is removed at a time. The procedure is usually successful if the amount of excess fat is limited and skin elas-ticity is good. The procedure is most effective if integrated into a program of dietary restriction and exercise. Side effects include infection, dimpling, and wavy skin contours. Although serious complications are rare, liposuction, like any surgical procedure, can lead to blood clots, shock, bleeding, impaired blood flow to vital organs, and even death. Liposuction is not an effective way to lose large amounts of fat, nor should it be a substitute for a healthy weight-management program.

What is cellulite, and how do I get rid of it? Cellulite is the name commonly given to ripply, wavy fat deposits that collect just under the skin. However, these rippling fat deposits are really the same as fat deposited anywhere else in the body. The only way to control them is to create a negative energy balance—burn up more calories than are taken in. There are no creams or lotions that will rub away surface (subcutaneous) fat deposits, and spot reducing is also ineffective. The only solution is sensible eating habits and exercise.

SUMMARY

- The human body is composed of fat-free mass (which includes bone, muscle, organ tissues, and connective tissues) and body fat (essential and nonessential).

- Having too much body fat has negative health consequences, especially in terms of cardiovascular disease. Distribution of fat is also a significant factor in health.

- A fit and healthy-looking body, with the right body composition for a particular person, develops from habits of proper nutrition and exercise.

- Measuring body weight is not an accurate way to assess body composition because it does not differentiate between muscle weight and fat weight.

- Two measurements of body composition are body mass index (formulated through weight and height measurements) and percent body fat (formulated through skinfold measurements).

- Hydrostatic weighing, the most accurate indirect measure of body composition, is based on body density; muscle has a higher density and fat a lower density than water. Bioelectrical impedance analysis estimates the amount of body water (and thereby fat-free tissue) by measuring the body's resistance to a small electrical current.

- Body fat distribution can be assessed through the waist-to-hip ratio or the total waist measurement.

- Recommended body weight can be determined by choosing a target BMI or target body fat percentage. Keep heredity in mind when setting a goal.

FOR MORE INFORMATION

Underwater weighing and bioelectrical impedance analysis are often available through campus adult fitness programs, and health clubs may also provide tests for percent body fat.

Books

American Diabetes Association. 1997. *American Diabetes Association Complete Guide to Diabetes: The Ultimate Home Diabetes Reference.* Alexandria, Va.: American Diabetes Association. *Explains the symptoms, causes, diagnosis, treatment, and self-care of diabetes.*

Brooks, G. A., T. D. Fahey, and T. P. White. 1996. *Exercise Physiology: Human Bioenergetics and Its Applications,* 2d ed. Mountain View, Calif.: Mayfield. *A basic exercise physiology textbook that describes principles of metabolism and body composition.*

Heyward, V. H., and L. M. Stolarczyk. 1996. *Applied Body Composition Assessment.* Champaign, Ill.: Human Kinetics. *Describes different methods of measuring and assessing body composition.*

Roche, A. F., S. T. Heymsfield, and T. G. Lohman. 1996. *Human Body Composition.* Champaign, Ill.: Human Kinetics. *This book discusses the theory and measurement of human body composition. Although it is mainly directed at sports scientists, people who are seriously interested in exercise might also be interested.*

Organizations and Web Sites

American Diabetes Association. Provides information, a free newsletter, and referrals to local support groups; the Web site includes an online diabetes risk assessment.

800-342-2383

http://www.diabetes.org

Healthy Body Calculator. Calculates and evaluates BMI, body weight, and waist-to-hip ratio.

http://www.dietitian.com/ibw

Shape Up America. A site devoted to promoting healthy weight management; calculates and rates BMI and looks at why BMI is an important measure of health.

http://shapeup.org

National Heart, Lung, and Blood Institute. Provides information on the latest federal obesity standards and a BMI calculator.

http://www.nhlbi.nih.gov/nhlbi/nhlbi.htm

National Institute of Diabetes and Digestive and Kidney Diseases Health Information/Nutrition and Obesity. Provides information about adult obesity: how it is defined and assessed, the risk factors associated with it, and its causes.

800-WIN-8090

http://www.niddk.nih.gov/health/nutrit/nutrit.htm

See also the listings for Chapters 2 and 9.

SELECTED BIBLIOGRAPHY

American College of Sports Medicine. 1995. *Guidelines for Exercise Testing and Prescription.* Baltimore: Williams & Wilkins.

American Heart Association. 1998. Press Release: Obesity Joins American Heart Association's List of Major Risk Factors for Heart Attack (retrieved June 2, 1998; http:www.american heart.org/whats_News/AHA_News_Releases/obesity.html).

Bender, R., C. Trautner, M. Spraul, and M. Berger. 1998. Assessment of excess mortality in obesity. *American Journal of Epidemiology* 147:42–48.

Broeder, C. E., et al. 1997. Assessing body composition before and after resistance or endurance training. *Medicine and Science in Sports and Exercise* 29(5): 705–712.

Center for Disease Control and Prevention. 1997. Trends in the prevalence and incidence of self-reported diabetes mellitus—United States, 1980–1994. *Morbidity and Mortality Weekly Report* 46(43): 1014–1018.

Chow, W. H., et al. 1998. Body mass index and risk of adenocarcinomas of the esophagus and gastric cardia. *Journal of the National Cancer Institute* 90(2): 150–155.

De Lorenzo, A., et al. 1997. Predicting body cell mass with bioimpedance by using theoretical methods: A technological review. *Journal of Applied Physiology* 82:1542–1558.

Diabetes: Weight control and exercise may keep you off the road to high blood sugar. 1998. *Mayo Clinic Health Letter Supplement,* February.

Ellis, K. J. 1997. Body composition of a young, multiethnic, male population. *American Journal of Clinical Nutrition* 66:1323–1331.

Guo, S. S., et al. 1997. Age- and maturity-related changes in body composition during adolescence into adulthood: The Fels Longitudinal Study. *International Journal of Obesity Related Metabolic Disorders* 21:1167–1175.

Han, T. S., et al. 1996. Waist circumference as a screening tool for cardiovascular risk factors: Evaluation of receiver operating characteristics (ROC). *Obesity Research* 4:533–547.

Huddy, D. C., et al. 1997. Relationship between body image and percent body fat among male and female college students enrolled in an introductory 14-week weight-training course. *Perceptual and Motor Skills* 85(3 Pt 1): 1075–1078.

Keller, C., and K. T. Thomas. 1997. Assessment of overweight and obese patients. *Nurse Pract Forum* 8:99–104.

Lemieux, S., et al. 1996. A single threshold value of waist girth identifies normal-weight and overweight subjects with excess visceral adipose tissue. *American Journal of Clinical Nutrition* 64:685–693.

Manson, J. E., et al. 1995. Body weight and mortality among women. *New England Journal of Medicine* 333(11): 677–685.

National Heart, Lung, and Blood Institute. 1998. *Clinical Guidelines on the Identification, Evaluation, and Treatment of Overweight and Obesity in Adults: The Evidence Report.* Bethesda, Md.: National Institutes of Health.

Nguyen, T. V., et al. 1998. Bone mass, lean mass, and fat mass: Same genes or same environments? *American Journal of Epidemiology* 147(1): 3–16.

Norgan, N. G. 1997. The beneficial effects of body fat and adipose tissue in humans. *International Journal of Obesity Related Metabolic Disorders* 21:738–746.

Otis, C. L., et al. 1997. American College of Sports Medicine position stand. The Female Athlete Triad. *Medicine and Science in Sports and Exercise* 29:I–IX.

Pichard, C., et al. 1997. Body composition by x-ray absorptiometry and bioelectrical impedance in female runners. *Medicine and Science in Sports and Exercise* 29(11): 1527–1534.

Salmeró, J., et al. 1997. Dietary fiber, glycemic load, and risk of non-insulin-dependent diabetes mellitus in women. *Journal of the American Medical Association* 277(6): 472–477.

Snyder, K. A., et al. 1997. The effects of long-term, moderate intensity, intermittent exercise on aerobic capacity, body composition, blood lipids, insulin and glucose in overweight females. *International Journal of Obesity Related Metabolic Disorders* 21:1180–1189.

Stevens, J., et al. 1998. The effect of age on the association between body-mass index and mortality. *New England Journal of Medicine* 338(1): 1–7.

Taylor, R. W., et al. 1998. Body mass index, waist girth, and waist-to-hip ratio as indexes of total and regional adiposity in women: Evaluation using receiver operating characteristic curves. *American Journal of Clinical Nutrition* 67:44–49.

To, W. W., M. W. Wong, and K. M. Chan. 1997. Association between body composition and menstrual dysfunction in collegiate dance students. *Journal of Obstetrics and Gynaecology Research* 23:529–535.

Wallberg-Henriksson, H., J. Rincon, and J. R. Zierath. 1998. Exercise in the management of non-insulin-dependent diabetes mellitus. *Sports Medicine* 25(1): 25–35.

Zannolli, R., and G. Morgese. 1996. Waist percentiles: A simple test for atherogenic disease? *Acta Paediatrica* 85:1368–1369.

Percent Body Fat Estimate for Men: Sum of Chest, Abdomen, and Thigh Skinfolds

Sum of Skinfolds (mm)	Age								
	Under 22	23–27	28–32	33–37	38–42	43–47	48–52	53–57	Over 57
8–10	1.3	1.8	2.3	2.9	3.4	3.9	4.5	5.0	5.5
11–13	2.2	2.8	3.3	3.9	4.4	4.9	5.5	6.0	6.5
14–16	3.2	3.8	4.3	4.8	5.4	5.9	6.4	7.0	7.5
17–19	4.2	4.7	5.3	5.8	6.3	6.9	7.4	8.0	8.5
20–22	5.1	5.7	6.2	6.8	7.3	7.9	8.4	8.9	9.5
23–25	6.1	6.6	7.2	7.7	8.3	8.8	9.4	9.9	10.5
26–28	7.0	7.6	8.1	8.7	9.2	9.8	10.3	10.9	11.4
29–31	8.0	8.5	9.1	9.6	10.2	10.7	11.3	11.8	12.4
32–34	8.9	9.4	10.0	10.5	11.1	11.6	12.2	12.8	13.3
35–37	9.8	10.4	10.9	11.5	12.0	12.6	13.1	13.7	14.3
38–40	10.7	11.3	11.8	12.4	12.9	13.5	14.1	14.6	15.2
41–43	11.6	12.2	12.7	13.3	13.8	14.4	15.0	15.5	16.1
44–46	12.5	13.1	13.6	14.2	14.7	15.3	15.9	16.4	17.0
47–49	13.4	13.9	14.5	15.1	15.6	16.2	16.8	17.3	17.9
50–52	14.3	14.8	15.4	15.9	16.5	17.1	17.6	18.2	18.8
53–55	15.1	15.7	16.2	16.8	17.4	17.9	18.5	19.1	19.7
56–58	16.0	16.5	17.1	17.7	18.2	18.8	19.4	20.0	20.5
59–61	16.9	17.4	17.9	18.5	19.1	19.7	20.2	20.8	21.4
62–64	17.6	18.2	18.8	19.4	19.9	20.5	21.1	21.7	22.2
65–67	18.5	19.0	19.6	20.2	20.8	21.3	21.9	22.5	23.1
68–70	19.3	19.9	20.4	21.0	21.6	22.2	22.7	23.3	23.9
71–73	20.1	20.7	21.2	21.8	22.4	23.0	23.6	24.1	24.7
74–76	20.9	21.5	22.0	22.6	23.2	23.8	24.4	25.0	25.5
77–79	21.7	22.2	22.8	23.4	24.0	24.6	25.2	25.8	26.3
80–82	22.4	23.0	23.6	24.2	24.8	25.4	25.9	26.5	27.1
83–85	23.2	23.8	24.4	25.0	25.5	26.1	26.7	27.3	27.9
86–88	24.0	24.5	25.1	25.7	26.3	26.9	27.5	28.1	28.7
89–91	24.7	25.3	25.9	26.5	27.1	27.6	28.2	28.8	29.4
92–94	25.4	26.0	26.6	27.2	27.8	28.4	29.0	29.6	30.2
95–97	26.1	26.7	27.3	27.9	28.5	29.1	29.7	30.3	30.9
98–100	26.9	27.4	28.0	28.6	29.2	29.8	30.4	31.0	31.6
101–103	27.5	28.1	28.7	29.3	29.9	30.5	31.1	31.7	32.3
104–106	28.2	28.8	29.4	30.0	30.6	31.2	31.8	32.4	33.0
107–109	28.9	29.5	30.1	30.7	31.3	31.9	32.5	33.1	33.7
110–112	29.6	30.2	30.8	31.4	32.0	32.6	33.2	33.8	34.4
113–115	30.2	30.8	31.4	32.0	32.6	33.2	33.8	34.5	35.1
116–118	30.9	31.5	32.1	32.7	33.3	33.9	34.5	35.1	35.7
119–121	31.5	32.1	32.7	33.3	33.9	34.5	35.1	35.7	36.4
122–124	32.1	32.7	33.3	33.9	34.5	35.1	35.8	36.4	37.0
125–127	32.7	33.3	33.9	34.5	35.1	35.8	36.4	37.0	37.6

SOURCE: Jackson, A. S., and M. L. Pollock. 1985. Practical assessment of body composition. *The Physician and Sportsmedicine* 13(5): 76–90. Reproduced by permission of McGraw-Hill, Inc.

Percent Body Fat Estimate for Women: Sum of Triceps, Suprailium, and Thigh Skinfolds

Sum of Skinfolds (mm)	Age								
	Under 22	23–27	28–32	33–37	38–42	43–47	48–52	53–57	Over 57
23–25	9.7	9.9	10.2	10.4	10.7	10.9	11.2	11.4	11.7
26–28	11.0	11.2	11.5	11.7	12.0	12.3	12.5	12.7	13.0
29–31	12.3	12.5	12.8	13.0	13.3	13.5	13.8	14.0	14.3
32–34	13.6	13.8	14.0	14.3	14.5	14.8	15.0	15.3	15.5
35–37	14.8	15.0	15.3	15.5	15.8	16.0	16.3	16.5	16.8
38–40	16.0	16.3	16.5	16.7	17.0	17.2	17.5	17.7	18.0
41–43	17.2	17.4	17.7	17.9	18.2	18.4	18.7	18.9	19.2
44–46	18.3	18.6	18.8	19.1	19.3	19.6	19.8	20.1	20.3
47–49	19.5	19.7	20.0	20.2	20.5	20.7	21.0	21.2	21.5
50–52	20.6	20.8	21.1	21.3	21.6	21.8	22.1	22.3	22.6
53–55	21.7	21.9	22.1	22.4	22.6	22.9	23.1	23.4	23.6
56–58	22.7	23.0	23.2	23.4	23.7	23.9	24.2	24.4	24.7
59–61	23.7	24.0	24.2	24.5	24.7	25.0	25.2	25.5	25.7
62–64	24.7	25.0	25.2	25.5	25.7	26.0	26.7	26.4	26.7
65–67	25.7	25.9	26.2	26.4	26.7	26.9	27.2	27.4	27.7
68–70	26.6	26.9	27.1	27.4	27.6	27.9	28.1	28.4	28.6
71–73	27.5	27.8	28.0	28.3	28.5	28.8	29.0	29.3	29.5
74–76	28.4	28.7	28.9	29.2	29.4	29.7	29.9	30.2	30.4
77–79	29.3	29.5	29.8	30.0	30.3	30.5	30.8	31.0	31.3
80–82	30.1	30.4	30.6	30.9	31.1	31.4	31.6	31.9	32.1
83–85	30.9	31.2	31.4	31.7	31.9	32.2	32.4	32.7	32.9
86–88	31.7	32.0	32.2	32.5	32.7	32.9	33.2	33.4	33.7
89–91	32.5	32.7	33.0	33.2	33.5	33.7	33.9	34.2	34.4
92–94	33.2	33.4	33.7	33.9	34.2	34.4	34.7	34.9	35.2
95–97	33.9	34.1	34.4	34.6	34.9	35.1	35.4	35.6	35.9
98–100	34.6	34.8	35.1	35.3	35.5	35.8	36.0	36.3	36.5
101–103	35.3	35.4	35.7	35.9	36.2	36.4	36.7	36.9	37.2
104–106	35.8	36.1	36.3	36.6	36.8	37.1	37.3	37.5	37.8
107–109	36.4	36.7	36.9	37.1	37.4	37.6	37.9	38.1	38.4
110–112	37.0	37.2	37.5	37.7	38.0	38.2	38.5	38.7	38.9
113–115	37.5	37.8	38.0	38.2	38.5	38.7	39.0	39.2	39.5
116–118	38.0	38.3	38.5	38.8	39.0	39.3	39.5	39.7	40.0
119–121	38.5	38.7	39.0	39.2	39.5	39.7	40.0	40.2	40.5
122–124	39.0	39.2	39.4	39.7	39.9	40.2	40.4	40.7	40.9
125–127	39.4	39.6	39.9	40.1	40.4	40.6	40.9	41.1	41.4
128–130	39.8	40.0	40.3	40.5	40.8	41.0	41.3	41.5	41.8

SOURCE: Jackson, A. S., and M. L. Pollock. 1985. Practical assessment of body composition. *The Physician and Sportsmedicine* 13(5): 76–90. Reproduced by permission of McGraw-Hill, Inc.

*Body Composition Ratings**

| | Percent Body Fat | | | | | |
Men	Very Lean	Excellent	Good	Fair	Poor	Very Poor
Age: 18–29	Below 5.3	5.3–9.4	9.5–14.1	14.2–17.4	17.5–22.4	Above 22.4
30–39	Below 9.2	9.2–13.9	14.0–17.5	17.6–20.5	20.6–24.2	Above 24.2
40–49	Below 11.5	11.5–16.3	16.4–19.6	19.7–22.5	22.6–26.1	Above 26.1
50–59	Below 13.0	13.0–17.9	18.0–21.3	21.4–24.1	24.2–27.5	Above 27.5
60 and over	Below 13.2	13.2–18.4	18.5–22.0	22.1–25.0	25.1–28.5	Above 28.5
Women						
Age: 18–29	Below 10.9	10.9–17.1	17.2–20.6	20.7–23.7	23.8–27.7	Above 27.7
30–39	Below 13.5	13.5–18.0	18.1–21.6	21.7–24.9	25.0–29.3	Above 29.3
40–49	Below 16.2	16.2–21.3	21.4–24.9	25.0–28.1	28.2–32.1	Above 32.1
50–59	Below 18.9	18.9–25.0	25.1–28.5	28.6–31.6	31.7–35.6	Above 35.6
60 and over	Below 16.9	16.9–25.1	25.2–29.3	29.4–32.5	32.6–36.6	Above 36.6

*These ratings are derived from norms based on the measurement of thousands of individuals. In evaluating your body composition, also consider the health-related recommendations for body fat given in Table 6-1 (p. 139). Obesity is defined as having more than 25% of body weight as fat for men and more than 33% of body weight as fat for women. Norms reflect the status of the population, while recommendations represent a more healthy and desirable status.

SOURCE: Based on norms from the Cooper Institute for Aerobics Research, Dallas, Texas; used with permission.

Other Methods of Assessing Percent Body Fat

Other methods of assessing percent body fat, including underwater weighing and bioelectrical impedance analysis, may be available on your campus or in your community. If you use one of these alternative methods, record the name of the method and the result below and in the chart at the end of this lab. Find your body composition rating on the table above.

Method used: _____

Percent body fat: _____ %

Rating (from table above): _____

Waist Circumference and Waist-to-Hip Ratio

Equipment

1. Tape measure
2. Partner to take measurements

Preparation

Wear clothes that will not add significantly to your measurements.

Instructions

Stand with your feet together and your arms at your sides. Raise your arms only high enough to allow for taking the measurements. Your partner should make sure the tape is horizontal around the entire circumference and pulled snugly against your skin. The tape shouldn't be pulled so tight that it causes indentations in your skin. Record measurements to the nearest millimeter or one-sixteenth of an inch.

Waist. Measure at the smallest waist circumference. If you don't have a natural waist, measure at the level of your navel.

Waist measurement: _____

Hip. Measure at the largest hip circumference.

Hip measurement: _____

Waist-to-Hip Ratio: You can use any unit of measurement (for example, inches or centimeters), as long as you're consistent. Waist-to-hip ratio equals waist measurement divided by hip measurement.

Waist-to-hip ratio: _____ ÷ _____ = _____
                                  waist measurement   hip measurement

Determining Your Risk

The table below indicates values for waist circumference and waist-to-hip ratio above which the risk of health problems increases significantly. If your measurement or ratio is above either cutoff point, put a check on the appropriate line below and in the chart on the final page of this lab.

Waist circumference: _____ (✔ high risk)

Waist-to-hip ratio: _____ (✔ high risk)

Body Fat Distribution

Cutoff Points for High Risk

	Waist Circumference	Waist-to-Hip Ratio
Men	more than 40 in. (102 cm)	more than 0.95
Women	more than 35 in. (88 cm)	more than 0.86

SOURCES: National Heart, Lung, and Blood Institute. 1998. *Clinical Guidelines on the Identification, Evaluation, and Treatment of Overweight and Obesity in Adults: The Evidence Report.* Bethesda, Md.: National Institutes of Health. American College of Sports Medicine. 1995. *Guidelines for Exercise Testing and Prescription.* Baltimore, Md9.: Williams & Wilkins.

Rating Your Body Composition

Assessment	Value	Classification
BMI	_____ kg/m²	_____
Skinfold measurements or alternative method of determining percent body fat. Specify method: _____	_____ % body fat	_____
Waist circumference Waist-to-hip ratio	_____ in. or cm _____ (ratio)	_____ (✔ high risk) _____ (✔ high risk)

Enter the results of this lab in the Preprogram Assessment column of Appendix D. After several weeks of a program to improve body composition, do this lab again, and enter the results in the Postprogram Assessment column of Appendix D. How do the results compare?

Putting Together a Complete Fitness Program

7

LOOKING AHEAD

After reading this chapter, you should be able to answer these questions about putting together a complete personalized exercise program:

- What are the steps for putting together a successful personal fitness program?

- What strategies can help maintain a fitness program over the long term?

- How can a fitness program be tailored to accommodate special health concerns?

Understanding the physiological basis and wellness benefits of health-related physical fitness, as explained in Chapters 1–6, is the first step toward creating a well-rounded exercise program. The next challenge is to combine activities into a program that develops all the fitness components and maintains motivation.

This chapter presents a step-by-step procedure for creating and maintaining a well-rounded program. Following the chapter, you'll find sample programs based on popular activities. The structure these programs provide can be helpful if you're beginning an exercise program for the first time.

Weight training does little to develop cardiorespiratory endurance but is excellent for developing muscular strength and endurance. An overall fitness program includes exercises to develop all the components of physical fitness.

DEVELOPING A PERSONAL FITNESS PLAN

If you're ready to create a complete fitness program based around the activities you enjoy most, begin by preparing the program plan and contract in Lab 7-1. By carefully developing your plan and signing a contract, you'll increase your chances of success. The step-by-step procedure outlined here (adapted from *Your Guide to Getting Fit,* by Ivan Kusinitz and Morton Fine) will guide you through the steps of Lab 7-1 to the creation of an exercise program that's right for you. Refer to Figure 7-1 for a sample personal fitness program plan and contract.

If you'd like additional help in setting up your program, choose one of the sample programs at the end of this chapter (pp. 170–178). Sample programs are provided for walking/jogging/running, cycling, swimming, and in-line skating; they include detailed instructions for starting a program and developing and maintaining fitness.

1. Set Goals

Setting goals to reach through exercise is a crucial first step. Ask yourself, "What do I want from my fitness program?" Develop different types of goals—general and specific, long term and short term. General or long-term goals might include things like lowering your risk for chronic disease, improving posture, and having more energy. It's a good idea to also develop some specific, short-term goals based on measurable factors. Specific goals might be raising $\dot{V}O_{2max}$ by 10%, reducing the time it takes you to jog 2 miles from 22 minutes to 19 minutes, increasing the number of push-ups you can do from 15 to 25, and lowering BMI from 26 to 24. Having specific goals will allow you to track your progress and enjoy the measurable changes brought about by your fitness program. Refer to the results of the assessment tests you completed in the labs for Chapters 3–6 for help in setting specific goals.

You'll find it easier to stick with your program if you choose goals that are both important to you and realistic. Remember that heredity, your current fitness level, and other individual factors influence the amount of improve-

ment and the ultimate level of fitness you can expect to obtain through physical training. Fitness improves most quickly during the first 6 months of an exercise program. After that, gains come more slowly and usually require a higher-intensity program. So don't expect to improve indefinitely. Improve your fitness to a reasonable target level, and then train consistently to maintain it.

Think carefully about your reasons for exercising, and then fill in the goals portion of your program plan in Lab 7-1.

2. Select Activities

If you have already chosen activities and created separate program plans for different fitness components in Chapters 3, 4, and 5, you can put those plans together into a single program. It's usually best to include exercises to develop each of the health-related components of physical fitness.

- Cardiorespiratory endurance is developed by activities such as walking, cycling, and aerobic dance that involve continuous rhythmic movements of large muscle groups like those in the legs (see Chapter 3).

A. I ___Tracie Kaufman___ am contracting with myself to follow a physical
                (name)
fitness program to work toward the following goals:

Specific or short-term goals

1. Improving cardiorespiratory fitness by raising my $\dot{V}O_{2max}$ to 37 ml/kg/min
2. Improving upper body muscular strength and endurance
3. Improving body composition (from 30% to 25% body fat)
4. Improving my tennis game (hitting 20 playable shots in a row against the ball machine)

General or long-term goals

1. Developing a more positive attitude about myself
2. Reducing my risk for diabetes and heart disease
3. Building and maintaining bone mass to reduce my risk of osteoporosis
4. Increasing my life expectancy

B. My program plan is as follows:

Activities	Components (Check ✓) CRE	MS	ME	F	BC	Intensity*	Duration	Frequency (Check ✓) M	Tu	W	Th	F	Sa	Su
Swimming	✓	✓	✓	✓	✓	140-150 bpm	35min	✓		✓		✓		
Tennis	✓	✓	✓	✓	✓	RPE = 14	90min						✓	
Weight training		✓	✓	✓	✓	see Lab 4-3	30min		✓		✓		✓	
Stretching				✓		—	25min	✓		✓		✓	✓	

*List your target heart rate range or an RPE value if appropriate.

C. My program will begin on __Sept. 21__. My program includes the following schedule
of mini-goals. For each step in my program, I will give myself the reward listed.

Completing 2 full weeks of program (mini-goal 1)	Oct 5 (date)	movie with friends (reward)
$\dot{V}O_{2max}$ of 34 ml/kg/min (mini-goal 2)	Nov 2 (date)	new CD (reward)
Completing 10 full weeks of program (mini-goal 3)	Nov 30 (date)	new sweater (reward)
Percent body fat of 28% (mini-goal 4)	Dec 22 (date)	weekend away (reward)
$\dot{V}O_{2max}$ of 36 ml/kg/min (mini-goal 5)	Jan 18 (date)	new CD (reward)

D. My program will include the addition of physical activity to my daily routine (such
as climbing stairs or walking to class):

1. Walking to and from campus job
2. Taking the stairs to dorm room instead of elevator
3. Bicycling to the library instead of driving
4. _____
5. _____

E. I will use the following tools to monitor my program and my progress toward
my goals: I'll use a chart that lists the number of laps and minutes I swim and the
charts for strength and flexibility from Labs 4-3 & 5-2.

I sign this contract as an indication of my personal commitment to reach my goal.

___Tracie Kaufman___   ___Sept 10___
(your signature)   (date)

I have recruited a helper who will witness my contract and _____
swim with me three days per week
(list any way your helper will participate in your program)

___Russell Walker___   ___Sept 10___
(witness's signature)   (date)

Figure 7-1 A sample personal fitness program plan and contract.

TABLE 7-1 **A Summary of Sports and Fitness Activities**

This table classifies sports and activities as high (H), moderate (M), or low (L) in terms of their ability to develop each of the five components of physical fitness: cardiorespiratory endurance (CRE), muscular strength (MS), muscular endurance (ME), flexibility (F), and body composition (BC). The skill level needed to obtain fitness benefits is noted: Low (L) means little or no skill is required to obtain fitness benefits; moderate (M) means average skill is needed to obtain fitness benefits; and high (H) means much skill is required to obtain fitness benefits. The fitness prerequisite, or conditioning needs of a beginner, is also noted: Low (L) means no fitness prerequisite is required, moderate (M) means some preconditioning is required, and high (H) means substantial fitness is required. The last two columns list the calorie cost of each activity when performed moderately and vigorously. To determine how many calories you burn, multiply the value in the appropriate column by your body weight and then by the number of minutes you exercise. Work up to using 300 or more calories per workout.

| Sports and Activities | Components | | | | | Skill Level | Fitness Prerequisite | Approximate Calorie Cost (cal/lb/min) | |
	CRE	MS*	ME*	F*	BC			Moderate	Vigorous
Aerobic dance	H	M	H	H	H	L	L	.046	.062
Backpacking	H	M	H	M	H	L	M	.032	.078
Badminton, skilled, singles	H	M	M	M	H	M	M	—	.071
Ballet (floor combinations)	M	M	H	H	M	M	L	—	.058
Ballroom dancing	M	L	M	L	M	M	L	.034	.049
Baseball (pitcher and catcher)	M	M	H	M	M	H	M	.039	—
Basketball, half court	H	M	H	M	H	M	M	.045	.071
Bicycling	H	M	H	M	H	M	L	.049	.071
Bowling	L	L	L	L	L	L	L	—	—
Calisthenic circuit training	H	M	H	M	H	L	L	—	.060
Canoeing and kayaking (flat water)	M	M	H	M	M	M	M	.045	—
Cheerleading	M	M	M	M	M	M	L	.033	.049
Fencing	M	M	H	H	M	M	L	.032	.078
Field hockey	H	M	H	M	H	M	M	.052	.078
Folk and square dancing	M	L	M	L	M	L	L	.039	.049
Football, touch	M	M	M	M	M	M	M	.049	.078
Frisbee, ultimate	H	M	H	M	H	M	M	.049	.078
Golf (riding cart)	L	L	L	M	L	L	L	—	—
Handball, skilled, singles	H	M	H	M	H	M	M	—	.078
Hiking	H	M	H	L	H	L	M	.051	.073
Hockey, ice and roller	H	M	H	M	H	M	M	.052	.078
Horseback riding	M	M	M	L	M	M	M	.052	.065
Interval circuit training	H	H	H	M	H	L	L	—	.062
Jogging and running	H	M	H	L	H	L	L	.060	.104

*Ratings are for the muscle groups involved.

- Muscular strength and endurance are developed by training against resistance (see Chapter 4).
- Flexibility is developed by stretching the major muscle groups (see Chapter 5).
- Healthy body composition can be developed by combining a sensible diet and a program of regular exercise, including cardiorespiratory endurance exercise to burn calories and resistance training to build muscle mass (see Chapter 6).

Table 7-1 rates many popular activities for their ability to develop each of the health-related components of fitness. Check the ratings of the activities you're considering to make sure the program you put together will develop all fitness components and help you achieve your goals. One strategy is to select one activity for each component of fitness—bicycling, weight training, and stretching, for example. Another strategy applies the principle of **cross-training,** using several different activities to develop a particular fitness component—aerobic dance, swimming, and volleyball for cardiorespiratory endurance, for example. Cross-training is discussed in the next section.

If you select activities that support your commitment rather than activities that turn exercise into a chore, the right program will be its own incentive for continuing. Consider the following factors in making your choices.

TABLE 7-1 *A Summary of Sports and Fitness Activities (continued)*

Sports and Activities	Components					Skill Level	Fitness Prerequisite	Approximate Calorie Cost (cal/lb/min)	
	CRE	MS*	ME*	F*	BC			Moderate	Vigorous
Judo	M	H	H	M	M	M	L	.049	.090
Karate	H	M	H	H	H	L	M	.049	.090
Lacrosse	H	M	H	M	H	H	M	.052	.078
Modern dance (moving combinations)	M	M	H	H	M	L	L	—	.058
Orienteering	H	M	H	L	H	L	M	.049	.078
Outdoor fitness trails	H	M	H	M	H	L	L	—	.060
Popular dancing	M	L	M	M	M	M	L	—	.049
Racquetball, skilled, singles	H	M	M	M	H	M	M	.049	.078
Rock climbing	M	H	H	H	M	H	M	.033	.033
Rope skipping	H	M	H	L	H	M	M	.071	.095
Rowing	H	H	H	H	H	L	L	.032	.097
Rugby	H	M	H	M	H	M	M	.052	.097
Sailing	L	L	M	L	L	M	L	—	—
Skating, ice, roller, and in-line	M	M	H	M	M	H	M	.049	.095
Skiing, alpine	M	H	H	M	M	H	M	.039	.078
Skiing, cross-country	H	M	H	M	H	M	M	.049	.104
Soccer	H	M	H	M	H	M	M	.052	.097
Squash, skilled, singles	H	M	M	M	H	M	M	.049	.078
Stretching	L	L	L	H	L	L	L	—	—
Surfing (including swimming)	M	M	M	M	M	H	M	—	.078
Swimming	H	M	H	M	H	M	L	.032	.088
Synchronized swimming	M	M	H	H	M	H	M	.032	.052
Table tennis	M	L	M	M	M	M	L	—	.045
Tennis, skilled, singles	H	M	M	M	H	M	M	—	.071
Volleyball	M	L	M	M	M	M	M	—	.065
Walking	H	L	M	L	H	L	L	.029	.048
Water polo	H	M	H	M	H	H	M	—	.078
Water skiing	M	M	H	M	M	H	M	.039	.055
Weight training	L	H	H	H	M	L	L	—	—
Wrestling	H	H	H	H	H	H	H	.065	.094
Yoga	L	L	M	H	L	H	L	—	—

*Ratings are for the muscle groups involved.

SOURCE: Kusinitz, I., and M. Fine. 1995. *Your Guide to Getting Fit,* 3d ed. Mountain View, Calif.: Mayfield.

• *Fun and interest.* Your fitness program is much more likely to be successful if you choose activities that you enjoy doing. Start by considering any activities you currently engage in and enjoy. Often you can modify your current activities to fit your fitness program. As you consider new activities, ask yourself, "Is this activity fun?" "Will it hold my interest over time?" For new activities, it is a good idea to undertake a trial period before making a final choice. Figure 7-2 shows popular fitness activities among Americans.

• *Your current skill and fitness level.* Although many activities are appropriate for beginners, some sports and

activities require participants to have a moderate level of skill in order to obtain fitness benefits. For example, a beginning tennis player will probably not be able to sustain rallies long enough to develop cardiorespiratory endurance. Refer to the skill level column in Table 7-1 to determine the level of skill needed for full participation in the activities you're considering. If your current skill

cross-training Alternating two or more activities to improve **TERMS**
a single component of fitness.

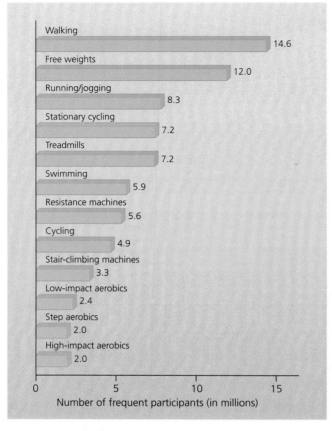

Figure 7-2   Popular fitness activities among Americans.
Frequent participants in the activities shown here are those who engage in the activity at least 100 days per year (52 days for swimming).   DATA SOURCE: Sporting Goods Manufacturers Association. *Tracking the Fitness Movement —1997 Edition* (http://www.sportlink.com).

level doesn't meet the requirement, you may want to begin your program with a different activity. For example, a beginning tennis player may be better off with a walking program while improving his or her tennis game. To build skill for a particular activity, consider taking a class or getting some instruction from a coach or fellow participant.

Your current fitness level may also limit the activities that are appropriate for your program. For example, if you have been inactive, a walking program would be more appropriate than a jogging program. Activities in which participants control the intensity of effort—walking, cycling, and swimming, for example—are more appropriate for a beginning fitness program than sports and activities that are primarily "other paced"—soccer, basketball, and tennis, for example. Refer to the fitness prerequisite column of Table 7-1 to determine the minimum level of fitness required for participation in the activities you're considering.

• *Time and convenience.* Unless exercise fits easily into your daily schedule, you are unlikely to maintain your program over the long term. As you consider activities, think about whether a special location or facility is required. Can you participate in the activity close to your residence, school, or job? Are the necessary facilities open and available at times convenient to you? Do you need a partner or a team to play? Can you participate in the activity year-round, or will you need to find an alternative during the summer or winter?

• *Cost.* Some sports and activities require equipment, fees, or some type of membership investment. If you are on a tight budget, limit your choices to activities that are inexpensive or free. Investigate the facilities on your campus, which you may be able to use at little or no cost. Many activities require no equipment beyond an appropriate pair of shoes (see the box "Choosing Exercise Footwear" for more information). Refer back to Chapters 2 and 3 for consumer guidelines for evaluating exercise equipment and facilities.

• *Special health needs.* If you have special exercise needs due to a particular health problem, choose activities that will conform to your needs and enhance your ability to cope. If necessary, consult your physician about how best to tailor an exercise program to your particular needs and goals. Guidelines and safety tips for exercisers with common chronic conditions are provided later in the chapter.

3. Set a Target Intensity, Duration, and Frequency for Each Activity

The next step in planning your fitness program is to set a target intensity, duration, and frequency for each activity you've chosen (see the sample in Figure 7-1). Refer to the calculations and plans you completed in Chapters 3, 4, and 5.

Cardiorespiratory Endurance Exercise   For intensity, note your target heart rate zone or RPE value. Your target total duration should be about 20–60 minutes, depending on the intensity of the activity (shorter durations are appropriate for high-intensity activities, longer durations for activities of more moderate intensity). You can exercise in a single session or in multiple sessions of 10 or more minutes. One way to check whether the total duration you've set is appropriate is to use the **calorie costs** (calories per minute per pound of body weight) given in Table 7-1. Your goal should be to work up to burning about 300 calories per workout; beginners should start with a calorie cost of about 100–150 calories per workout. You can calculate the calorie cost of your activities by multiplying the appropriate factor from Table 7-1 by your body weight and the duration of your workout. For example, walking at a moderate pace burns about 0.029 calorie per minute per pound of body weight. A person

Name Tracie Kaufman

Enter duration, distance, or other factor to track your progress.

Activity/Date	M	Tu	W	Th	F	S	S	Weekly Total	M	Tu	W	Th	F	S	S	Weekly Total
1 Swimming	800 yd		725 yd		800 yd			2325 yd	800 yd		800 yd		850 yd			2450 yd
2 Tennis				90 min				90 min					95 min			95 min
3 Weight training		✓		✓		✓				✓		✓		✓	✓	
4 Stretching	✓		✓		✓	✓			✓			✓	✓	✓	✓	
5																
6																

Figure 7-3 A sample program log.

weighing 150 pounds could begin her exercise program by walking for 30 minutes, burning about 130 calories. Once her fitness improves, she might choose to start cycling for her cardiorespiratory endurance workouts. Cycling at a moderate pace has a higher calorie cost than walking (0.049 calorie per minute per pound), and if she cycled for 40 minutes, she would burn the target 300 calories during her workout.

An appropriate frequency for cardiorespiratory endurance exercise is 3–5 times per week.

Muscular Strength and Endurance Training   As described in Chapter 4, a general fitness strength training program includes 1 or more sets of 8–12 repetitions of 8–10 exercises that work all major muscle groups. For intensity, choose a weight that is heavy enough to fatigue your muscles but not so heavy that you cannot complete the full number of repetitions with proper form. A frequency of 2–3 days per week is recommended.

Flexibility Training   Stretches should be performed for all major muscle groups. For each exercise, stretch to the point of slight tension or mild discomfort and hold the stretch for 10–30 seconds; do at least 4 repetitions of each exercise. Stretches should be performed at least 2–3 days per week, preferably when muscles are warm.

4. Set Up a System of Mini-Goals and Rewards

To keep your program on track, it is important to set up a system of goals and rewards. Break your specific goals into several steps, and set a target date for each step. For example, if one of the goals of an 18-year-old male student's program is to improve upper body strength and endurance, he could use the push-up test in Lab 4-2 to set intermediate goals. If he can currently perform 15 push-ups (for a rating of "very poor"), he might set intermedi-

ate goals of 20, 25, and 30 push-ups (for a final rating of "fair"). By allowing 4–6 weeks between mini-goals and specifying rewards, he'll be able to track his progress and reward himself as he moves toward his final goal. For more on choosing appropriate rewards, refer to p. 11 in Chapter 1 and Activity 4 in the Behavior Change Workbook at the end of the text.

5. Include Lifestyle Physical Activity in Your Program

As described in Chapter 2, daily physical activity is an important part of a fit and well lifestyle. As part of your fitness program plan, specify ways that you will be more active during your daily routine. You may find it helpful to first use your health journal to track your activities for several days. Review the records in your journal, identify routine opportunities to be more active, and add these to your program plan in Lab 7-1.

6. Develop Tools for Monitoring Your Progress

A record that tracks your daily progress will help remind you of your ongoing commitment to your program and give you a sense of accomplishment. Lab 7-2 shows you how to create a general program log and record the activity type, frequency, and durations (a sample is shown in Figure 7-3). Or if you wish, complete specific activity logs like those in Labs 3-2, 4-3, and 5-2 in addition to, or instead of, a general log. Post your log in a place where you'll see it often as a reminder and as an incentive for improvement. If you have specific, measurable goals, you

calorie cost   The amount of energy used to perform a particular activity, usually expressed in calories per minute per pound of body weight.   **TERMS**

Footwear is perhaps the most important item of equipment for almost any activity. Shoes protect and support your feet and improve your traction. When you jump or run, you place as much as six times more force on your feet than when you stand still. Shoes can help cushion against the stress that this additional force places on your lower legs and thus prevent injuries. Some athletic shoes are also designed to help prevent ankle rollover, another common source of injury.

Shoe Terminology

Understanding the structural features of athletic shoes can help you make sound choices.

Outsole: The bottom of the shoe that touches the ground and provides traction. The shape and composition of an outsole depend on the activity for which the shoe is designed.

Midsole: The layer of shock-absorbing material located between the insole and the outsole; typically composed of polyurethane, ethyl vinyl acetate (EVA), or another cushioning material. For improved durability, some shoe midsoles include encapsulated air or gel.

Insole: The insert or sock lining that the foot rests on inside the shoe, usually contoured to fit the foot and containing additional cushioning and arch and heel support.

Collar: The opening of the shoe where the foot goes in.

Upper: The top part of the shoe, usually made of nylon, canvas, or leather.

Toe box: The front part of the upper, which surrounds the toes.

Heel counter: The stiff cup in the back of the inside of the shoe that provides support and stability.

Notched heel: Some shoes have raised heel padding to support the Achilles tendon.

Stabilizers: Bars or strips of rubber, polyurethane, or nylon near the heel or forefoot area of some shoes; they provide additional stability.

Wedge: The thick portion of the midsole that makes the heel higher than the ball of the foot in some shoes.

General Guidelines

When choosing athletic shoes, first consider the activity you've chosen for your exercise program. Shoes appropriate for different activities have very different characteristics. For example, running shoes typically have highly cushioned midsoles, rubber outsoles with elevated heels, and a great deal of flexibility in the forefoot. The heels of walking shoes tend to be lower, less padded, and more beveled than those designed for running. For aerobic dance, shoes must be flexible in the forefoot and have straight, nonflared heels to allow for safe and easy lateral movements. Court shoes also provide substantial support for lateral movements; they typically have outsoles made from white rubber that will not damage court surfaces.

Also consider the location and intensity of your workouts. If you plan to walk or run on trails, you should choose shoes with water-resistant, highly durable uppers and more outsole traction. If you work out intensely or have a relatively high body weight, you'll need thick, firm midsoles to avoid bottoming-out the cushioning system of your shoes.

Foot type is another important consideration. If your feet tend to roll in excessively (overpronate), you may need shoes with additional stability features on the inner side of the shoe to counteract this movement. If your feet tend to roll outward excessively (oversupinate), you may need highly flexible and cushioned shoes that promote foot motion. For aerobic dancers

---

can also graph your weekly or monthly progress toward your goal (Figure 7-4).

7. Make a Commitment

Your final step in planning your program is to make a commitment by signing a contract. Find a witness for your contract—preferably one who will be actively involved in your program. Keep your contract in a visible spot to remind you of your commitment.

PUTTING YOUR PLAN INTO ACTION

Once you've developed a detailed plan and signed your contract, you are ready to begin your fitness program. Refer to the specific training suggestions provided in Chapters 2–5 for advice on beginning and maintaining your program. Some key guidelines are summarized below.

• *Start slowly and increase intensity and duration gradually.* Overzealous exercising can result in discouraging with feet that tend to pronate or supinate, mid-cut to high-cut shoes may be more appropriate than low-cut aerobic shoes or cross-trainers (shoes designed to be worn for several different activities). Compared with men, women have narrower feet overall and narrower heels relative to the forefoot. Most women will get a better fit if they choose shoes that are specifically designed for women's feet rather than those that are down-sized versions of men's shoes.

For successful shoe shopping, keep these strategies in mind:

- Shop at an athletic shoe or specialty store that has personnel trained to fit athletic shoes and a large selection of styles and sizes.

- Shop late in the day or, ideally, following a workout. Your foot size increases over the course of the day and as a result of exercise.

- Wear socks like those you plan to wear during exercise. If you have an old pair of athletic shoes, bring them with you. The wear pattern on your old shoes can help you select a pair with extra support or cushioning in the places you need it the most.

- Ask for help. Trained salespeople know which shoes are designed for your foot type and your level of activity. They can also help fit your shoes properly.

- Don't insist on buying shoes in what you consider to be your typical shoe size. Sizes vary from shoe to shoe. In addition, foot sizes change over time, and many people have one foot that is larger or wider than the other. Try several sizes in several widths if necessary. Don't buy shoes that are too small.

- Try on both shoes, and wear them around for at least 10 minutes. Try walking on a noncarpeted surface. Approximate the movements of your activity: walk, jog, run, jump, and so on.

- Check the fit and style carefully.

  Is the toe box roomy enough? Your toes will spread out when your foot hits the ground or you push off. There should be at least one thumb's width of space from the longest toe to the end of the toe box.

  Do they have enough cushioning? Do your feet feel cushioned and supported when you bounce up and down? Try bouncing on your toes and on your heels.

  Do your heels fit snugly into the shoe? Do they stay put when you walk, or do they rise up?

  Are the arches of your feet right on top of the shoes' arch supports?

  Do the shoes feel stable when you twist and turn on the balls of your feet? Try twisting from side to side while standing on one foot.

  Do you feel any pressure points?

- If the shoe isn't comfortable in the store, don't buy it. Don't expect athletic shoes to stretch over time in order to fit your feet properly.

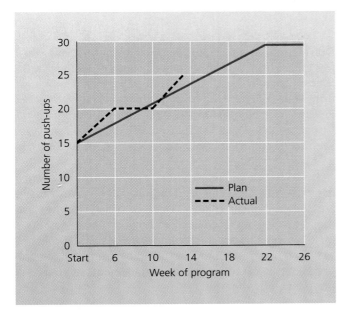

Figure 7-4   A sample program progress chart.

discomforts and injuries. Your program is meant to last a lifetime. The important first step is to break your established pattern of inactivity. Be patient and realistic. Once your body has adjusted to your starting level of exercise, slowly increase the amount of overload. Small increases are the key—achieving a large number of small improvements will eventually result in substantial gains in fitness. It's usually best to increase duration and frequency before increasing intensity.

- *Find an exercise buddy.* The social side of exercise is an important factor for many regular exercisers. Working out with a friend will make exercise more enjoyable and increase your chances of sticking with your program. Find an exercise partner who shares your goals and general fitness level.

- *Vary your program.* You can make your program more fun over the long term if you participate in a variety of different activities that you enjoy. You can also add interest by strategies such as varying the routes you take when walking, running, biking, or in-line skating;

Troublesome technique. Exercise technique is critical, even for activities that you take for granted, like walking. When increasing the pace of walking, for example, it's natural to take longer strides. But this can overstress your shins. Proper technique entails taking more rapid strides without increasing their length. If necessary, take a class or get other expert help to ensure proper technique for the activities you participate in.

A small breath of air. Novice exercisers tend to breathe rapidly and shallowly because it feels right. But with this type of breathing, oxygen does not make its way to the depths of the lungs where it's needed. This contributes to a sense of breathlessness. Instead, consciously take longer and deeper breaths.

Beginner's pluck. If you have not been active, your body is ill prepared for demanding exercise. Even so, you are likely to make rapid gains in the beginning stages of an exercise program, which can inspire you to do too much too soon. Resist the temptation. Working out like a veteran can easily lead to injury.

Veteran's overconfidence. Even if you are a seasoned exerciser, don't advance more quickly than your body will allow, and avoid overconfidence. Those who were once in shape but have quit exercising and want to start again are particularly likely to increase too rapidly—advancing, for instance, from a 2-mile run to a 6-mile run in a few weeks. Whether you are starting from scratch or restarting from a higher level, progress slowly.

Feel the burnout. Your abilities and drive may inspire you to keep adding to your exercise workload. But even small and slow increases can become too much. If you find yourself dreading exercise sessions or dragging through the day because of exhausting workouts, you may be overtraining. If so, cut back to where your workouts are comfortable again and you look forward to them. Take a few days off completely and then return at a much reduced level.

Not easing in and out. Take time to warm up and ease into exercise. Even if you walk or do other forms of mild exercise, your body needs an adjustment period. Start with a slow, comfortable walk before progressing to faster speeds. At the end of a workout, don't stop abruptly, but rather slow your pace gradually until you quit. Finish with stretching exercises.

Leave it for weekends. Many people use sports as a means of getting in shape. They push themselves on weekends in demanding sports like basketball that can stress the body to its limits. This "weekend warrior" approach is backward. Instead, get in shape first so you can enjoy sports safely. This is especially important if you do not participate regularly.

Fair-weather exercise. Regardless of your goals or the type of exercise you choose, little will be accomplished by sporadic exercise. The key to success is consistency. On occasion, you won't have time to exercise as much as you would like. On those days, it's important to do something, no matter how small. A little exercise performed daily will produce much greater results than sporadic, lengthy workouts.

Adapted from Stamford, B. 1997. Exercise adviser: Dodging common exercise pitfalls. *The Physician and Sportsmedicine* 25(7).

finding a new tennis or racquetball partner; changing your music for aerobic dance; or switching to a new volleyball or basketball court.

Varying your activities, a strategy known as cross-training, has other benefits. It can help you develop balanced, total body fitness. For example, by alternating running with swimming, you build both upper and lower body strength. Cross-training can thus prepare you for a wider range of activities and physical challenges. It can also reduce the risk of injury and overtraining because the same muscles, bones, and joints are not continuously subjected to the stresses of the same activity. Cross-training can be done either by choosing different activities on different days or by alternating activities within a single workout.

• *Expect fluctuations and lapses.* On some days, your progress will be excellent, but on others, you'll barely be able to drag yourself through your scheduled activities.

Don't let off-days or lapses discourage you or make you feel guilty. Instead, feel a renewed commitment for your fitness program. Focus on the improvements you obtain from your program and how good you feel after exercise. Reward yourself often for sticking with your program. Visualize what it will be like to reach your goals, and keep these pictures in your mind as an incentive to stick with your program.

If you notice you're slacking off, use your health journal to identify the negative thoughts and behaviors that are causing noncompliance. Devise a strategy to decrease the frequency of these negative thoughts and behaviors. Make changes in your program plan and reward system to help renew your enthusiasm and commitment to your program. Expect to make many adjustments in your program along the way.

See the box "Dodging Common Exercise Pitfalls" for additional suggestions.

Regular, appropriate exercise is safe and beneficial for many people with chronic conditions or other special health concerns. For example, people with heart disease or hypertension who exercise may lower their blood pressure and improve their cholesterol levels. For people with diabetes, exercise can improve insulin sensitivity and body composition. For people with asthma, regular exercise may reduce the risk of acute attacks during exertion. For many people with special health concerns, the risks associated with *not* exercising are far greater than those associated with a moderate program of regular exercise.

The fitness recommendations for the general population presented in this text can serve as a general guideline for any exercise program. However, for people with chronic health conditions, special precautions and monitoring may be required. Anyone with special health concerns should consult a physician before beginning an exercise program. Guidelines and cautions for some common health conditions are described below.

An individual with special health concerns can develop a safe and effective fitness program by choosing activities carefully and making appropriate modifications in the program. Swimming is an excellent activity choice for this man with asthma because breathing warm, moist air reduces the risk of asthma attacks during exercise.

Arthritis

- Begin an exercise program as early as possible in the course of the disease.
- Warm up thoroughly before each exercise session to loosen stiff muscles and lower the risk of injury.
- For cardiorespiratory endurance exercise, avoid high-impact activities that may damage arthritic joints; consider a swimming program or another type of exercise in a warm pool.
- Perform strength training exercises for the whole body; pay special attention to muscles that support and protect affected joints (for example, build quadriceps, hamstring, and calf strength for the knee). Start with small loads and build intensity gradually.
- Perform flexibility exercises regularly to maintain joint mobility.

Asthma

- Exercise regularly. Acute attacks are more likely if you exercise only occasionally.
- Carry medication during workouts, and avoid exercising alone.
- Warm up and cool down slowly to reduce the risk of acute attacks.
- When starting an exercise program, choose self-paced endurance activities, especially those involving **interval training** (short bouts of exercise followed by a rest period). Increase intensity of cardiorespiratory endurance exercise gradually.
- Cold, dry air can trigger or worsen an attack. Drink water before, during, and after a workout to moisten your airways. In cold weather, cover your mouth with a mask or scarf to warm and humidify the air your breathe. Swimming in a heated pool is an excellent activity choice for people with asthma.
- Avoid outdoor activities during pollen season or when the air is polluted. Avoid exercise in dry or dusty indoor environments.

Diabetes

- Don't begin an exercise program unless your diabetes is under control and you have checked about exercise safety with your physician. Because diabetics have an increased risk for heart disease, an exercise stress test may be recommended.
- Don't exercise alone. Wear a bracelet identifying yourself as a diabetic.
- If you are taking insulin or another medication, you may need to adjust the timing and amount of each dose. Work with your physician and check your blood sugar levels regularly so you can learn to balance your energy intake and output and your medication dosage.

interval training A training technique that alternates exercise intervals with rest intervals or intense exercise intervals with low to moderate intervals. **TERMS**

- To prevent abnormally rapid absorption of injected insulin, inject it over a muscle that won't be exercised and wait at least an hour before exercising.

- Check blood sugar levels before, during, and after exercise, and adjust your diet or insulin dosage if needed. Carry high-carbohydrate foods during a workout.

- If you have poor circulation or numbness in your extremities, check your skin regularly for blisters and abrasions, especially on your feet. Avoid high-impact activities, and wear comfortable shoes.

- For maximum benefit and minimum risk, choose low-to-moderate-intensity activities.

Heart Disease and Hypertension

- Check with your physician about exercise safety before increasing your activity level.

- Exercise at a moderate rather than a high intensity. Keep your heart rate below the level at which abnormalities appear on an exercise stress test.

- Warm-up and cool-down sessions should be gradual and last at least 10 minutes.

- Monitor your heart rate during exercise, and stop if you experience dizziness or chest pain.

- If prescribed, carry nitroglycerin with you during exercise. If you are taking beta-blockers for hypertension, use RPE rather than heart rate to monitor exercise intensity (beta-blockers reduce heart rate). Exercise at an RPE level of "somewhat hard"; your breathing should be unlabored and you should be able to talk.

- Don't hold your breath when exercising. Doing so can cause sudden, steep increases in blood pressure. Take special care during weight training; don't lift extremely heavy loads.

- Increase exercise intensity, duration, and frequency very gradually.

Obesity

- For maximum benefit and minimum risk, choose low-to-moderate-intensity activities.

- Choose non- or low-weight-bearing activities such as cycling, swimming, or walking. Low-impact activities are less likely to lead to joint problems or injuries.

- Stay alert for symptoms of heat-related problems during exercise (see Chapter 3). People who are obese are particularly vulnerable to problems with heat intolerance.

- Ease into an exercise program, and increase overload gradually. Increase duration and frequency of exercise before increasing intensity.

- Include strength training in your fitness program to build or maintain fat-free mass.

Osteoporosis

- For cardiorespiratory endurance activities, exercise at the maximum intensity that causes no significant discomfort. If possible, choose low-impact weight-bearing activities to help safely maintain bone density (see Chapter 8 for more strategies for building and maintaining bone density).

- To prevent fractures, avoid any activity or movement that stresses the back or carries a risk of falling.

- Include weight training in your exercise program to improve strength and balance and reduce the risk of falls and fractures. Avoid lifting heavy loads.

Exercise guidelines for people with other special health concerns have been discussed in other chapters: disabilities (Chapter 2), pregnancy (Chapter 3), and low-back pain (Chapter 5).

COMMON QUESTIONS ANSWERED

Should I exercise every day?   Some daily exercise is beneficial, and health experts recommend that you engage in at least 30 minutes of moderate physical activity over the course of every day. However, if you train intensely every day without giving yourself a rest, you will likely get injured or become overtrained. When strength training, for example, rest at least 1 day between workouts before exercising the same muscle group. For cardiorespiratory endurance exercise, rest or exercise lightly the day after an intense or long-duration workout. Balancing the proper amount of rest and exercise will help you feel better and improve your fitness faster.

I'm just starting an exercise program; how much activity should I do at first?   Be conservative. Walking is a good way

to begin almost any fitness program. At first, walk for approximately 10 minutes, and then increase the distance and pace. After several weeks, you can progress to something more vigorous. Let your body be your guide. If the intensity and duration of a workout seem easy, increase them a little the next time. The key is to be progressive; don't try to achieve physical fitness in one or two workouts. Build your fitness gradually.

I'm concerned about my safety when I go for a jog or walk. What can I do to make sure that my training sessions are safe and enjoyable?   A person exercising alone in the park can be a tempting target for criminals. Don't exercise alone. You are much less likely to be a crime victim if you are training in a group or with a partner. Another alternative is to take an exercise class. Classes are fun and much more safe than exercising by yourself. If you must train alone, try to exercise where there are plenty of people. A good bet is the local high school or college track.

Make sure you're wearing proper safety equipment. If you're riding a bike, wear a helmet. If you're playing racquetball or handball, wear eye protectors. Don't go in-line skating unless you're wearing the proper pads and protective equipment. If jogging at night, wear reflective clothing that can be seen easily.

Refer to Appendix A for more information on personal safety.

SUMMARY

- Steps for putting together a complete fitness program include (1) setting realistic goals, (2) selecting activities to develop all the health-related components of fitness, (3) setting a target intensity, duration, and frequency for each activity, (4) setting up a system of mini-goals and rewards, (5) making lifestyle physical activity a part of the daily routine, (6) developing tools for monitoring progress, and (7) making a commitment.

- In selecting activities, consider fun and interest, your current skill and fitness level, time and convenience, cost, and any special health concerns.

- Keys to putting a successful plan into action are starting slowly, increasing intensity and duration gradually, finding a buddy, varying the program, and expecting fluctuations and lapses.

- Regular exercise is appropriate and highly beneficial for people with special health concerns; program modifications may be necessary to maximize safety.

FOR MORE INFORMATION

See the listings for Chapters 2–6.

SELECTED BIBLIOGRAPHY

American College of Sports Medicine. 1998. ACSM Position Stand: The Recommended Quantity and Quality of Exercise for Developing and Maintaining Cardiorespiratory and Muscular Fitness, and Flexibility in Healthy Adults. *Medicine and Science in Sports and Exercise* 30(6): 975–991.

American College of Sports Medicine and American Diabetes Association. 1997. Joint position statement: Diabetes mellitus and exercise. *Medicine and Science in Sports and Exercise* 29(12): I–VI.

Ballas, M. T., J. Tytko, and D. Cookson. 1997. Common overuse running injuries: Diagnosis and management. *American Family Physician* 77(7): 2473–2484.

Buckwalter, J. A., and N. E. Lane. 1997. Athletics and osteoarthritis. *American Journal of Sports Medicine* 25(6): 873–881.

Halbert, J. A., et al. 1997. The effectiveness of exercise training in lowering blood pressure: A meta-analysis of randomised controlled trials of 4 weeks or longer. *Journal of Human Hypertension* 11(10): 641–649.

International Inline Skating Association. *Gear Up! Guide to Inline Skating. Health Benefits* (retrieved February 11, 1998; http://www.iisa.org).

Katz, W. A. 1998. Exercise for osteoporosis. *The Physician and Sportsmedicine* 26(2).

Martin, D. R. 1997. Athletic shoes: Finding a good match. *The Physician and Sportsmedicine* 25(9): 138–144.

Morris, J. N., and A. E. Hardman. 1997. Walking to health. *Sports Medicine* 23(5): 306–332.

Nguyen, M. N., L. Potvin, and J. Otis. 1997. Regular exercise in 30- to 60-year-old men: Combining the stages-of-change model and the theory of planned behavior to identify determinants for targeting heart health interventions. *Journal of Community Health* 22:233–246.

Powell, M., and J. Svensson. 1993. *In-Line Skating.* Champaign, Ill.: Human Kinetics.

Scheiber, R. A., et al. 1996. Risk factors for injuries from in-line skating and the effectiveness of safety gear. *New England Journal of Medicine* 355(22): 1630–1635.

Stamford, B. 1996. Cross-training: Giving yourself a whole-body workout. *The Physician and Sportsmedicine* 24(9): 103.

Tan, R. A., and S. L. Spector. 1998. Exercise-induced asthma. *Sports Medicine* 25(1): 1–6.

Thompson, D. C., R. P. Rivera, and R. S. Thompson. 1996. Effectiveness of bicycle safety helmets in preventing head injuries: A case-controlled study. *Journal of the American Medical Association* 276(24): 1968–1973.

Thordarson, D. B. 1997. Running biomechanics. *Clinics in Sports Medicine* 16:239–247.

Wallberg-Henriksson, H., J. Rincon, and J. R. Zierath. 1998. Exercise in the management of non-insulin-dependent diabetes mellitus. *Sports Medicine* 25(1): 25–35.

Wallick, M. E., et al. 1995. Physiological responses to in-line skating compared to treadmill running. *Medicine and Science in Sports and Exercise* 27(2): 242–248.

Young, J. C. 1998. Exercise for clients with type 2 diabetes. *ACSM's Health and Fitness Journal* 2(3): 24–29.

Zachwieja, J. J. 1996. Exercise as treatment for obesity. *Endocrinology and Metabolism Clinics of North America* 25: 965–988.

Sample fitness programs begin on p. 170.

Sample programs based on four different types of cardiorespiratory activities—walking/jogging/running, bicycling, swimming, and in-line skating—are presented below. Each sample program includes regular cardiorespiratory endurance exercise, resistance training, and stretching. To choose a sample program, first compare your fitness goals with the benefits of the different types of endurance exercise featured in the sample programs (see Table 7-1). Identify the programs that meet your fitness needs. Next, read through the descriptions of the programs you're considering and decide which will work best for you based on your present routine, the potential for enjoyment, and adaptability to your lifestyle. If you choose one of these programs, complete the personal fitness program plan in Lab 7-1, just as if you had created a program from scratch.

No program will bring about enormous changes in your fitness level in the first few weeks. Give your program a good chance. Follow the specifics of the program for 3–4 weeks. Then if the exercise program doesn't seem suitable, make adjustments to adapt it to your particular needs. But retain the basic elements of the program that make it effective for developing fitness.

General Guidelines

The following guidelines can help make the activity programs more effective for you.

- *Intensity.* To work effectively for cardiorespiratory endurance training or to improve body composition, you must raise your heart rate into its target zone. Monitor your pulse, or use rates of perceived exertion to monitor your intensity.

  If you've been sedentary, begin very slowly. Give your

muscles a chance to adjust to their increased workload. It's probably best to keep your heart rate below target until your body has had time to adjust to new demands. At first you may not need to work very hard to keep your heart rate in its target zone, but as your cardiorespiratory endurance improves, you will probably need to increase intensity.

- *Duration and frequency.* To experience training effects, you should exercise for 20–60 minutes at least three times per week.

- *Interval training.* Some of the sample programs involve continuous activity. Others rely on interval training, which calls for alternating a relief interval with exercise (walking after jogging, for example, or coasting after biking uphill). Interval training is an effective way to achieve progressive overload: When your heart rate gets too high, slow down to lower your pulse rate until you're at the low end of your target zone. Interval training can also prolong the total time you spend in exercise and delay the onset of fatigue.

- *Warm-up and cool-down.* Begin each exercise session with a 10-minute warm-up. Begin your activity at a slow pace, and work up gradually to your target heart rate. Always slow down gradually at the end of your exercise session to bring your system back to its normal state. It's a good idea to do stretching exercises to increase your flexibility after cardiorespiratory exercise or strength training because your muscles will be warm and ready to stretch.

- *Record keeping.* After each exercise session, record your daily distance or time on a progress chart like the one shown in Lab 7-2.

WALKING/JOGGING/RUNNING SAMPLE PROGRAM

Walking, jogging, and running are the most popular forms of training for people who want to improve cardiorespiratory endurance; they also improve body composition and muscular endurance of the legs. It's not always easy to distinguish among these three endurance activities. For clarity and consistency, we'll consider walking to be any on-foot exercise of less than 5 miles per hour, jogging any pace between 5 and 7.5 miles per hour, and running any pace faster than that. Table 1 divides walking, jogging, and running into nine categories, with rates of speed (in both miles per hour and minutes per mile) and calorie costs for each. The faster your pace or the longer you exercise, the more calories you burn. The greater the number of calories burned, the higher the potential training effects of these activities.

Equipment and Technique

These activities require no special skills, expensive equipment, or unusual facilities. Comfortable clothing, well-fitted walking or running shoes, and a stopwatch or ordinary watch with a second hand are all you need.

Developing Cardiorespiratory Endurance

The four variations of the basic walking/jogging/running sam-

ple program that follow are designed to help you regulate the intensity, duration, and frequency of your program. Use the following guidelines to choose the variation that is right for you.

- *Variation 1: Walking (Starting).* Choose this program if you have medical restrictions, are recovering from illness or surgery, tire easily after short walks, are obese, or have a sedentary lifestyle, and if you want to prepare for the advanced walking program to improve cardiorespiratory endurance, body composition, and muscular endurance.

- *Variation 2: Advanced Walking.* Choose this program if you already can walk comfortably for 30 minutes and if you want to develop and maintain cardiorespiratory fitness, a lean body, and muscular endurance.

- *Variation 3: Preparing for a Jogging Program.* Choose this program if you already can walk comfortably for 30 minutes and if you want to prepare for the jogging/running program to improve cardiorespiratory endurance, body composition, and muscular endurance.

- *Variation 4: Jogging/Running.* Choose this program if you already can jog comfortably without muscular discomfort, if you already can jog for 15 minutes without stopping or 30 minutes with brief walking intervals within your target

SAMPLE PROGRAM TABLE I
Calorie Costs for Walking/Jogging/Running

This table gives the calorie costs of walking, jogging, and running for slow, moderate, and fast paces. Calculations for calorie costs are approximate and assume a level terrain. A hilly terrain would result in higher calorie cost. To get an estimate of the number of calories you burn, multiply your weight by the calories per minute per pound for the speed at which you're doing the activity (listed in the right-hand column), and then multiply that by the number of minutes you exercise.

	Speed		
Activity	Miles per Hour	Minutes: Seconds per Mile	Calories per Minute per Pound
Walking			
Slow	2.0	30:00	.020
	2.5	24:00	.023
Moderate	3.0	20:00	.026
	3.5	17:08	.029
Fast	4.0	15:00	.037
	4.5	13:20	.048
Jogging			
Slow	5.0	12:00	.060
	5.5	11:00	.074
Moderate	6.0	10:00	.081
	6.5	9:00	.088
Fast	7.0	8:35	.092
	7.5	8:00	.099
Running			
Slow	8.5	7:00	.111
Moderate	9.0	6:40	.116
Fast	10.0	6:00	.129
	11.0	5:30	.141

SOURCE: Kusinitz, I., and M. Fine. 1995. *Your Guide to Getting Fit*, 3d ed. Mountain View, Calif.: Mayfield.

heart rate range, and if you want to develop and maintain a high level of cardiorespiratory fitness, a lean body, and muscular endurance.

Variation 1: Walking (Starting)

Intensity, duration, and frequency: Walk at first for 15 minutes at a pace that keeps your heart rate below your target zone. Gradually increase to 30-minute sessions. The distance you travel will probably be 1–2 miles. At the beginning, walk every other day. You can gradually increase to daily walking if you want to burn more calories (helpful if you want to change body composition).

Calorie cost: Work up to using 90–135 calories in each session (see Table 1). To increase calorie costs to the target level, walk for a longer time or for a longer distance rather than sharply increasing speed.

At the beginning: Start at whatever level is most comfortable. Maintain a normal easy pace, and stop to rest as often as you need to. Never prolong a walk past the point of comfort. When walking with a friend (a good motivation), let a comfortable conversation be your guide to pace.

As you progress: Once your muscles have become adjusted to the exercise program, increase the duration of your sessions—but by no more than 10% each week. Increase your intensity only enough to keep your heart rate just below your target. When you're able to walk 1.5 miles in 30 minutes, using 90–135 calories per session, you should consider moving on to Variation 2 or 3. Don't be discouraged by lack of immediate progress, and don't try to speed things up by overdoing. Remember that pace and heart rate can vary with the terrain, the weather, and other factors.

Variation 2: Advanced Walking

Intensity, duration, and frequency: Start at a pace at the lower end of your target heart rate zone, and begin soon afterward to increase your pace. This might boost your heart rate into the upper levels of your target zone, which is fine for brief periods. But don't overdo the intervals of fast walking. Slow down after a short time to drop your pulse rate. Vary your pattern to allow for intervals of slow, medium, and fast walking. Walk at first for 30 minutes and gradually increase your walking time until eventually you reach 60 minutes, all the while maintaining your target heart rate. The distance you walk will probably be 2–4 miles. Walk at least every other day.

Calorie cost: Work up to using about 200–350 calories in each session (see Table 1).

At the beginning: Begin by walking somewhat faster than you did in Variation 1. Check your pulse to make sure you keep your heart rate within your target zone. Slow down when necessary to lower your heart rate when going up hills or when extending the duration of your walks.

As you progress: As your heart rate adjusts to the increased workload, gradually increase your pace and your total walking time. Gradually lengthen the periods of fast walking and shorten the relief intervals of slow walking, always maintaining target heart rate. Eventually, you will reach the fitness level you would like to maintain. And to maintain that level of fitness, continue to burn the same amount of calories in each session.

Vary your program by changing the pace and distance walked, or by walking routes with different terrains and views. Gauge your progress toward whatever calorie goal you've set by using Table 1.

Variation 3: Preparing for a Jogging Program

Intensity, duration, and frequency: Start by walking at a moderate pace (3–4 miles per hour or 15–20 minutes per mile). Staying within your target heart rate zone, begin to add brief intervals of slow jogging (5–6 miles per hour or 10–12 minutes per mile). Keep the walking intervals constant at 60 seconds or at 110 yards, but gradually increase the jogging intervals until eventually you jog 4 minutes for each minute of walking. You'll probably cover between 1.5 and 2.5 miles. Each exercise session should last 15–30 minutes. Exercise every other day. If your goals include changing body composition and you want to exercise more frequently, walk on days you're not jogging.

SAMPLE PROGRAM TABLE 2 *Walking/Jogging Progression by Time*

This table is based on a walking interval of 3.75 miles per hour, measured in seconds, and a jogging interval of 5.5 miles per hour, measured in minutes:seconds. The combination of the two intervals equals a single set. In the Number of Sets column, the higher figure represents the maximum number of sets to be completed.

	Walk Interval (sec)	Jog Interval (min:sec)	Number of Sets	Total Distance (mi)	Total Time (min:sec)
Stage 1	:60	:30	10–15	1.0–1.7	15:00–22:30
Stage 2	:60	:60	8–13	1.2–2.0	16:00–26:00
Stage 3	:60	2:00	5–19	1.3–2.3	15:00–27:00
Stage 4	:60	3:00	5–7	1.6–2.4	16:00–28:00
Stage 5	:60	4:00	3–6	1.5–2.7	15:00–30:00

SOURCE: Kusinitz, I., and M. Fine. 1995. *Your Guide to Getting Fit,* 3d ed. Mountain View, Calif.: Mayfield.

SAMPLE PROGRAM TABLE 3 *Walking/Jogging Progression by Distance*

This table is based on a walking interval of 3.75 miles per hour, measured in yards, and a jogging interval of 5.5 miles per hour, also measured in yards. The combination of the two intervals equals a singe set. (One lap around a typical track is 440 yards.)

	Walk Interval (yd)	Jog Interval (yd)	Number of Sets	Total Distance (mi)	Total Time (min:sec)
Stage 1	110	55	11–21	1.0–2.0	15:00–28:12
Stage 2	110	110	16	2.0	26:56
Stage 3	110	220	11	2.0	26:02
Stage 4	110	330	8	2.0	24:24
Stage 5	110	440	7	2.2	26:05
Stage 6	110	440	8	2.5	29:49

SOURCE: Kusinitz, I., and M. Fine. 1995. *Your Guide to Getting Fit,* 3d ed. Mountain View, Calif.: Mayfield.

Calorie cost: Work up to using 200–350 calories in each session (see Table 1).

At the beginning: Start slowly. Until your muscles adjust to jogging, you may need to exercise at less than your target heart rate. At the outset, expect to do two to four times as much walking as jogging, even more if you're relatively inexperienced. Be guided by how comfortable you feel—and by your heart rate—in setting the pace for your progress. Follow the guidelines presented in Chapter 3 for exercising in hot or cold weather. Drink enough liquids to stay adequately hydrated, particularly in hot weather. In addition, use the proper running technique described below.

- Run with your back straight and your head up. Look straight ahead, not at your feet. Shift your pelvis forward, and tuck your buttocks in.

- Hold your arms slightly away from your body. Your elbows should be bent so that your forearms are parallel to the ground. You may cup your hands, but do not clench your fists. Allow your arms to swing loosely and rhythmically with each stride.

- Your heel should hit the ground first in each stride. Then roll forward onto the ball of your foot and push off for the next stride. If you find this difficult, you can try a more flat-footed style, but don't land on the balls of your feet.

- Keep your steps short by allowing your foot to strike the ground just below your knee. Keep your knees bent at all times.

- Breathe deeply through your mouth. Try to use your abdominal muscles rather than just your chest muscles to take deep breaths.

- Stay relaxed.

As you progress: Adjust your ratio of walking to jogging to keep within your target heart rate zone as much as possible. When you have progressed to the point where most of your 30-minute session is spent jogging, consider moving on to Variation 4. To find a walking/jogging progression that suits you, refer to Tables 2 and 3 (one uses time, the other distance). Which one you choose will depend, to some extent, on where you work out. If you have access to a track or can use a measured distance with easily visible landmarks to indicate yardage covered, you may find it convenient to use distance as your organizing principle. If you'll be using parks, streets, or woods, time intervals (measured with a watch) would probably work better. The suggested progressions in Tables 2 and 3 are not meant to be rigid; they are guidelines to help you develop your own rate of progress. Let your progress be guided by your heart rate, and increase your intensity and duration only to achieve your target zone.

Variation 4: Jogging/Running

Intensity, duration, and frequency: The key is to exercise within your target heart rate zone. Most people who sustain a continuous jog/run program will find that they can stay within their target heart rate zone with a speed of 5.5–7.5 miles per hour (8–11 minutes per mile). Start by jogging steadily for 15 minutes. Gradually increase your jog/run session to a regular 30–60 minutes (or about 2.5–7 miles). Exercise at least every other day. Increasing frequency by doing other activities on alternate days will place less stress on the weight-bearing parts of your lower body than will a daily program of jogging/running.

Calorie cost: Use about 300–750 calories in each session (see Table 1).

At the beginning: The greater number of calories you burn per minute makes this program less time-consuming for altering body composition than the three other variations in the walking/jogging/running program.

As you progress: If you choose this variation, you probably already have a moderate-to-high level of cardiorespiratory fitness. To stay within your target heart rate zone, increase your distance or both pace and distance as needed. Add variety to your workouts by varying your route, intensity, and duration. Alternate short runs with long ones. If you run for 60 minutes one day, try running for 30 minutes the next session. Or try doing sets that alternate hard and easy intervals—even walking, if you feel like it. You can also try a road race now and then, but be careful not to do too much too soon.

Developing Muscular Strength and Endurance

Walking, jogging, and running provide muscular endurance workouts for your lower body; they also develop muscular strength of the lower body to a lesser degree. To develop muscular strength and endurance of the upper body, and to make greater and more rapid gains in lower-body strength, you need to include resistance training in your fitness program. Use the general wellness weight training program from Chapter 4, or tailor one to fit your personal fitness goals. If you'd like to in-crease your running speed and performance, you might want to focus your program on lower-body exercises. (Don't neglect upper-body strength, however; it is important for overall wellness.) Regardless of what strength training exercises you choose, follow the guidelines for successful training:

- Train 2–3 days per week
- Perform 1 or more sets of 8–12 repetitions of 8–10 exercises.
- Include exercises that work all the major muscle groups: neck, shoulders, chest, arms, upper and lower back, abdomen, thighs, and calves.

Depending on the amount of time you are able to set aside for exercise, you may find it more convenient to alternate between your cardiorespiratory endurance workouts and your muscular strength and endurance workouts. In other words, walk or jog one day and strength train the next day.

Developing Flexibility

To round out your fitness program, you also need to include exercises that develop flexibility. The best time for a flexibility workout is when your muscles are warm, as they are immediately following cardiorespiratory endurance exercise or strength training. Perform the stretching routine presented in Chapter 5 or one that you have created to meet your own goals and preferences. Be sure to pay special attention to the hamstrings and quadriceps, which are not worked through their complete range of motion during walking or jogging. As you put your program together, remember the basic structure of a successful flexibility program:

- Stretch at least 2–3 days per week, preferably when muscles are warm.
- Stretch all the major muscle groups.
- Stretch to the point of mild discomfort, and hold for 10–30 seconds.
- Repeat each stretch at least 4 times.

BICYCLING SAMPLE PROGRAM

Bicycling can also lead to large gains in physical fitness. For many people, cycling is a pleasant and economical alternative to driving and a convenient way to build fitness.

Equipment and Technique

Cycling has its own special array of equipment, including head-gear, lighting, safety pennants, and special shoes. The bike is the most expensive item, ranging from about $100 to well over $1000. Avoid making a large investment until you're sure you'll use your bike regularly. While investigating what the market-place has to offer, rent or borrow a bike. Consider your intended use of the bike. Most cyclists who are interested primarily in fitness are best served by a sturdy 10-speed rather than a mountain bike or sport bike. Stationary cycles are good for rainy days and areas that have harsh winters.

Clothing for bike riding shouldn't be restrictive or binding, nor should it be so loose-fitting or so long that it might get caught in the chain. Clothing worn on the upper body should be comfortable but not so loose that it catches the wind and slows you down. Always wear a helmet to help prevent injury in case of a fall or crash. Wearing glasses or goggles can protect the eyes from dirt, small objects, and irritation from wind.

To avoid saddle soreness and injury, choose a soft or padded saddle, and adjust it to a height that allows your legs to almost reach full extension while pedaling. Wear a pair of well-padded gloves if your hands tend to become numb while riding or if you begin to develop blisters or calluses. To prevent backache and neck strain, warm up thoroughly, and periodically shift the position of your hands on the handlebars and your body in the saddle. Keep your arms relaxed, and don't lock your elbows. To protect your knees from strain, pedal with your feet pointed straight ahead or very slightly inward, and don't pedal in high gear for long periods.

Bike riding requires a number of precise skills that practice makes automatic. If you've never ridden before, consider taking a course. In fact, many courses are not just for beginners.

They'll help you develop skills in braking, shifting, and handling emergencies, as well as teach you ways of caring for and repairing your bike.

The National Injury Information Clearinghouse classifies bicycle riding as the nation's most dangerous sport. Many injuries are the result of the cyclist's carelessness. For safe cycling, follow these rules:

- Always wear a helmet.

- Keep on the correct side of the road. Bicycling against traffic is usually illegal and always dangerous.

- Obey all traffic signs and signals.

- On public roads, ride in single file, except in low-traffic areas (if the law permits). Ride in a straight line; don't swerve or weave in traffic.

- Be alert; anticipate the movements of other traffic and pedestrians. Listen for approaching traffic that is out of your line of vision.

- Slow down at street crossings. Check both ways before crossing.

- Use hand signals—the same as for automobile drivers—if you intend to stop or turn. Use audible signals to warn those in your path.

- Maintain full control. Avoid anything that interferes with your vision. Don't jeopardize your ability to steer by carrying anything (including people) on the handlebars.

- Keep your bicycle in good shape. Brakes, gears, saddle, wheels, and tires should always be in good condition.

- See and be seen. Use a headlight at night, and equip your bike with rear reflectors. Use side reflectors on pedals, front and rear. Wear light-colored clothing or use reflective tape at night and bright colors or fluorescent tape by day.

- Be courteous to other road users. Anticipate the worst, and practice preventive cycling.

- Use a rear-view mirror.

Developing Cardiorespiratory Endurance

Cycling is an excellent way to develop and maintain cardiorespiratory endurance and a healthy body composition.

Intensity, duration, and frequency: If you've been inactive for a long time, begin your cycling program at a heart rate that is 10–20% below your target zone. Once you feel at home on your bike, try 1 mile at a comfortable speed, and then stop and check your heart rate. Increase your speed gradually until you can cycle at 12–15 miles per hour (4–5 minutes per mile), a speed fast enough to bring most new cyclists' heart rate into their target zone. Allow your pulse rate to be your guide: More highly fit individuals may need to ride faster to achieve their target heart rate. Cycling for at least 20 minutes three times per week will improve your fitness.

Calorie cost: Use Table 4 to determine the number of calories you burn during each outing. You can increase the number of calories burned by cycling faster or for a longer duration (it's usually better to increase distance rather than to add speed).

At the beginning: It may require several outings to get the muscles and joints of your legs and hips adjusted to this new activity. Begin each outing with a 10-minute warm-up that includes stretches for your hamstrings and your back and neck muscles. Until you become a skilled cyclist, select routes with the fewest hazards, and avoid heavy automobile traffic.

As you progress: Interval training is also effective with bicycling. Simply increase your speed for periods of 4–8 minutes or for specific distances, such as 1–2 miles. Then coast for 2–3 minutes. Alternate the speed intervals and slow intervals for a total of 20–60 minutes, depending on your level of fitness. Hilly terrain is also a form of interval training.

Developing Muscular Strength and Endurance

Bicycling develops a high level of endurance and a moderate level of strength in the muscles of the lower body. To develop muscular strength and endurance of the upper body—and to make greater and more rapid gains in lower-body strength—you need to include resistance training as part of your fitness program. Use the general wellness weight training program from Chapter 4, or tailor one to fit your personal fitness goals. If one of your goals is to increase your cycling speed and performance, be sure to include exercises for the quadriceps, hamstrings, and buttocks muscles in your strength training program. No matter which exercises you include in your program, follow the general guidelines for successful and safe training:

- Train 2–3 days per week.

- Perform 1 or more sets of 8–12 repetitions of 8–10 exercises.

- Include exercises that work all the major muscle groups: neck, shoulders, chest, arms, upper and lower back, abdomen, thighs, and calves.

Depending on your schedule, you may find it more convenient to alternate between your cardiorespiratory endurance workouts and your muscular strength and endurance workouts. In other words, cycle one day and strength train the next day.

Developing Flexibility

A complete fitness program also includes exercises that develop flexibility. The best time for a flexibility workout is when your muscles are warm, as they are immediately following a session of cardiorespiratory endurance exercise or strength training. Perform the stretching routine presented in Chapter 5, or develop one that meets your own goals and preferences. Pay special attention to the hamstrings and quadriceps, which are not worked through their complete range of motion during bike riding, and to the muscles in your lower back, shoulders, and neck. As you put your stretching program together, remember these basic guidelines:

- Stretch at least 2–3 days per week, preferably when muscles are warm.

- Stretch all the major muscle groups.

- Stretch to the point of mild discomfort, and hold for 10–30 seconds.

- Repeat each stretch at least 4 times.

SAMPLE PROGRAM TABLE 4 *Calorie Costs for Bicycling*

This table gives the approximate calorie costs per pound of body weight for cycling from 5 to 60 minutes for distances of .50 mile up to 15 miles on a level terrain. To use the table, find on the horizontal line the time most closely approximating the number of minutes you cycle. Next, locate on the vertical column the approximate distance in miles you cover. The figure at the intersection represents an estimate of the calories used per minute per pound of body weight. Multiply this figure by your own body weight. Then multiply the product of these two figures by the number of minutes you cycle to get the total number of calories burned. For example, assuming you weigh 154 pounds and cycle 6 miles in 40 minutes, you would burn 260 calories: $154 \times .042$ (calories per pound, from table) $= 6.5 \times 40$ (minutes) $= 260$ calories burned.

Distance (mi)	Time (min)											
	5	10	15	20	25	30	35	40	45	50	55	60
.50	.032											
1.00	.062	.032										
1.50		.042	.032									
2.00		.062	.039	.032								
3.00			.062	.042	.036	.032						
4.00				.062	.044	.039	.035	.032				
5.00				.097	.062	.045	.041	.037	.035	.032		
6.00					.088	.062	.047	.042	.039	.036	.034	.032
7.00						.081	.062	.049	.043	.040	.038	.036
8.00							.078	.062	.050	.044	.041	.039
9.00								.076	.062	.051	.045	.042
10.00								.097	.074	.062	.051	.045
11.00									.093	.073	.062	.052
12.00										.088	.072	.062
13.00											.084	.071
14.00												.081
15.00												.097

SOURCE: Kusinitz, I., and M. Fine. 1995. *Your Guide to Getting Fit,* 3d ed. Mountain View, Calif.: Mayfield.

SWIMMING SAMPLE PROGRAM

Swimming is one of the best activities for developing all-around fitness. Because water supports the body weight of the swimmer, swimming places less stress than weight-bearing activities on joints, ligaments, and tendons and tends to cause fewer injuries.

Equipment and Safety Guidelines

Aside from having access to a swimming pool, the only equipment required for a swimming program is a swimsuit and a pair of swimming goggles to protect the eyes from irritation in chlorinated pools.

Following these few simple rules can help keep you safe and healthy during your swimming sessions:

- Swim only in a pool with a qualified lifeguard on duty.
- Always walk carefully on wet surfaces.
- Dry your ears well after swimming. If you experience the symptoms of swimmer's ear (itching, discharge, or even a partial hearing loss), consult your physician. If you swim while recovering from swimmer's ear, protect your ears with a few drops of lanolin on a wad of lamb's wool.
- To avoid back pain, try not to arch your back excessively when you swim.
- Be courteous to others in the pool.

If you swim in a setting other than a pool with a lifeguard, remember the following important rules:

- Don't swim beyond your skill and endurance limits.
- Avoid being chilled by water colder than 70°F.
- Never drink alcohol before going swimming.
- Never swim alone.

Developing Cardiorespiratory Endurance

Any one or any combination of common swimming strokes—front crawl stroke, breaststroke, backstroke, butterfly stroke, sidestroke, or elementary backstroke—can help develop and maintain cardiorespiratory fitness. (Swimming may not be as helpful as walking, jogging, or cycling for body fat loss.)

Intensity, duration, and frequency: Because swimming is not a weight-bearing activity and is not done in an upright position, it elicits a lower heart rate per minute. Therefore, you need to adjust your target heart rate zone. To calculate your target heart rate for swimming, use this formula:

Maximum swimming heart rate (MSHR) $= 205 -$ age
Target heart rate zone $= 65–90\%$ of MSHR

SAMPLE PROGRAM TABLE 5 *Calorie Costs for Swimming*

To use this table, find on the top horizontal row the distance in yards that most closely approximates the distance you swim. Next, locate on the appropriate vertical column (below the distance in yards) the time it takes you to swim the distance. Then locate in the first column on the left the approximate number of calories burned per minute per pound for the time and distance. To find the total number of calories burned, multiply your weight by the calories per minute per pound. Then multiply the product of these two numbers by the time it takes you to swim the distance (minutes:seconds). For example, assuming you weigh 130 pounds and swim 500 yards in 20 minutes, you would burn 106 calories: 130 × .041 (calories per pound, from table) = 5.33 × 20 (minutes) = 106 calories burned.

Calories per Minute per Pound	Distance (yd)					
	25	100	150	250	500	750
.033	1:15	5:00	7:30	12:30	25:00	30:30
.041	1:00	4:00	6:00	10:00	20:00	30:00
.049	0:50	3:20	5:00	8:20	18:40	25:00
.057	0:43	2:52	4:18	7:10	17:20	21:30
.065	0:37.5	2:30	3:45	6:15	10:00	
.073	0:33	2:13	3:20	5:30	8:50	
.081	0:30	2:00	3:00	5:00	8:00	
.090	0:27	1:48	2:42	4:30	7:12	
.097	0:25	1:40	2:30	4:10	6:30	

SOURCE: Kusinitz, I., and M. Fine. 1995. *Your Guide to Getting Fit*, 3d ed. Mountain View, Calif.: Mayfield.

For example, a 19-year-old would calculate her target heart rate zone for swimming as follows:

MSHR = 205 − 19 = 186 bpm

Target heart rate zone for swimming:

at 65% intensity: 0.65 × 186 = 121 bpm

at 90% intensity: 0.90 × 186 = 167 bpm

Base your duration of swimming on your intensity and target calorie costs. Swim at least three times per week.

Calorie cost: Calories burned while swimming are the result of the pace: how far you swim and how fast (see Table 5). Work up to using at least 300 calories per session.

At the beginning: If you don't have much experience swimming, invest the time and money for instruction. You'll make more rapid gains in fitness if you learn correct swimming technique. If you've been sedentary and haven't done any swimming for a long time, begin your program with 2–3 weeks, three times per week, of leisurely swimming at a pace that keeps your heart rate 10–20% below your target zone. Start swimming laps of the width of the pool if you can't swim the length. To keep your heart rate below target, take rest intervals as needed. Swim one lap, then rest 15–90 seconds as needed. Start with 10 minutes of swim/rest intervals and work up to 20 minutes. How long it takes will depend on your swimming skills and muscular fitness.

As you progress: Gradually increase the duration, or the intensity, or both duration and intensity of your swimming to raise your heart rate to a comfortable level within your target zone. Gradually increase your swimming intervals and decrease your rest intervals as you progress. Once you can swim the length of the pool at a pace that keeps your heart rate on target, continue swim/rest intervals for 20 minutes. Your rest intervals should be 30–45 seconds. You may find it helpful to get out of the pool during your rest intervals and walk until you've lowered your heart rate. Next, swim two laps of the pool length per swim interval and continue swim/rest intervals for 30 minutes. For the 30-second rest interval, walk (or rest) until you've lowered your heart rate. Gradually increase the number of laps you swim consecutively and the total duration of your session until you reach your target calorie expenditure and fitness level. But take care not to swim at too fast a pace: It can raise your heart rate too high and limit your ability to sustain your swimming. Alternating strokes can rest your muscles and help prolong your swimming time. A variety of strokes will also let you work more muscle groups.

Developing Muscular Strength and Endurance

The swimming program outlined in this section will result in moderate gains in strength and large gains in endurance in the muscles used during the strokes you've chosen. To develop strength and endurance in all the muscles of the body, you need to include resistance training as part of your fitness program. Use the general wellness weight training program from Chapter 4, or tailor one to fit your personal fitness goals. To improve your swimming performance, include exercises that work key muscles. For example, if you swim primarily front crawl, include exercises to increase strength in your shoulders, arms, and upper back. (Training the muscles you use during swimming can also help prevent injuries.) Regardless of which strength training exercise you include in your program, follow the general guidelines for successful training:

- Train 2–3 days per week.
- Perform 1 or more sets of 8–12 repetitions of 8–10 exercises.
- Include exercises that work all the major muscle groups: neck, shoulders, chest, arms, upper and lower back, abdomen, thighs, and calves.

Depending on the amount of time you have for exercise, you might want to schedule your cardiorespiratory endurance workouts and your muscular strength and endurance workouts on alternate days. In other words, swim one day and strength train the next day.

Developing Flexibility

For a complete fitness program, you also need to include exercises that develop flexibility. The best time for a flexibility workout is when your muscles are warm, as they are immediately following cardiorespiratory endurance exercise or strength training. Perform the stretching routine presented in Chapter 5 or one you have created to meet your own goals and preferences. Be sure to pay special attention to the muscles you use during swimming, particularly the shoulders and back. As you put your program together, remember the basic structure of a successful flexibility program:

- Stretch at least 2–3 days per week, preferably when muscles are warm.
- Stretch all the major muscle groups.
- Stretch to the point of mild discomfort, and hold for 10–30 seconds.
- Repeat each stretch at least 4 times.

IN-LINE SKATING SAMPLE PROGRAM

In-line skating is currently the fastest growing sport in the United States. Skating is convenient and inexpensive (after the initial outlay for equipment); it can be done on city streets, on paved bike paths and trails, and in parks. If done intensively enough, skating can provide a cardiorespiratory endurance workout comparable to the workouts provided by jogging and cycling. Studies indicate that skating consumes about as many calories as jogging.

An advantage of skating over jogging is that skating is low impact, so it is less harmful to the knees and ankles. An advantage of skating over bicycling is that it works the hamstring muscle in the back of the thigh. Skating develops lower-body strength and endurance, working all the muscles of the leg and hip and strengthening the muscles and connective tissues surrounding the ankles, knees, and hips.

Equipment

To skate safely and enjoyably, you will need a pair of comfortable, sturdy, quality skates and adequate safety equipment. The skate consists of a hard polyurethane shell or outer boot; a padded foam liner; and a frame or chassis that holds the wheels, bearings, spacers, and brake. If you want to try out the sport before making a commitment, rent your skates and equipment from a skate shop. If you are buying, plan to spend about $110–$200 for skates that meet the basic needs of most recreational skaters. Shop for the best combination of price, quality, comfort, and service.

Essential safety equipment includes a helmet, elbow pads, knee pads, and wrist guards. (Wrist injuries are the most common in-line skating injury.) You may want to put reflective tape on your skates for those occasions when you don't get home before dark. Carry moleskin or adhesive bandages with you in case you start to develop a blister while skating. (For more on safety, see Appendix A.)

Technique

In-line skating uses many of the skills and techniques of ice skating, roller skating, and skiing, so if you have ever participated in any of those activities, you will probably take to in-line skating fairly readily. Many people begin in-line skating without instruction, but instruction will allow you to progress more quickly.

To begin, center your weight equally over both skates, bend your knees slightly so your nose, knees, and toes are all in the same line, and look straight ahead. Keep your weight forward over the balls of your feet; don't lean back.

To skate, use a stroke, glide, stroke, glide rhythm (rather than a series of quick, short strokes). Push with one leg while gliding with the other. Shift your body weight back and forth so it is always centered over the gliding skate.

To stop, use your brake, located on the back of the right skate in most skates. With knees bent and arms extended in front of your body, move the right foot forward, shift your weight to your left leg, and lift your right toe until the brake pad touches the ground and stops you. An alternative stop is the T-stop, in which you drag one skate behind the other at a 90-degree angle to the direction of your forward motion.

If you lose your balance and are about to fall, lower your center of gravity by bending at the waist and putting your hands on your knees. If you can't regain your balance, try to fall forward, directing the impact to your wrist guards and knee pads. Try not to fall backward.

Again, instruction can help you learn many moves and techniques that will make the sport safer and more enjoyable.

Developing Cardiorespiratory Endurance

Studies have shown that in-line skaters raise their heart rates and oxygen consumption comparably to joggers, bicyclers, and walkers. Skaters reached 60–75% of $\dot{V}O_{2max}$ by skating continuously (not pushing off and gliding for several seconds) at 10.6–12.5 mph for 20–30 minutes. It may be difficult for recreational skaters to safely skate this fast for this long, however, given the typical constraints of city and suburban streets. Experts suggest skating uphill as much as possible to reach the level of intensity that builds cardiorespiratory endurance. If you can reach and maintain higher speeds in parks or on paved paths, do so, but always skate safely. (If you belong to a gym or fitness club and want to do some indoor skating, Nautilus has introduced a new piece of equipment called the Skate Machine.)

SAMPLE PROGRAM TABLE 6
Calorie Costs for In-Line Skating

To estimate the number of calories you burn, first determine your approximate speed (use the minutes per mile column if necessary), multiply the calories per minute per pound by your weight, and then multiply that figure by the number of minutes you skate. For example: assuming you weigh 145 pounds and skate at 10 mph for 30 minutes, you would burn 273 calories: 145 × .063 (calories per pound, from table) = 9.1 × 30 (minutes) = 273 calories burned. Calculations are approximate.

| | Speed | |
Miles per Hour	Minutes: Seconds per Mile	Calories per Minute per Pound
8	7:30	.041
9	6:40	.053
10	6:00	.063
11	5:25	.072
12	5:00	.084
13	4:35	.095
14	4:20	.105
15	4:00	.115

Intensity, duration, and frequency: Start your early skating sessions at a pace that keeps your heart rate about 10–20% below your target zone. Skate for 5–10 minutes, and then check your heart rate. Increase your speed gradually until you can skate at about 10 miles per hour (6 minutes per mile). Use your pulse as a guide to speed, aiming for 65% of your target heart rate zone. To achieve cardiorespiratory benefits, you will have to skate at a continuous and relatively intense pace for at least 20 minutes three times a week. The more fit you are, the more intensively you will need to skate to reach your target heart rate.

Calorie cost: Use Table 6 to determine the approximate number of calories you burn during each outing. You can increase the number of calories burned by skating faster, for a longer time, or uphill.

At the beginning: If you are a beginner, practice skating in an empty schoolyard or parking lot. As you become confident with the basic techniques, you can move on to streets, parks, and paved bike trails. Maintain an easy pace, alternating stroking and gliding.

Begin each outing with a 5- to 10-minute warm-up of walking, jogging, or even slow skating. Once your muscles are warm, you can do some stretches to help loosen and warm up the primary muscles used during skating—the quadriceps, hamstrings, buttocks, hips, groin, ankles, calves, and lower back. You can also save the stretches for the end of the workout.

To launch an in-line skating fitness program, aim for slow, long-distance workouts. Start by skating for 15 minutes, and gradually increase your session to 20–30 minutes of continuous skating (or about 3.5–5 miles). Try to skate about 20 miles a week, or 5 miles a day (about 30 minutes) 4 days a week.

As you progress: After the first week or two, add about a mile a day, up to 40 miles per week (60 minutes a day). To increase intensity, add some hills, sprints (bursts of short, rapid striding), and interval training (periods of intensive exercise at your target heart rate alternating with timed rest periods when your heart rate drops below your target zone). Try to skate 30–60 minutes a day four or more times a week.

The harder and faster you skate, the more intensive your workout will be and the more your cardiorespiratory endurance and muscular strength will improve. The longer and more often you skate, the more your endurance will increase.

Developing Muscular Strength and Endurance

In-line skating develops the muscles in the entire upper leg, buttocks, and hip; lower back; and upper arms and shoulders when arms are swung vigorously. To make greater gains in lower-body strength and to develop the entire upper body, include resistance training in your overall fitness program. Use the general wellness weight training program from Chapter 4, or tailor one to fit your personal fitness goals. No matter which exercises you include in your program, follow the general guidelines for successful and safe training:

- Train 2–3 days per week.
- Perform 1 or more sets of 8–12 repetitions of 8–10 exercises.
- Include exercises that work all the major muscle groups: neck, shoulders, chest, arms, upper and lower back, thighs, and calves.

Depending on your schedule, you may find it more convenient to skate and weight train on alternate days.

Developing Flexibility

The best times for a flexibility workout are when your muscles are warm, so stretch after a short warm-up at the beginning of your skating session, or after your skating session, or after a weight training session. Use the stretching routine presented in Chapter 5, or develop one that meets your own goals and preferences. Pay particular attention to your quadriceps, hamstrings, buttocks, hips, groin, ankles, calves, and lower back. Remember these basic guidelines:

- Stretch at least 2–3 days per week, preferably when muscles are warm.
- Stretch all the major muscle groups.
- Stretch to the point of mild discomfort, and hold for 10–30 seconds.
- Repeat each stretch at least 4 times.

Name _____ **Section** _____ **Date** _____

LAB 7-1 A Personal Fitness Program Plan and Contract

A. I, _____, am contracting with myself to follow a physical fitness
(name)

program to work toward the following goals:

Specific or short-term goals

1. _____

2. _____

3. _____

4. _____

General or long-term goals

1. _____

2. _____

3. _____

4. _____

B. My program plan is as follows:

Activities	Components (Check ✓)					Intensity*	Duration	Frequency (Check ✓)						
	CRE	MS	ME	F	BC			M	Tu	W	Th	F	Sa	Su

*Conduct activities for achieving CRE goals at your target heart rate or RPE value.

C. My program will begin on _____. My program includes the following schedule of mini-goals. For each step
(date)

in my program, I will give myself the reward listed.

_____	_____	_____
(mini-goal 1)	(date)	(reward)
(mini-goal 2)	(date)	(reward)
(mini-goal 3)	(date)	(reward)
(mini-goal 4)	(date)	(reward)
(mini-goal 5)	(date)	(reward)

D. My program will include the addition of physical activity to my daily routine (such as climbing stairs or walking to class):

1. _____

2. _____

3. _____

4. _____

5. _____

E. I will use the following tools to monitor my program and my progress toward my goals:

_____

(list any charts, graphs, or journals you plan to use)

_____

_____

I sign this contract as an indication of my personal commitment to reach my goal.

_____   _____

(your signature)   (date)

I have recruited a helper who will witness my contract and _____

_____

(list any way your helper will participate in your program)

_____

_____   _____

(witness's signature)   (date)

LAB 7-2 *Monitoring Your Program Progress*

Track your adherence to your program and your progress by filling out a program log. Use the one below, or make one specifically designed to match your program. If you prefer detailed program logs for each of your fitness components, use the logs in Labs 3-2, 4-3, and 5-2. (A more extensive series of logs is included in the Daily Fitness Log booklet and in the Lab Activities and Fitness Log software.)

To use the log below, fill in the activities that are part of your program. Each day, note the distance and/or time for each activity. For flexibility or strength training workouts, you may prefer just to enter a check mark each time you complete a workout. At the end of each week, total your distances and/or times.

Activity/Date	M	Tu	W	Th	F	Sa	Su	Weekly Total	M	Tu	W	Th	F	Sa	Su	Weekly Total
1																
2																
3																
4																
5																
6																

Activity/Date	M	Tu	W	Th	F	Sa	Su	Weekly Total	M	Tu	W	Th	F	Sa	Su	Weekly Total
1																
2																
3																
4																
5																
6																

Activity/Date	M	Tu	W	Th	F	Sa	Su	Weekly Total	M	Tu	W	Th	F	Sa	Su	Weekly Total
1																
2																
3																
4																
5																
6																

Activity/Date	M	Tu	W	Th	F	Sa	Su	Weekly Total	M	Tu	W	Th	F	Sa	Su	Weekly Total
1																
2																
3																
4																
5																
6																

Activity/Date	M	Tu	W	Th	F	Sa	Su	Weekly Total	M	Tu	W	Th	F	Sa	Su	Weekly Total
1																
2																
3																
4																
5																
6																

Nutrition

8

LOOKING AHEAD

After reading this chapter, you should be able to answer these questions about nutrition:

- What are the different kinds of essential nutrients, and what functions do they perform in the body?

- What guidelines have been developed to help people choose a healthy diet, avoid nutritional deficiencies, and protect themselves from diet-related chronic diseases?

- What special nutritional guidelines apply to vegetarian diets?

- How can people adapt nutritional information to their own lives and circumstances?

183

Nutrition is a vital component of wellness. What you eat affects your energy levels, well-being, and overall health. Eating habits can also be closely linked with certain diseases, disabling conditions, and other health problems. Of particular concern is the connection between lifetime nutritional habits and the risk of the major chronic diseases, including heart disease, cancer, stroke, and diabetes. On the more positive side, however, a well-planned diet in conjunction with a fitness program can help prevent such conditions and even reverse some of them.

Creating a diet plan to support maximum fitness and protect against disease is a two-part project. First, you have to know which nutrients are necessary and in what amounts. Second, you have to translate those requirements into a diet consisting of foods you like to eat that are both available and affordable. Once you have an idea of what constitutes a healthy diet for you, you may also have to make adjustments in your current diet to bring it into line with your goals.

This chapter provides the basic principles of nutrition. It introduces the six classes of essential nutrients, explaining their role in the functioning of the body. It also provides different sets of guidelines that are available to help you design a healthy diet plan. Finally, it offers practical tools and advice to help you apply the guidelines to your own life, whether you are eating at home, at school, or in a restaurant. Diet is an area of your life in which you have almost total control. Using your knowledge and understanding of nutrition to create a healthy diet plan is a significant step toward wellness.

COMPONENTS OF A HEALTHY DIET

When you think about your diet, you probably do so in terms of the foods you like to eat—a turkey sandwich and a glass of milk, or a steak and a baked potato. What's important for your health, though, are the nutrients contained in those foods. Your body requires proteins, fats, carbohydrates, vitamins, minerals, and water—about 45 **essential nutrients.** The word *essential* in this context means that you must get these substances from food because your body is unable to manufacture them at all, or at least not fast enough to meet your physiological needs. The six classes of nutrients, along with their functions and major sources, are listed in Table 8-1.

Nutrients are released into the body by the process of **digestion,** which breaks them down into compounds that the gastrointestinal tract can absorb and the body can use (Figure 8-1). In this form, the essential nutrients provide energy, build and maintain body tissues, and regulate body functions.

Providing energy is the most immediate function of nutrients. The energy in foods is measured in **kilocalories** (abbreviated **kcalories**). One kcalorie represents the amount of heat it takes to raise the temperature of 1 kilogram of water 1°C. The average adult requires about 2000 kcalories per day to meet energy needs. Kilocalories consumed in excess of energy needs are stored as body fat. In common usage, the term *kilocalorie* is generally shortened to **calorie,** although a calorie is actually a very small energy unit—a kilocalorie contains 1000 calories. For convenience, this chapter will use the more familiar term, *calorie,* to stand for the larger energy unit.

Three of the six classes of nutrients supply energy: proteins, carbohydrates, and fats. Fats provide the most energy—9 calories per gram; protein and carbohydrates each provide 4 calories per gram. (Alcohol, although it is not an essential nutrient, also supplies energy, providing 7 calories per gram.) Experts advise against high fat consumption, in part because fats provide so many calories. Given the typical American diet, most Americans do not need the extra calories to meet energy needs.

Meeting our energy needs is only one of the functions of food. All the nutrients perform numerous other vital functions. In terms of quantity, water is the most significant nutrient: The body is approximately 60% water and can survive only a few days without it. Vitamins and minerals are needed in much smaller quantities, but they are still vital.

Practically all foods contain mixtures of nutrients, although foods are commonly classified according to their predominant nutrients. For example, spaghetti is considered a carbohydrate food although it contains small amounts of other nutrients. Let's take a closer look at the functions and sources of the six classes of nutrients.

Proteins

Protein is an important component of muscle, bone, blood, enzymes, cell membranes, and some hormones. As mentioned above, protein can also provide energy at 4 calories per gram of protein weight. Proteins are composed of **amino acids.** Twenty common amino acids are found in food; nine of these are essential to an adult diet:

TERMS **essential nutrients** Vitamins, minerals, some amino acids, linoleic and alpha-linolenic acid, carbohydrate, water, and other substances the body must obtain from food because it can't manufacture them in sufficient quantity for its physiological needs.

digestion The process of breaking down foods in the gastrointestinal tract into nutrients the body can absorb.

kilocalorie (kcalorie) The unit of fuel potential in a food. One kcalorie represents the amount of heat required to raise the temperature of 1 kilogram of water 1°C.

calorie The amount of heat required to raise the temperature of 1 gram of water 1°C; the word commonly used when kilocalorie is meant.

amino acids The components of proteins used to build muscle and other tissue.

TABLE 8-1	*The Six Classes of Essential Nutrients*	
Nutrient	**Function**	**Major Sources**
Proteins (4 calories/gram)	Form important parts of muscles, bone, blood, enzymes, some hormones, and cell membranes; repair tissue; regulate water and acid-base balance; help in growth; supply energy	Meat, fish, poultry, eggs, milk products, legumes, nuts
Carbohydrates (4 calories/gram)	Supply energy to cells in brain, nervous system, and blood; supply energy to muscles during exercise	Grains (breads and cereals), fruits, vegetables, milk
Fats (9 calories/gram)	Supply energy; insulate, support, and cushion organs; provide medium for absorption of fat-soluble vitamins	Saturated fats primarily from animal sources, palm and coconut oils, and hydrogenated vegetable fats; unsaturated fats from grains, nuts, seeds, fish, vegetables
Vitamins	Promote (initiate or speed up) specific chemical reactions within cells	Abundant in fruits, vegetables, and grains; also found in meat and dairy products
Minerals	Help regulate body functions; aid in the growth and maintenance of body tissues; act as catalysts for the release of energy	Found in most food groups
Water	Makes up 50–70% of body weight; provides a medium for chemical reactions; transports chemicals; regulates temperature; removes waste products	Fruits, vegetables, and other liquids

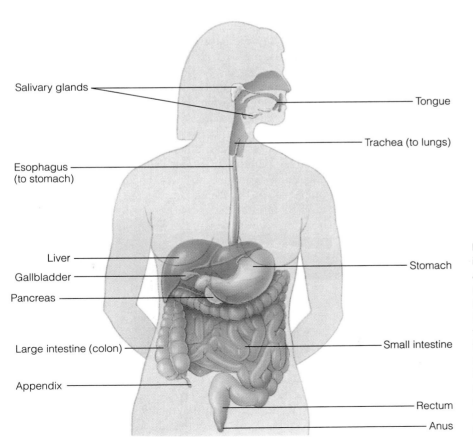

Salivary glands
Tongue
Trachea (to lungs)
Esophagus (to stomach)
Liver
Gallbladder
Pancreas
Stomach
Large intestine (colon)
Small intestine
Appendix
Rectum
Anus

Figure 8-1 The digestive system. Food is partially broken down by being chewed and mixed with saliva in the mouth. As food moves through the digestive tract, it is mixed by muscular contractions and broken down by chemicals. After traveling to the stomach via the esophagus, food is broken down further by stomach acids. Most absorption of nutrients occurs in the small intestine, aided by secretions from the pancreas, gallbladder, and intestinal lining. The large intestine reabsorbs excess water; the remaining solid wastes are collected in the rectum and excreted through the anus.

histidine, isoleucine, leucine, lysine, methionine, phenyl-alanine, threonine, tryptophan, and valine. "Essential," again, means that they are required for normal health and growth but must be provided in the diet because the body manufactures them in insufficient quantities, if at all. The other eleven amino acids can be produced by the body as long as the necessary ingredients are supplied by foods.

Foods are rated as "complete" protein sources if they supply all nine essential amino acids in adequate amounts; they are classified as "incomplete" protein sources if they supply only some. Meat, fish, poultry, eggs, milk, cheese, and other foods from animal sources provide complete proteins. Incomplete proteins come from plant sources such as beans, peas, and nuts; these are good sources of most essential amino acids but are usually low in one or two. Different vegetable proteins are low in different amino acids, so combinations can provide complete proteins. Vegetarians who eat no foods from animal sources can obtain all essential amino acids by eating a wide variety of foods each day.

The leading sources of protein in the American diet are (1) beef, steaks, and roasts; (2) hamburgers and meatloaf; (3) white bread, rolls, and crackers; (4) milk; and (5) pork. About two-thirds of the protein in the American diet comes from animal sources, which means the nation's diet is rich in amino acids. About 10–15% of the total calories in a well-balanced diet should come from protein. However, many Americans consume more than that amount every day. This excess protein is synthesized into fat for energy storage or burned for energy. For most people, extra protein in the diet is not harmful, but it does contribute fat to the diet because protein-rich foods are often fat-rich as well.

Fats

At 9 calories per gram, fats (also known as lipids) are the most concentrated source of energy. The fats stored in your body represent usable energy, help insulate your body, and support and cushion your organs. Fats in the diet help your body absorb fat-soluble vitamins and add important flavor and texture to foods. During periods of rest and light activity, fats are the major body fuel. The nervous system, brain, and red blood cells are fueled by carbohydrates, but most of the rest of the body's organs are fueled by fats. Two fats—linoleic acid and alpha-linolenic acid—are essential to the diet; they are key regulators of such body functions as the maintenance of blood pressure and the progress of a healthy pregnancy.

Types and Sources of Fats　Most of the fats in food and in your body are in the form of **triglycerides,** which are composed of a glycerine molecule (an alcohol) plus three fatty acids. A fatty acid is made up of a chain of carbon atoms with oxygen attached at the end and hydrogen atoms attached along the length of the chain. Fatty acids differ in the length of their carbon atom chains and in

Figure 8-2　Chemical structures of saturated and unsaturated fatty acids.　This example of a triglyceride consists of a molecule of glycerol with three fatty acids attached. Fatty acids can differ in the length of their carbon chains and their degree of saturation.

their degree of saturation (the number of hydrogens attached to the chain). If every available bond from each carbon atom in a fatty acid chain is attached to a hydrogen atom, the fatty acid is said to be **saturated** (Figure 8-2). If not all the available bonds are taken up by hydrogens, the carbon atoms in the chain will form double bonds with each other. Such fatty acids are called unsaturated fats. If there is only one double bond, the fatty acid is called **monounsaturated.** If there are two or more double bonds, the fatty acid is called **polyunsaturated.** The essential fatty acids, linoleic and alpha-linolenic acids, are both polyunsaturated.

Foods fats are often composed of both saturated and unsaturated fatty acids; the dominant type of fatty acid determines the fat's characteristics. Food fats containing large amounts of saturated fatty acids are usually solid at room temperature (these are called "fats"); they are generally found in animal products. The leading sources of saturated fat in the American diet are unprocessed animal flesh (hamburger, steak, roasts), whole milk, cheese, and hot dogs and lunch meats. Food fats containing large amounts of monounsaturated and polyunsaturated fatty acids are usually from plant sources and are liquid at room temperature (these are called "oils"). Olive, canola, and peanut oils contain mostly monounsaturated fatty acids. Sunflower, corn, and safflower oils contain mostly polyunsaturated fatty acids. For the relative amounts of fatty acids in common dietary fats, see Figure 8-3.

There are notable exceptions to these generalizations. When unsaturated vegetable oils undergo the process of **hydrogenation,** a mixture of saturated and unsaturated fatty acids is produced. Hydrogenation turns many of the double bonds in unsaturated fatty acids into single bonds, increasing the degree of saturation and producing a more solid fat from a liquid oil. Hydrogenation also produces

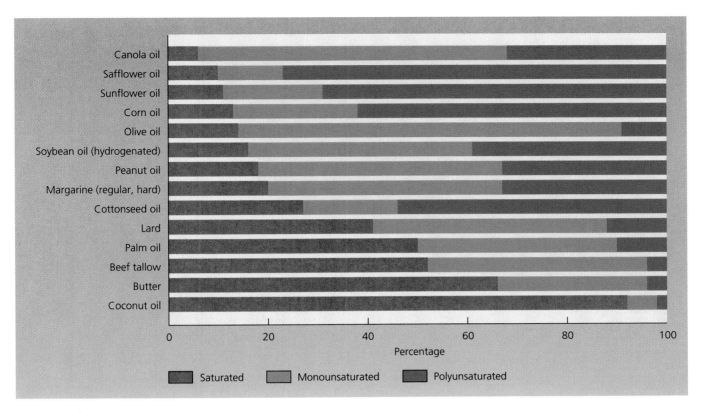

Figure 8-3 Comparisons of dietary fats.

trans fatty acids, unsaturated fatty acids with an atypical shape that affects their behavior during cooking and in the body. Food manufacturers use hydrogenation to increase the stability of an oil so it can be reused for deep frying; to improve the texture of certain foods (to make pastries and pie crusts flakier, for example); to keep oil from separating out of peanut butter; and to extend the shelf life of foods made with oil. Hydrogenation is the process used to transform a liquid oil into margarine or vegetable shortening.

Many baked and fried foods are prepared with hydrogenated vegetable oils, so they can be relatively high in saturated and trans fatty acids. Leading sources of trans fatty acids in the American diet are deep-fried fast foods such as french fries and fried chicken or fish (typically fried in vegetable shortening rather than oil); baked and snack foods such as pot pies, cakes, cookies, pastries, doughnuts, and chips; and stick margarine. In general, the more solid a hydrogenated oil is, the more saturated and trans fats it contains; for example, stick margarines typically contain more saturated and trans fatty acids than do tub or squeeze margarines. Smaller amounts of trans fats are found naturally in meat and milk.

Hydrogenated vegetable oils are not the only plant fats that contain saturated fats. Palm and coconut oils, although derived from plants, are also highly saturated. On the other hand, fish oils, derived from an animal source, are rich in polyunsaturated fats.

Recommended Fat Intake   You need only about 1 tablespoon (15 grams) of vegetable oil per day incorporated into your diet to supply the essential fats. The average American diet supplies considerably more than this amount; in fact, fats make up about 33% of our calorie intake. (This is the equivalent of about 75 grams, or 5 tablespoons, of fat per day.) Health experts recommend that we reduce our fat intake to 30%, but not less than 10%, of total daily calories, with less than 10% coming from

triglyceride   The most common lipid found in fatty tissues; composed of a glycerol molecule and three fatty acids.   **TERMS**

saturated fatty acid   A fatty acid that has no double bonds between carbon atoms; solid at room temperature.

monounsaturated fatty acid   A fatty acid that has one double bond between carbon atoms; liquid at room temperature.

polyunsaturated fatty acid   A fatty acid that has two or more double bonds between carbon atoms; liquid at room temperature.

hydrogenation   A process by which hydrogens are added to unsaturated fats, increasing the degree of saturation and turning liquid oils into solid fats. Hydrogenation produces a mixture of saturated fatty acids and standard and trans forms of unsaturated fatty acids.

trans fatty acid   A type of unsaturated fatty acid produced during the process of hydrogenation; trans fats have an atypical shape that changes their chemical activity.

	0–10%	10–30%	30–50%	50–75%	75–100%
Breads, cereals, rice, and pasta	Many dry cereals and breads, rice, pasta, tortillas, pretzels	Plain popcorn, hot cereals, some breads	Granola, buttered popcorn, crackers, biscuit, muffin	Croissant	
Vegetables and fruits	Most fresh, frozen, canned, and dried fruits and vegetables		French fries, onion rings	Potato chips, coconut	Avocado, olives
Milk, yogurt, and cheese	Nonfat milk, yogurt, and cottage cheese	Low-fat cottage cheese and yogurt, 1% and 2% milk, buttermilk	Whole milk, regular ice cream	Most cheeses, rich ice cream	Half and half, cream cheese, sour cream, heavy cream
Meat, poultry, fish, dry beans, eggs, nuts	Skinless turkey breast, haddock, cod, most dry beans, egg whites	Skinless white meat chicken, halibut, shrimp, clams, tuna in water, red snapper, trout, low-fat tofu	Beef top round, broiled steak, ham, skinless dark meat poultry, salmon, mackerel, swordfish	Roast beef, ground chuck; pork, lamb and veal chops; poultry with skin; tuna in oil; regular tofu; eggs	Salami, bacon, hot dogs, spare ribs, most nuts and seeds, peanut butter, egg yolks
Combination foods	Clear soup (bouillon)	Most broth-based soups; vegetarian chili	Hamburger, lasagna, chili with meat, potato salad, vegetable and cheese pizza, macaroni and cheese, enchilada	Cheeseburger; meat pizza; large meat, poultry, or cheese sandwich, taco salad	
Fats, oils, and sweets	Hard candy, chewing gum			Chocolate bar	Butter, margarine, vegetable oil, mayonnaise, salad dressing

Figure 8-4   Percent of total calories from fat for selected foods.

saturated fat. The fat content of many common foods is given in Figure 8-4; the box "Setting Goals for Fat, Protein, and Carbohydrate Intake" explains how to set a daily goal for fat consumption.

Fats and Health   Different types of fats have very different effects on health. Many studies have examined the effects of dietary fat intake on blood **cholesterol** levels and the risk of heart disease. Saturated and trans fatty acids have been found to raise blood levels of **low-density lipoprotein (LDL),** or "bad" cholesterol, thereby increasing a person's risk of heart disease. Unsaturated fatty acids, on the other hand, lower LDL and may increase levels of **high-density lipoprotein (HDL),** or

"good" cholesterol. Thus, to reduce the risk of heart disease, it is important to substitute unsaturated fats for saturated and trans fats. (A heart-healthy diet is described in Chapter 11.)

Most Americans consume more saturated fat (11% of total calories) than trans fat (2–4% of total calories). The best way to reduce saturated fat in your diet is to lower your intake of meat and full-fat dairy products (whole milk, cream, butter, cheese, ice cream). To lower trans fats, decrease your intake of deep-fried foods and baked goods made with hydrogenated vegetable oils; use liquid oils rather than margarine and favor tub or squeeze margarines over stick margarines. (Remember, the softer or more liquid a fat is, the less saturated and trans fat it is likely to contain.) Saturated fats are listed on the nutrition label of prepared foods. Trans fats are not, but you can check for the presence of hydrogenated oils on the ingredient list; if "partially hydrogenated" oils or fats or "vegetable shortening" appears near the top of the list, the product may be high in trans fats.

Research has indicated that certain forms of polyunsaturated fatty acids—known as **omega-3 fatty acids** and found in fish—may have a particularly positive effect on cardiovascular health. If the endmost double bond of a polyunsaturated fat occurs three carbons from the end of the fatty acid chain, an omega-3 form is produced. (The polyunsaturated fatty acid shown in Figure 8-2 is an omega-3 form.) If the endmost double bond occurs at the

Setting Daily Goals

To meet the recommendations for nutrient intakes, start by setting some overall daily goals.

1. Determine approximately how many calories you consume each day. Depending on your activity level, daily needs range from about 2200 to 3500 calories for men and from about 1600 to 2500 for women.

2. Set percentage goals or limits for your intake of fat, protein, and carbohydrate. Those recommended for the general public are 30% or less of total daily calories from fat, 10–15% of total daily calories from protein, and 55% of total daily calories from carbohydrate. If your diet already meets these goals, you may want to set more challenging marks, such as raising your daily carbohydrate consumption to 60% of total calories.

3. Change your limits or goals from percentages to grams for easy tracking. A person who eats about 2200 calories per day could calculate her or his goals as follows:

Fat: 2200 calories per day $\times$ 30% = 660 calories of fat per day

660 calories $\div$ 9 calories per gram = **73 g of fat per day**

Protein: 2200 calories per day $\times$ 15% = 330 calories of protein per day

330 calories $\div$ 4 calories per gram = **83 g of protein per day**

Carbohydrate: 2200 calories per day $\times$ 55% = 1210 calories of carbohydrate per day

1210 calories $\div$ 4 calories per gram = **303 g of carbohydrate per day**

(Remember, there are 9 calories per gram of fat and 4 calories per gram of protein and carbohydrate.)

Evaluating an Individual Food Item

You can do the same type of calculations to evaluate a particular food item, to determine whether it is high or low in protein, fat, or carbohydrate. For example, suppose you want to determine how high in fat peanut butter is. First, you need to know the total number of calories and grams of fat it contains. Multiply the grams of fat by 9 (because there are 9 calories in a gram of fat), and then divide that number by the total calories. For a tablespoon of peanut butter (8 grams of fat and 95 calories), you would calculate as follows: 8 $\times$ 9 = 72; 72 $\div$ 95 = 0.76, or 76% of calories from fat. This means peanut butter is relatively high in fat. If your overall daily fat consumption goal is 70 grams of fat, a tablespoon of peanut butter would represent 11% of your daily target.

Of course, you can still eat high-fat foods. But it makes good sense to limit the size of your portions and to balance your intake with low-fat foods. For example, a tablespoon of peanut butter eaten on whole-wheat bread and served with a banana, carrot sticks, and a glass of nonfat milk makes a nutritious lunch—high in protein and carbohydrate, low in fat. Three tablespoons of peanut butter on high-fat crackers with potato chips, cookies, and whole milk is a less healthy combination. So while it's important to evaluate individual food items, it is more important to look at them in the context of your overall diet.

Monitoring Your Progress

Depending on your current diet and health needs, you may choose to focus on a particular goal, such as that for fat or protein. For prepared foods, food labels list the number of grams of fat, protein, and carbohydrate. The breakdown for many common foods and for popular fast-food items can be found in Appendixes B and C. Nutrition information is also posted in many grocery stores, published in inexpensive nutrition guides, and available online. By checking these resources, you can keep a running total of the grams of fat, protein, and carbohydrate you eat and determine how close you are to meeting your goals.

---

sixth carbon atom, an omega-6 form is produced. Most of the polyunsaturated fats currently consumed by Americans are omega-6 forms, primarily from corn oil and soybean oil. However, the consumption of omega-3 fatty acids in fish has been shown to reduce the tendency of blood to clot, to decrease inflammatory responses in the body, and to raise levels of HDL. It even appears to lower the risk of heart disease in some people. Because of these benefits, nutritionists now recommend that Americans increase the proportion of omega-3 polyunsaturated fats in their diet by increasing their consumption of fish to two or more times a week. Mackerel, herring, salmon, sardines, anchovies, tuna, and trout are all good sources of omega-3 fatty acids.

Dietary fat can affect health in other ways. Diets high in fat are associated with an increased risk of certain forms of cancer, especially colon cancer. A high-fat diet can also make weight management more difficult. Because fat is a concentrated source of calories (9 calories per gram versus 4 calories per gram for protein and carbohydrate), a high-fat diet is often a high-calorie diet that can lead to weight gain. In addition, there is some evidence that calories from fat are more easily converted to body fat than calories from protein or carbohydrate.

Although more research is needed on the precise effects of different types and amounts of fat on overall health, a great deal of evidence points to the fact that most people benefit from lowering their overall fat intake to recommended levels and substituting unsaturated fats for saturated and trans fats.

Carbohydrates

Carbohydrates function primarily to supply energy to body cells. Some cells, such as those in the brain and other parts of the nervous system and in the blood, use only carbohydrates for fuel. During high-intensity exercise, muscles also get most of their energy from carbohydrates. When we don't eat enough carbohydrates to satisfy the needs of the brain and red blood cells, our bodies synthesize carbohydrates from proteins. In situations of extreme deprivation, when the diet lacks sufficient amounts of both carbohydrates and proteins, the body turns to its own proteins, resulting in severe muscle wasting. This rarely occurs, however, because the body's daily carbohydrate requirement is filled by just three or four slices of bread.

Simple and Complex Carbohydrates Carbohydrates are classified into two groups: simple and complex. Simple carbohydrates contain only one or two sugar units in each molecule. A one-sugar carbohydrate is called a **monosaccharide;** a two-sugar carbohydrate, a **disaccharide.** Simple carbohydrates include sucrose (table sugar),

fructose (fruit sugar, honey), maltose (malt sugar), and lactose (milk sugar); they provide much of the sweetness in foods. Simple carbohydrates are found naturally in fruits and milk and are added to soft drinks, fruit drinks, candy, and sweet desserts. There is no evidence that any type of simple sugar is more nutritious than others.

Starches and most types of dietary fiber are complex carbohydrates; they consist of chains of many sugar molecules and are called **polysaccharides.** Starches are found in a variety of plants, especially grains (wheat, rye, rice, oats, barley, millet), **legumes,** and tubers (potatoes and yams). Most other vegetables contain a mix of starches and simple carbohydrates. Dietary fiber, discussed in the next section, is found in fruits, vegetables, and grains.

Many nutritionists also distinguish between refined (processed) and unrefined carbohydrates. The refinement of wheat flour, rice, and cereal grains transforms whole-wheat flour to white flour, brown rice to white rice, and so on. Refined carbohydrates usually retain all the calories of their unrefined counterparts, but they tend to be much lower in fiber, vitamins, and minerals. In general, unrefined carbohydrates tend to take longer to chew and digest than refined ones; they also enter the bloodstream more slowly. This slower digestive pace tends to make people feel full sooner and for a longer period, lessening the chance that they will overeat and gain weight. It also helps keep blood sugar and insulin levels low, which may decrease the risk of diabetes and heart disease. For all these reasons, unrefined carbohydrates are recommended over those that have been refined.

During digestion in the mouth and small intestine, the body breaks down starches and disaccharides into monosaccharides, such as **glucose,** for absorption into the bloodstream. Once the glucose is absorbed, cells take it up and use it for energy. The liver and muscles also take up glucose and store it in the form of a starch called **glycogen.** The muscles use glycogen as fuel during endurance events or long workouts. Carbohydrates consumed in excess of the body's energy needs are changed into fat and stored. Whenever calorie intake exceeds calorie expenditure, fat storage can lead to weight gain. This is true whether the excess calories come from carbohydrates, proteins, fat, or alcohol.

Recommended Carbohydrate Intake On average, Americans consume over 250 grams of carbohydrates per day, well above the minimum of 50–100 grams of essential carbohydrate required by the body. However, health experts recommend that Americans increase their consumption of carbohydrates—particularly complex carbohydrates—to 55% of total daily calories.

Experts also recommend that Americans alter the proportion of simple and complex carbohydrates in the diet, lowering simple carbohydrate intake from 25% to 15% or less of total daily calories. To accomplish this change, reduce your intake of foods like candy, sweet desserts, soft

TERMS **monosaccharide** A simple carbohydrate consisting of one sugar molecule.

disaccharide A simple carbohydrate consisting of two single-sugar molecules (monosaccharides) linked together.

polysaccharide A complex carbohydrate composed of many sugar molecules (monosaccharides) linked together.

legumes Vegetables such as peas and beans that are high in fiber and are also important sources of protein; examples include pinto beans, kidney beans, chickpeas, black-eyed peas, and soybeans.

glucose A simple sugar that is the body's basic fuel.

glycogen A complex carbohydrate stored principally in the liver and skeletal muscles; the major fuel source during most forms of exercise.

dietary fiber Carbohydrates and other substances in plants that are difficult or impossible for humans to digest.

soluble fiber Dietary fiber that dissolves in water or is broken down by bacteria in the large intestine. It tends to absorb cholesterol-containing compounds in the intestine.

insoluble fiber Fiber that does not dissolve in water and is not broken down by bacteria in the large intestine; it binds water and increases bulk in the stool.

Our bodies require adequate amounts of all essential nutrients—water, proteins, carbohydrates, fats, vitamins, and minerals—in order to grow and function properly. Choosing foods to satisfy these nutritional requirements is an important part of a healthy lifestyle.

drinks, and sweetened fruit drinks, which are high in simple sugars but low in other nutrients. The bulk of the simple carbohydrates in your diet should come from fruits, which are excellent sources of vitamins and minerals, and milk, which is high in protein and calcium. Instead of prepared foods high in added sugars, choose a variety of foods rich in complex, unrefined carbohydrates.

Athletes in training can especially benefit from high-carbohydrate diets (60–70% of total daily calories), which enhance the amount of carbohydrates stored in their muscles (as glycogen) and therefore provide more carbohydrate fuel for use during endurance events or long workouts. In addition, carbohydrates consumed during prolonged athletic events can help fuel muscles and extend the availability of the glycogen stored in muscles. (For more on the special nutritional needs of athletes, see pp. 209–210.)

Dietary Fiber   **Dietary fiber** consists of carbohydrate plant substances that are difficult or impossible for humans to digest. Instead, fiber passes through the intestinal tract and provides bulk for feces in the large intestine, which in turn facilitates elimination. In the large intestine, some types of fiber are broken down by bacteria into acids and gases, which explains why consuming too much fiber can lead to intestinal gas. Because humans cannot digest dietary fiber, fiber is not a source of carbohydrate in the diet; however, the consumption of dietary fiber is necessary for good health.

Nutritionists classify dietary fiber as soluble or insoluble. **Soluble fiber** slows the body's absorption of glucose and binds cholesterol-containing compounds in the intestine, lowering blood cholesterol levels and reducing the risk of cardiovascular disease. **Insoluble fiber** binds water, making the feces bulkier and softer so they pass more quickly and easily through the intestines.

Both kinds of fiber contribute to disease prevention. A diet high in soluble fiber can help people manage diabetes and high blood cholesterol levels. A diet high in insoluble fiber can help prevent a variety of health problems, including constipation, hemorrhoids, and diverticulitis (a painful condition in which abnormal pouches form and become inflamed in the wall of the large intestine). Some studies have linked high levels of insoluble fiber in the diet with a decreased incidence of colon and rectal cancer; conversely, a low-fiber diet may increase the risk of colon cancer. There is even some evidence that high levels of insoluble fiber can suppress and reverse precancerous changes that can lead to colon and rectal cancer.

All plant foods contain some dietary fiber, but fruits, legumes, oats (especially oat bran), barley, and psyllium (found in some laxatives) are particularly rich in it. Wheat (especially wheat bran), cereals, grains, and vegetables are all good sources of insoluble fiber (see Table 8-2). However, the processing of packaged foods can remove fiber, so it's important to depend on fresh fruits and vegetables and foods made from whole (unrefined) grains as sources of dietary fiber.

Although it is not yet clear precisely how much and what types of fiber are ideal, most experts believe the average American would benefit from an increase in daily fiber intake. Currently, most Americans consume about 15 grams of fiber a day, whereas the recommended daily amount is 20–35 grams of food fiber—not from supplements, which should be taken only under medical supervision. However, too much fiber—more than 40–60 grams a day—can cause health problems, such as overlarge stools or the malabsorption of important minerals. In fiber intake, as in all aspects of nutrition, balance and moderation are key principles.

To increase the amount of fiber in your diet, try the following:

TABLE 8-2	Foods High in Fiber	
Food Item	Serving Size	Fiber (g)
Fruits		
Apple, with skin	1	4.0
Apricot, with skin	3	2.0
Avocado	¼ cup	2.7
Banana	1	2.3
Cantaloupe	½	2.0
Dried fruit	¼ cup	2.4
Kiwi	1	2.1
Nectarine	1	3.3
Orange	1	3.8
Pear	1	4.8
Prunes, uncooked	5	3.9
Raisins	¼ cup	2.5
Raspberries	½ cup	3.0
*Grains and Cereals**		
Bread, mixed-grain	1 slice	1.4
Bread, whole-wheat	1 slice	2.5
Oatmeal, cooked	⅔ cup	3.0
Pasta, whole-wheat, cooked	½ cup	3.0
Rice, brown, cooked	½ cup	1.8
Legumes		
Kidney beans, cooked	½ cup	4.6
Lima beans, cooked	½ cup	4.3
Pinto beans, cooked	½ cup	4.3
Tofu	½ cup	1.5
Vegetables		
Artichoke, cooked	1	4.0
Beans, green, cooked	½ cup	2.0
Beets, cooked	½ cup	2.5
Broccoli, cooked	½ cup	2.1
Brussels sprouts, cooked	½ cup	2.2
Carrot, raw	½ cup	2.2
Corn, cooked	½ cup	4.6
Eggplant, cooked	1 cup	2.0
Peas, green, cooked	½ cup	3.5
Potato, baked, with skin	1	5.0
Spinach, cooked	½ cup	3.5
Squash, winter, cooked	½ cup	3.0
Sweet potato, cooked	½ cup	4.0
Tomato, medium	1	1.8

*Many breakfast cereals contain significant amounts of dietary fiber (2–5 grams per serving). Check the labels for exact amounts.

- Choose whole-grain bread instead of white bread, brown rice instead of white rice, and whole-wheat pasta instead of regular pasta. Select high-fiber breakfast cereals. Look for breads, crackers, and cereals that list a whole grain first in the ingredient list: Whole-wheat flour, whole-grain oats, and whole-grain rice are whole grains; wheat flour is not.
- Eat whole fruits rather than drinking fruit juice. Top cereals, yogurt, and desserts with berries, apple slices, or other fruit.
- Include beans in soups and salads. Prepare salads that combine raw vegetables with pasta, rice, or beans.
- Substitute bean dip for cheese-based or sour cream–based dips or spreads. Use raw vegetables rather than chips for dipping.

Vitamins

Vitamins are organic (carbon-containing) substances required in very small amounts to promote specific chemical reactions within living cells (Table 8-3). Humans need 13 vitamins. Four are fat-soluble (A, D, E, and K), and nine are water-soluble (C and the eight B-complex vitamins: thiamin, riboflavin, niacin, vitamin B-6, folate, vitamin B-12, biotin, and pantothenic acid). Solubility affects how a vitamin is absorbed, transported, and stored in the body. The water-soluble vitamins are absorbed directly into the bloodstream, where they travel freely; excess water-soluble vitamins are detected by the kidneys and excreted in urine. Fat-soluble vitamins require a more complex digestive process; they are usually carried in the blood by special proteins and are stored in the body in fat tissues rather than excreted.

Functions of Vitamins Vitamins help chemical reactions take place. They provide no energy to the body directly but help unleash the energy stored in carbohydrates, proteins, and fats. Vitamins are critical in the production of red blood cells and the maintenance of the nervous, skeletal, and immune systems. Some vitamins also form substances that act as **antioxidants,** which help preserve healthy cells in the body. Key vitamin antioxidants include vitamin E, vitamin C, and the vitamin A derivative beta-carotene. (The actions of antioxidants will be described later in the chapter.)

Sources of Vitamins The human body does not manufacture most of the vitamins it requires and must obtain them from foods. Vitamins are abundant in fruits, vegetables, and grains. In addition, many processed foods, such as flour and breakfast cereals, are enriched with certain vitamins during the manufacturing process. On the other hand, both vitamins and minerals can be lost or destroyed during the storage and cooking of foods. For tips on

| TABLE 8-3 | *Facts About Vitamins* | | | |

Vitamin	Important Dietary Sources	Major Functions	Signs of Prolonged Deficiency	Toxic Effects of Megadoses
Fat-Soluble				
Vitamin A	Liver, milk, butter, cheese, and fortified margarine; carrots, spinach, and other orange and deep-green vegetables and fruits	Maintenance of vision, skin, linings of the nose, mouth, digestive and urinary tracts, immune function	Night blindness; dry, scaling skin; increased susceptibility to infection; loss of appetite; anemia; kidney stones	Headache, vomiting and diarrhea, vertigo, double vision, bone abnormalities, liver damage, miscarriage and birth defects
Vitamin D	Fortified milk and margarine, fish liver oils, butter, egg yolks (sunlight on skin also produces vitamin D)	Development and maintenance of bones and teeth, promotion of calcium absorption	Rickets (bone deformities) in children; bone softening, loss, and fractures in adults	Kidney damage, calcium deposits in soft tissues, depression, death
Vitamin E	Vegetable oils, whole grains, nuts and seeds, green leafy vegetables, asparagus, peaches	Protection and maintenance of cellular membranes	Red blood cell breakage and anemia, weakness, neurological problems, muscle cramps	Relatively nontoxic, but may cause excess bleeding or formation of blood clots
Vitamin K	Green leafy vegetables; smaller amounts widespread in other foods	Production of factors essential for blood clotting	Hemorrhaging	None observed
Water-Soluble				
Vitamin C	Peppers, broccoli, spinach, brussels sprouts, citrus fruits, strawberries, tomatoes, potatoes, cabbage, other fruits and vegetables	Maintenance and repair of connective tissue, bones, teeth, and cartilage; promotion of healing; aid in iron absorption	Scurvy, anemia, reduced resistance to infection, loosened teeth, joint pain, poor wound healing, hair loss, poor iron absorption	Urinary stones in some people, acid stomach from ingesting supplements in pill form, nausea, diarrhea, headache, fatigue
Thiamin	Whole-grain and enriched breads and cereals, organ meats, lean pork, nuts, legumes	Conversion of carbohydrates into usable forms of energy, maintenance of appetite and nervous system function	Beriberi (symptoms include muscle wasting, mental confusion, anorexia, enlarged heart, abnormal heart rhythm, nerve changes)	None reported
Riboflavin	Dairy products, enriched breads and cereals, lean meats, poultry, fish, green vegetables	Energy metabolism; maintenance of skin, mucous membranes, and nervous system structures	Cracks at corners of mouth, sore throat, skin rash, hypersensitivity to light, purple tongue	None reported
Niacin	Eggs, poultry, fish, milk, whole grains, nuts, enriched breads and cereals, meats, legumes	Conversion of carbohydrates, fats, and protein into usable forms of energy	Pellagra (symptoms include diarrhea, dermatitis, inflammation of mucous membranes, dementia)	Flushing of the skin, nausea, vomiting, diarrhea, liver dysfunction, glucose intolerance
Vitamin B-6	Eggs, poultry, fish, whole grains, nuts, soybeans, liver, kidney, pork	Protein and neurotransmitter metabolism; red blood cell synthesis	Anemia, convulsions, cracks at corners of mouth, dermatitis, nausea, confusion	Neurological abnormalities and damage
Folate	Green leafy vegetables, yeast, oranges, whole grains, legumes, liver	Amino acid metabolism, synthesis of RNA and DNA, new cell synthesis	Anemia, weakness, fatigue, irritability, shortness of breath, swollen tongue	Masking of vitamin B-12 deficiency
Vitamin B-12	Eggs, milk, meats, other animal foods	Synthesis of red and white blood cells; other metabolic reactions	Anemia, fatigue, nervous system damage, sore tongue	None reported
Biotin	Cereals, yeast, egg yolks, soy flour, liver; widespread in foods	Metabolism of fats, carbohydrates, and proteins	Rash, nausea, vomiting, weight loss, depression, fatigue, hair loss	None reported
Pantothenic acid	Animal foods, whole grains, legumes; widespread in foods	Metabolism of fats, carbohydrates, and proteins	Fatigue, numbness and tingling of hands and feet, gastrointestinal disturbances	None reported

SOURCES: Food and Nutrition Board. 1998. *Dietary Reference Intakes for Thiamin, Riboflavin, Niacin, Vitamin B₆, Folate, Vitamin B₁₂, Pantothenic Acid, and Choline.* Washington, D.C.: National Academy Press. National Research Council. 1989. *Recommended Dietary Allowances,* 10th ed. Washington, D.C.: National Academy Press. Copyright © 1989 by the National Academy of Sciences. Adapted with permission from the National Academy Press, Washington, D.C. Shils, M. E., and V. R. Young, eds. 1993. *Modern Nutrition in Health and Disease,* 8th ed. Baltimore: Williams & Wilkins.

1. *Consume or process vegetables immediately after purchasing (or harvesting).* The longer vegetables are kept before they are eaten or processed, the more vitamins are lost.

2. *Store vegetables and fruits properly.* If you can't eat fruits and vegetables immediately after purchasing (or harvesting) but plan to do so within a few days, keep them in the refrigerator. Place them in covered containers or plastic bags to minimize moisture loss. Freezing is the best method for longer-term preservation.

3. *Minimize the preparation and cooking of vegetables and other foods.* The more preparation and cooking of foods that is done before eating, the greater the nutrient loss. To reduce the losses:

   • When possible, cook vegetables, such as potatoes, in their skins.

• Don't soak and rinse rice before cooking.

• Cook in as little water as possible.

• Don't add baking soda to vegetables to enhance the green color.

• Bake, steam, broil, or microwave vegetables.

• When boiling, use tight-fitting lids to minimize evaporation of water.

• Cook vegetables as little as possible. Develop a taste for a more crunchy texture.

• Don't thaw frozen vegetables before cooking.

• Prepare lettuce salads right before eating.

---

minimizing such losses, see the box "Keeping the Nutrient Value in Food."

A few vitamins are made in certain parts of the body: The skin makes vitamin D when it is exposed to sunlight, and intestinal bacteria make biotin and vitamin K.

Vitamin Deficiencies and Excesses

If your diet lacks sufficient amounts of a particular vitamin, characteristic symptoms of deficiency develop (see Table 8-3). For example, vitamin A deficiency can cause blindness and vitamin B-6 deficiency can cause seizures. Vitamin deficiency diseases are most often seen in developing countries; they are relatively rare in the United States because vitamins are readily available from our food supply. However, intakes below recommended levels can have adverse effects on health even if they are not low enough to cause a deficiency disease. For example, low intake of folate increases a woman's chance of giving birth to a baby with a neural tube defect (a congenital malformation of the central nervous system).

Extra vitamins in the diet can be harmful, especially when taken as supplements. High doses of vitamin A are toxic and increase the risk of birth defects, for example. Vitamin B-6 can cause irreversible nerve damage when taken in large doses. Megadoses of fat-soluble vitamins are particularly dangerous because the excess will be stored in the body rather than excreted, increasing the risk of toxicity. Even when not taken in excess, relying on supplements for an adequate intake of vitamins can be a problem: There are many substances in foods other than vitamins and minerals, and some of these compounds may have important health effects. Later in the chapter we will discuss specific recommendations for vitamin intake and when a supplement is advisable. For now, keep in mind that it's best to obtain most of your vitamins from foods rather than supplements.

Minerals

Minerals are inorganic (non-carbon-containing) compounds you need in relatively small amounts to help regulate body functions, aid in the growth and maintenance of body tissues, and help release energy (Table 8-4). There are about 17 essential minerals. The major minerals, those that the body needs in amounts exceeding 100 milligrams, include calcium, phosphorus, magnesium, sodium, potassium, and chloride. The essential trace minerals, those that you need in minute amounts, include copper, fluoride, iodide, iron, selenium, and zinc.

Characteristic symptoms develop if an essential mineral is consumed in a quantity too small or too large for good health. The minerals most commonly lacking in the American diet are iron, calcium, zinc, and magnesium. Focus on good food choices for these nutrients (see Table 8-4). Lean meats are rich in iron and zinc, while low-fat or nonfat dairy products are excellent choices for calcium. Plant foods are good sources of magnesium. Iron-deficiency **anemia** is a problem in some age groups, and researchers fear poor calcium intakes are sowing the seeds for future **osteoporosis,** especially in women. See the box "Osteoporosis" to learn more.

Water

Water is the major component in both foods and the human body: You are composed of about 60% water. Your need for other nutrients, in terms of weight, is much less than your need for water. You can live up to 50 days without food, but only a few days without water.

Water is distributed all over the body, among lean and other tissues and in urine and other body fluids. Water is used in the digestion and absorption of food and is the medium in which most of the chemical reactions take place within the body. Some water-based fluids like blood

TABLE 8-4 *Facts About Selected Minerals*

Mineral	Important Dietary Sources	Major Functions	Signs of Prolonged Deficiency	Toxic Effects of Megadoses
Calcium	Milk and milk products, tofu, fortified orange juice and bread, green leafy vegetables, bones in fish	Maintenance of bones and teeth, control of nerve impulses and muscle contraction	Stunted growth in children, bone mineral loss in adults	Constipation, urinary stones, calcium deposits in soft tissues, inhibition of mineral absorption
Fluoride	Fluoride-containing drinking water, tea, marine fish eaten with bones	Maintenance of tooth (and possibly bone) structure	Higher frequency of tooth decay	Increased bone density, mottling of teeth, impaired kidney function
Iron	Meat, legumes, eggs, enriched flour, green vegetables, dried fruit, liver	Component of hemoglobin, muscle fiber, and enzymes	Iron-deficiency anemia, weakness, impaired immune function, gastrointestinal distress	Liver and kidney damage, joint pains, sterility, disruption of cardiac function, death
Iodine	Iodized salt, seafood	Essential part of thyroid hormones, regulation of body metabolism	Goiter (enlarged thyroid), cretinism (birth defect)	Depression of thyroid activity, hyperthyroidism in susceptible people
Magnesium	Widespread in foods and water (except soft water); especially found in grains, legumes, nuts, seeds, green vegetables	Transmission of nerve impulses, energy transfer, activation of many enzymes	Neurological disturbances, cardiovascular problems, kidney disorders, nausea, growth failure in children	Nausea, vomiting, diarrhea, central nervous system depression, coma; death in people with impaired kidney function
Phosphorus	Present in nearly all foods, especially milk, cereal, legumes, meat, poultry, fish	Bone growth and maintenance, energy transfer in cells	Weakness, bone loss, kidney disorders, cardiorespiratory failure	Drop in blood calcium levels, calcium deposits in soft tissues
Potassium	Meats, milk, fruits, vegetables, grains, legumes	Nerve function and body water balance	Muscular weakness, nausea, drowsiness, paralysis, confusion, disruption of cardiac rhythm	Cardiac arrest
Selenium	Seafood, meat, eggs, whole grains	Protection of cells from oxidative damage, immune response	Muscle pain and weakness, heart disorders	Hair loss, nausea and vomiting, weakness, irritability
Sodium	Salt, soy sauce, salted foods	Body water balance, acid-base balance, nerve function	Muscle weakness, loss of appetite, nausea, vomiting; sodium deficiency is rarely seen	Edema, hypertension in sensitive people
Zinc	Whole grains, meat, eggs, liver, seafood (especially oysters)	Synthesis of proteins, RNA, and DNA; wound healing; immune response; ability to taste	Growth failure, loss of appetite, impaired taste acuity, skin rash, impaired immune function, poor wound healing	Vomiting, impaired immune function, decline in blood HDL levels, impaired copper absorption

SOURCES: Food and Nutrition Board. 1997. Dietary Reference Intakes for Calcium, Phosphorus, Magnesium, Vitamin D, and Fluoride. Washington, D.C.: National Academy Press. National Research Council. 1989. *Recommended Dietary Allowances*, 10th ed. Washington, D.C.: National Academy Press. Copyright © 1989 by the National Academy of Sciences. Reprinted with permission from National Academy Press, Washington, D.C. Shils, M. E., and V. R. Young, eds. 1993. *Modern Nutrition in Health and Disease*, 8th ed. Baltimore: Williams & Wilkins.

transport substances around the body, while other fluids serve as lubricants or cushions. Water also helps regulate body temperature.

Water is contained in almost all foods, particularly in liquids, fruits, and vegetables. The foods and fluids you consume provide 80–90% of your daily water intake; the remainder is generated through metabolism. You lose water each day in urine, feces, and sweat and through

TERMS

minerals Inorganic compounds needed in relatively small amounts for regulation, growth, and maintenance of body tissues and functions.

anemia A deficiency in the oxygen-carrying material in the red blood cells.

osteoporosis A condition in which the bones become extremely thin and brittle; fractures of the wrist, spine, and hip commonly result.

Osteoporosis is a condition in which the bones become dangerously thin and fragile over time. It currently afflicts some 25 million Americans, 80% of them women, and results in 1.5 million bone fractures each year. The incidence of osteoporosis may double in the next 25 years as the population ages.

The bones in your body are continually being broken down and rebuilt in order to adapt to mechanical strain. About 20% of your body's bone mass is replaced each year. In the first few decades of life, bones become thicker and stronger as they are rebuilt. Most of your bone mass (95%) is built by age 18. After bone mass peaks between the ages of 25 and 35, the rate of bone loss exceeds the rate of replacement, and bones become less dense. In osteoporosis, this loss of density becomes so severe that bones become very fragile.

Fractures are the most serious consequences of osteoporosis; up to 25% of all people who suffer a hip fracture die within a year. Other problems associated with osteoporosis are loss of height and a stooped posture caused by vertebral fractures, severe back and hip pain, and breathing problems caused by changes in the shape of the skeleton.

Who Is at Risk?

Women are at greater risk than men for osteoporosis because they have 10–25% less bone in their skeleton. As they lose bone mass with age, women's bones become dangerously thin sooner than men's bones. More men will probably develop osteoporosis in the future as they live into their eighties and nineties. Bone loss accelerates in women during the first 5–10 years after the onset of menopause because of a drop in estrogen production. (Estrogen improves calcium absorption and reduces the amount of calcium the body excretes.)

Other risk factors for osteoporosis include a family history of osteoporosis, early menopause (before age 45), abnormal menstruation, a history of anorexia, a thin, small frame, and European or Asian background. Certain medications can also have a negative impact on bone mass, including thyroid medication and high doses of cortisonelike drugs for asthma or arthritis.

What Can You Do?

To prevent osteoporosis, the best strategy is to build as much bone as possible during your young years and then do everything you can to maintain it as you age. Up to 50% of bone loss is determined by controllable lifestyle factors.

- *Ensure an adequate intake of calcium.* Consuming an adequate amount of calcium is important throughout life to build and maintain bone mass. Americans consume an average of 400–600 mg of calcium per day, less than half of what is currently recommended. Milk, yogurt, and calcium-fortified orange juice, bread, and cereals are all good sources. Nutritionists suggest that you obtain calcium from foods first and then take supplements only if needed to make up the difference.

- *Ensure an adequate intake of vitamin D.* Vitamin D is necessary for bones to absorb calcium. It can be obtained from food (milk and fortified cereals, for example) and is manufactured by the skin when it is exposed to sunlight. Candidates for vitamin D supplements include people who don't eat many foods rich in vitamin D; those who don't expose their face, arms, and hands to the sun (without sunscreen) for 5–15 minutes each day; and people who live north of an imaginary line roughly between Boston and the Oregon-California border (the sun is weaker in northern latitudes). Many calcium supplements also contain vitamin D.

- *Exercise.* Weight-bearing aerobic activities help build and maintain bone mass throughout life, but they must be performed 5–15 minutes each day in order to have lasting effects. Strength training is also helpful: It improves bone density, muscle mass, strength, and balance, protecting against both bone loss and falls, a major cause of fractures.

- *Don't smoke.* Smoking reduces the body's estrogen levels and is linked to earlier menopause and more rapid post-menopausal bone loss.

- *Drink alcohol only in moderation.* Alcohol reduces the body's ability to absorb calcium and may interfere with estrogen's bone-protecting effects.

- *Monitor your consumption of caffeine.* The association between caffeine-containing beverages and osteoporosis isn't clear, but researchers recommend that heavy caffeine consumers take special care to include calcium-rich foods in their diet because calcium may counterbalance any caffeine-linked drop in bone mass.

- *Be moderate in your consumption of protein and sodium.* A high intake of protein and sodium has been shown to increase calcium loss in the urine and may lead to loss of calcium from the skeleton.

- *Manage depression and stress.* Some women who have depression experience significant bone loss that may increase their risk of fractures. Researchers haven't identified the mechanism, but it may be linked to increases in the stress hormone cortisol.

- *After menopause, consider hormone replacement therapy (HRT) or another drug treatment.* HRT combats bone loss as well as menopausal symptoms and heart disease. However, it is not without side effects and risks. A physician can review your risk factors and test your bone density to help you decide whether HRT is a wise choice for you. Other drug treatments include alendronate (Fosamax) and calcitonin (Miacalcin), which slow the resorption of bone by the body, and fluoride, which helps build bone in women who already have osteoporosis.

Scientists recently discovered a gene linked to bone density, so a test to identify people at high risk for osteoporosis may become available in the future. Although not helpful in treating the condition, such a test could alert those at greater risk.

evaporation in your lungs. To maintain a balance between water consumed and water lost, you need to take in about 1 milliliter of water for each calorie you burn—about 2 liters, or 8 cups, of fluid per day—more if you live in a hot climate or engage in vigorous exercise.

Thirst is one of the body's first signs of dehydration that we can actually recognize. However, by the time we are actually thirsty, our cells have been needing fluid for quite some time. A good motto to remember, especially when exercising, is: Drink *before* you're thirsty. If the thirst mechanism is faulty, as it may be during illness or vigorous exercise, hormonal mechanisms can help conserve water by reducing the output of urine. Severe dehydration causes weakness and can lead to death.

Other Substances in Food

There are many substances in food that are not essential nutrients but which may influence health.

Antioxidants When the body uses oxygen or breaks down certain fats as a normal part of metabolism, it gives rise to substances called **free radicals.** Environmental factors such as cigarette smoke, exhaust fumes, radiation, excessive sunlight, certain drugs, and stress can increase free radical production. A free radical is a chemically unstable molecule that is missing an electron; it will react with any molecule it encounters from which it can take an electron. In their search for electrons, free radicals react with fats, proteins, and DNA, damaging cell membranes and mutating genes. Because of this, free radicals have been implicated in aging, cancer, cardiovascular disease, and degenerative diseases like arthritis.

Antioxidants found in foods can help rid the body of free radicals, thereby protecting cells. Antioxidants react with free radicals and donate electrons, rendering them harmless. Some antioxidants, such as vitamin C, vitamin E, and selenium, are also essential nutrients; others, such as flavonoids, found in citrus fruits, are not. Obtaining a regular intake of these nutrients is vital for maintaining health. Many fruits and vegetables are rich in antioxidants.

Phytochemicals Antioxidants are a particular type of **phytochemical,** a substance found in plant foods that may help prevent chronic disease. Researchers have just begun to identify and study all the different compounds found in foods, and many preliminary findings are promising. For example, certain proteins found in soy foods may help lower cholesterol levels. Sulforaphane, a compound isolated from broccoli and other cruciferous vegetables, may render some carcinogenic compounds harmless. Allyl sulfides, a group of chemicals found in garlic and onions, appear to boost the activity of cancer-fighting immune cells. Further research on phytochemicals may extend the role of nutrition to the prevention and treatment of many chronic diseases.

If you want to increase your intake of phytochemicals, it is best to obtain them by eating a variety of fruits and vegetables rather than relying on supplements. Like many vitamins and minerals, isolated phytochemicals may be harmful if taken in high doses. In addition, it is likely that their health benefits are the result of chemical substances working in combination. The role of phytochemicals in disease prevention and strategies for increasing your intake of phytochemicals are discussed in Chapters 11 and 12.

NUTRITIONAL GUIDELINES

The second part of putting together a healthy food plan—after you've learned about necessary nutrients—is choosing foods that satisfy nutritional requirements and meet your personal criteria. Various tools have been created by scientific and government groups to help people design healthy diets. The **Recommended Dietary Allowances (RDAs), Dietary Reference Intakes (DRIs),** and related guidelines are standards for nutrient intake designed to prevent nutritional deficiencies and reduce the risk of chronic disease. The **Food Guide Pyramid** translates these nutrient recommendations into a balanced food group plan that includes all essential nutrients. To provide further guidance, **Dietary Guidelines for Americans** have been established to address the

TERMS

free radical An electron-seeking compound that can react with fats, proteins, and DNA, damaging cell membranes and mutating genes in its search for electrons; produced through chemical reactions in the body and by exposure to environmental factors such as sunlight and tobacco smoke.

phytochemical A naturally occurring substance found in plant foods that may help prevent and treat chronic diseases such as heart disease and cancer; *phyto* means plant.

Recommended Dietary Allowances (RDAs) Amounts of certain nutrients considered adequate to prevent deficiencies in most healthy people; will eventually be replaced by the Dietary Reference Intakes (DRIs).

Dietary Reference Intakes (DRIs) An umbrella term for four types of nutrient standards: Adequate Intake (AI), Estimated Average Requirement (EAR), and Recommended Dietary Allowance (RDA) set levels of intake considered adequate to prevent nutrient deficiencies and reduce the risk of chronic disease; Tolerable Upper Intake Level (UL) sets the maximum daily intake that is unlikely to cause health problems.

Food Guide Pyramid A food group plan that provides practical advice to ensure a balanced intake of the essential nutrients.

Dietary Guidelines for Americans General principles of good nutrition provided by the U.S. Department of Agriculture and the U.S. Department of Health and Human Services.

prevention of diet-related chronic diseases. Together, these tools make up a complete set of resources for dietary planning.

Recommended Dietary Allowances (RDAs) and Dietary Reference Intakes (DRIs)

The Food and Nutrition Board of the National Academy of Sciences establishes the RDAs, DRIs, and related guidelines. The RDAs were developed as standards to prevent nutritional deficiency diseases such as rickets, scurvy, and anemia (see Tables 8-3 and 8-4). First published in 1941, the RDAs have been updated periodically to keep pace with new research findings; the most recent version was published in 1989. RDAs include intake recommendations for individual nutrients in one of three categories: (1) the RDAs themselves, which give specific recommended intakes of nutrients that are well known and well researched; (2) the Estimated Safe and Adequate Daily Dietary Intakes (ESADDIs), which provide a range of values for nutrients about which our knowledge is still sketchy; and (3) Estimated Minimum Requirements, which provide minimum values for three minerals.

Scientific knowledge about nutrition has increased dramatically since the inception of the RDAs, and current research focuses not just on the prevention of nutrient deficiencies but also on the role of nutrients in preventing chronic diseases such as osteoporosis, cancer, and cardiovascular disease. This expanded focus is the basis for the development of a new system of recommendations, the Dietary Reference Intakes. The DRIs, which will eventually replace the RDAs, include standards for both recommended intakes and maximum safe intakes.

- Recommended nutrient intakes can be expressed as three different types of standards—Adequate Intake (AI), Estimated Average Requirement (EAR), and Recommended Dietary Allowance (RDA). The type of standard used for a particular nutrient or age group depends on the amount of scientific information available and the intended use of the standard. Regardless of the type of standard attached to a particular nutrient, the DRI represents the best available estimate of intake for optimal health.

- Maximum intake level guidelines are expressed as the Tolerable Upper Intake Level (UL), the maximum daily intake by a healthy person that is unlikely to cause health problems. Because of lack of suitable data, ULs have not been established for all nutrients. This does not mean that people can tolerate chronic intakes of these vitamins above recommended levels. Like all chemical agents, nutrients can produce adverse effects if intakes are excessive; when data are limited, extra caution may be warranted. There is no established benefit from consuming nutrients at levels above the AI or RDA.

The DRIs are being issued in stages, and they have not yet been established for all vitamins and minerals. Table 8-5 is an abridged version of the 1989 RDAs; it includes nutrients for which DRIs have not yet been set. Table 8-6 gives recommended intakes for the vitamins and minerals for which DRIs have been set. Table 8-7 lists the upper intake levels for adults; as described earlier, ULs have not been established for all nutrients.

Should You Take Supplements?   The aim of the RDAs and DRIs is to guide you in meeting your nutritional needs primarily with food, rather than with vitamin and mineral supplements. This goal is important because recommendations have not yet been set for some essential nutrients. Many supplements contain only nutrients with established recommendations, so using them to meet nutrient needs can leave you deficient in other nutrients. Supplements also lack potentially beneficial phytochemicals that are found only in whole foods. Nutrition scientists generally agree that most Americans can obtain most of the vitamins and minerals they need to prevent deficiencies by consuming a varied, nutritionally balanced diet. Ongoing research is examining whether supplements of particular vitamins and minerals should be recommended for their potential disease-fighting properties, as for the antioxidant vitamins C and E.

The question of whether or not to take supplements is a serious one. Some vitamins and minerals are dangerous when ingested in excess, as shown in Tables 8-3 and 8-4. Large doses of particular nutrients can also cause health problems by affecting the absorption of other vitamins and minerals. For all these reasons, you should think carefully about whether or not to take supplements; consider consulting a physician or registered dietitian.

In 1998, the Food and Nutrition Board of the National Academy of Sciences recommended supplements of particular nutrients for the following groups:

- Women who are capable of becoming pregnant should take 400 μg per day of folic acid from fortified foods and/or supplements in addition to folate from a varied diet. Research indicates that this level of folate intake will reduce the risk of neural tube defects. (This defect occurs early in pregnancy, before most women know they are pregnant; therefore, the recommendation for folate intake applies to all women of reproductive age rather than only to pregnant women.) Since 1998, enriched breads, flours, corn meals, rice, noodles, and other grain products have been fortified with small amounts of folic acid. Folate is found naturally in leafy green vegetables, legumes, citrus fruits and juices, and most berries.

- People over age 50 should consume foods fortified with vitamin B-12, B-12 supplements, or a combination of the two in order to meet the majority of the

TABLE 8-5 — Recommended Dietary Allowances, Revised 1989[a,b,c] (Abridged)

Category	Age (years) or Condition	Protein (g/kg)[d]	Vitamin A (μg RE)[e]	Vitamin E (mg α-TE)[f]	Vitamin K (μg)	Vitamin C (mg)	Iron (mg)	Zinc (mg)	Iodine (μg)	Selenium (μg)
Infants	0.0–0.5	2.2	375	3	5	30	6	5	40	10
	0.5–1.0	1.6	375	4	10	35	10	5	50	15
Children	1–3	1.2	400	6	15	40	10	10	70	20
	4–6	1.1	500	7	20	45	10	10	90	20
	7–10	1.0	700	7	30	45	10	10	120	30
Males	11–14	1.0	1000	10	45	50	12	15	150	40
	15–18	0.9	1000	10	65	60	12	15	150	50
	19–24	0.8	1000	10	70	60	10	15	150	70
	25–50	0.8	1000	10	80	60	10	15	150	70
	51+	0.8	1000	10	80	60	10	15	150	70
Females	11–14	1.0	800	8	45	50	15	12	150	45
	15–18	0.8	800	8	55	60	15	12	150	50
	19–24	0.8	800	8	60	60	15	12	150	55
	25–50	0.8	800	8	65	60	15	12	150	55
	51+	0.8	800	8	65	60	10	12	150	55
Pregnant		+10g	800	10	65	70	30	15	175	65
Lactating	1st 6 Months	+15g	1300	12	65	95	15	19	200	75
	2nd 6 Months	+12g	1200	11	65	90	15	16	200	75

[a]This table includes RDAs for those nutrients for which DRIs had not yet been established as of June 1998. The allowances, expressed as average daily intakes over time, are intended to provide for individual variations among most normal people as they live in the United States under usual environmental stresses. Diet should be based on a variety of common foods in order to provide other nutrients for which human requirements have been less well defined.

[b]Estimated Safe and Adequate Daily Dietary Intakes (ESADDIs) for adults: 1.5–3.0 mg copper; 2.0–5.0 mg manganese; 50–200 μg chromium; 75–250 mg molybdenum. (For information on other age groups, see National Research Council. 1989. Recommended Dietary Allowances, 10th ed. Washington, D.C.: National Academy Press.)

[c]Estimated Minimum Requirements of healthy adults: 500 mg sodium; 750 mg chloride; 2000 mg potassium. (For information on other age groups, see Recommended Dietary Allowances, 10th ed.)

[d]The RDA for protein is expressed as grams of protein per kilogram of body weight. To calculate the RDA, multiply body weight in kilograms (1 kilogram = 2.2 pounds) by the appropriate number from the protein column. For example, a 19-year-old male who weighs 165 pounds would calculate his protein RDA as follows: 165 lb ÷ 2.2 kg/lb = 75 kg × 0.8 g/kg (from table) = 60 g protein per day. For pregnant or lactating women, calculate RDA based on age and then add the appropriate number of additional grams listed in the table.

[e]Retinol equivalents: 1 retinol equivalent = 1 μg retinol or 6 μg β-carotene.

[f]α-Tocopherol equivalents: 1 mg d-α tocopherol = 1 α-TE.

SOURCE: Reprinted with permission from Recommended Dietary Allowances: 10th Edition. Copyright © 1989 by the National Academy of Sciences. Courtesy of the National Academy Press, Washington, D.C.

DRI of 2.4 mg of B-12 daily. Up to 30% of people over 50 may have problems absorbing vitamin B-12; the consumption of supplements and fortified foods can overcome this problem and help prevent a deficiency.

Supplements may also be recommended in the following cases:

- Women with heavy menstrual flows may need extra iron to compensate for the monthly loss.
- Some vegetarians may need extra calcium, iron, zinc, and vitamin B-12.
- Newborns need a single dose of vitamin K, which must be administered under the direction of a physician.
- People who are unable to consume adequate calories may need a range of vitamins and minerals.
- People who have certain diseases or who take certain medications may need specific vitamin and mineral supplements. Such supplement decisions must be made by a physician because some vitamins and minerals counteract the actions of certain medications.

In deciding whether to take a vitamin and mineral supplement, consider whether you already regularly consume

TABLE 8-6

Dietary Reference Intakes (DRIs): Recommended Levels for Individual Intake

Life Stage	Group	Calcium (mg/day)	Phosphorus (mg/day)	Magnesium (mg/day)	Vitamin D (μg/day)[a,b]	Fluoride (mg/day)	Thiamin (mg/day)	Riboflavin (mg/day)
Infants	0–5 months	210	100	30	5	0.01	0.2	0.3
	6–11 months	270	275	75	5	0.5	0.3	0.4
Children	1–3 years	500	460	80	5	0.7	0.5	0.5
	4–8 years	800	500	130	5	1	0.6	0.6
Males	9–13 years	1300	1250	240	5	2	0.9	0.9
	14–18 years	1300	1250	410	5	3	1.2	1.3
	19–30 years	1000	700	400	5	4	1.2	1.3
	31–50 years	1000	700	420	5	4	1.2	1.3
	51–70 years	1200	700	420	10	4	1.2	1.3
	>70 years	1200	700	420	15	4	1.2	1.3
Females	9–13 years	1300	1250	240	5	2	0.9	0.9
	14–18 years	1300	1250	360	5	3	1.0	1.0
	19–30 years	1000	700	310	5	3	1.1	1.1
	31–50 years	1000	700	320	5	3	1.1	1.1
	51–70 years	1200	700	320	10	3	1.1	1.1
	>70 years	1200	700	320	15	3	1.1	1.1
Pregnancy	≤18 years	1300	1250	400	5	3	1.4	1.4
	19–30 years	1000	700	350	5	3	1.4	1.4
	31–50 years	1000	700	360	5	3	1.4	1.4
Lactation	≤18 years	1300	1250	360	5	3	1.5	1.6
	19–30 years	1000	700	310	5	3	1.5	1.6
	31–50 years	1000	700	320	5	3	1.5	1.6

NOTE: This table includes Dietary Reference Intakes for those nutrients for which DRIs had been set through June 1998. The table includes values for the type of DRI standard—Adequate Intake (AI) or Recommended Dietary Allowance (RDA)—that has been established for that particular nutrient and life stage.

[a]As cholecalciferol. 1 μg cholecalciferol = 40 IU vitamin D.
[b]In the absence of adequate exposure to sunlight.
[c]As niacin equivalents. 1 mg of niacin = 60 mg of tryptophan.
[d]As dietary folate equivalents (DFE). 1 DFE = 1 μg food folate = 0.6 μg of folic acid (from fortified food or supplement) consumed with food = 0.5 μg of synthetic (supplemental) folic acid taken on an empty stomach.
[e]Although AIs have been set for choline, there are few data to assess whether a dietary supply of choline is needed at all stages of the life cycle, and it may be that the choline requirement can be met by endogenous synthesis at some of these stages.
[f]Since 10–30% of older people may malabsorb food-bound B-12, it is advisable for those older than 50 years to meet their RDA mainly by consuming foods fortified with B-12 or a B-12-containing supplement.
[g]In view of evidence linking folate intake with neural tube defects in the fetus, it is recommended that all women capable of becoming pregnant consume 400 μg of synthetic folic acid from fortified food and/or supplements in addition to intake of food folate from a varied diet.
[h]It is assumed that women will continue consuming 400 μg of folic acid until their pregnancy is confirmed and they enter prenatal care, which ordinarily occurs after the end of the periconceptional period—the critical time for formation of the neural tube.

SOURCES: Food and Nutrition Board. Institute of Medicine. National Academy of Sciences. 1997. *Dietary Reference Intakes for Calcium, Phosphorus, Magnesium, Vitamin D, and Fluoride.* Washington, D.C.: National Academy Press. Food and Nutrition Board. Institute of Medicine. National Academy of Sciences. 1998. *Dietary Reference Intakes for Thiamin, Riboflavin, Niacin, Vitamin B$_6$, Folate, Vitamin B$_{12}$, Pantothenic Acid, Biotin, and Choline.* Washington, D.C.: National Academy Press. Copyright © 1998 by the National Academy of Sciences. Reprinted with permission from National Academy Press, Washington, D.C.

a fortified breakfast cereal. If you do decide to take a supplement, choose a balanced formulation that contains 50–100% of the adult Daily Value for vitamins and minerals (see below). Avoid supplements containing large doses of particular nutrients.

Daily Values   Because the RDAs and DRIs are far too cumbersome to use as a basis for food labels, the U.S.

Food and Drug Administration developed another set of dietary standards, the **Daily Values.** The Daily Values are based on several different sets of guidelines and include standards for fat, cholesterol, carbohydrate, dietary fiber, and selected vitamins and minerals. On food labels, they are expressed as a percentage of a 2000-calorie diet, an average daily calorie intake for Americans. Using a single set of recommendations—the Daily Values—on food la-

TABLE 8-6 *Dietary Reference Intakes (DRIs) (continued)*

Niacin (mg/day)[c]	Vitamin B-6 (mg/day)	Folate (µg/day)[d]	Vitamin B-12 (µg/day)	Pantothenic Acid (mg/day)	Biotin (µg/day)	Choline[e] (mg/day)
2	0.1	65	0.4	1.7	5	125
3	0.3	80	0.5	1.8	6	150
6	0.5	150	0.9	2	8	200
8	0.6	200	1.2	3	12	250
12	1.0	300	1.8	4	20	375
16	1.3	400	2.4	5	25	550
16	1.3	400	2.4	5	30	550
16	1.3	400	2.4	5	30	550
16	1.7	400	2.4[f]	5	30	550
16	1.7	400	2.4[f]	5	30	550
12	1.0	300	1.8	4	20	375
14	1.2	400[g]	2.4	5	25	400
14	1.3	400[g]	2.4	5	30	425
14	1.3	400[g]	2.4	5	30	425
14	1.5	400[g]	2.4[f]	5	30	425
14	1.5	400	2.4[f]	5	30	425
18	1.9	600[h]	2.6	6	30	450
18	1.9	600[h]	2.6	6	30	450
18	1.9	600[h]	2.6	6	30	450
17	2.0	500	2.8	7	35	550
17	2.0	500	2.8	7	35	550
17	2.0	500	2.8	7	35	550

TABLE 8-7 *Tolerable Upper Intake Levels for Adults*

Nutrient	Upper Intake Level
Calcium	2500 mg/day
Phosphorus	4000 mg/day
Magnesium (nonfood sources)	350 mg/day
Vitamin D	50 µg/day
Fluoride	10 mg/day
Niacin	35 mg/day
Vitamin B-6	100 mg/day
Folate	1000 µg/day
Choline	3500 mg/day

This table includes the adult Tolerable Upper Intake Level (UL) standard of the Dietary Reference Intakes (DRIs). For some nutrients, there is insufficient data on which to develop a UL. This does not mean that there is no potential for adverse effects from high intake, and when data about adverse effects are limited, extra caution may be warranted. In healthy individuals, there is no established benefit from nutrient intakes above the RDA or AI.

SOURCES: Food and Nutrition Board. Institute of Medicine. National Academy of Sciences. 1997. *Dietary Reference Intakes for Calcium, Phosphorus, Magnesium, Vitamin D, and Fluoride.* Washington, D.C.: National Academy Press. Food and Nutrition Board. Institute of Medicine. National Academy of Sciences. 1998. *Dietary Reference Intakes for Thiamin, Riboflavin, Niacin, Vitamin B₆, Folate, Vitamin B₁₂, Pantothenic Acid, Biotin, and Choline.* Washington, D.C.: National Academy Press.

bels helps make nutrition information more accessible to the consumer. Food labels are described in more detail later in the chapter.

The Food Guide Pyramid

Many of us learned about food groups in grade school. We learned that by choosing foods from each group, we could have a healthy diet. The fundamental principles of this food guide are moderation, variety, and balance—a theme echoed throughout this chapter. A diet is balanced if it contains appropriate amounts of each nutrient, and choosing foods from each of the food groups helps ensure that balance.

The latest version of the food-group plan is the U.S. Department of Agriculture's Food Guide Pyramid (Figure 8-5). It is based on a recommended number of servings from six food groups. A range of servings is given for each group. The smaller number is for people who consume about 1600 calories a day, such as many sedentary women; the larger number is for those who consume

Daily Values A simplified version of the RDAs used on food labels; also included are values for nutrients with no RDA per se. **TERMS**

Figure 8-5   The Food Guide Pyramid: a guide to daily food choices.   The Pyramid is an outline of what to eat each day—not a rigid prescription, but a general guide that lets you choose a healthful diet that's right for you. It calls for eating a variety of foods to get the nutrients you need and at the same time the right amount of calories to maintain a healthy weight. The Pyramid also focuses on fat because many Americans eat too much fat, especially saturated fat.   SOURCE: U.S. Department of Agriculture, Human Nutrition Information Service. 1996. *Food Guide Pyramid.* Home and Garden Bulletin No. 252.

about 2800 calories a day, such as active men. Serving sizes and examples of foods are described below for each group.

It is important to choose a variety of foods within each group because different foods have different combinations of nutrients: for example, within the vegetable group, potatoes are high in vitamin C, while spinach is a rich source of vitamin A. Foods also vary in their amount of calories and nutrients, and people who do not need many calories should focus on nutrient-dense foods within each group (foods that are high in nutrients relative to the amount of calories they contain). Many foods you eat contain servings from more than one food group.

Bread, Cereals, Rice, and Pasta (6–11 Servings)

Foods from this group are usually low in fat and rich in complex carbohydrates, dietary fiber, and many vitamins and minerals, including thiamin, riboflavin, iron, niacin, folate, and zinc. Although 6–11 servings may seem like a large amount of food, many people eat several servings at a time. A single serving is the equivalent of the following:

- 1 slice of bread or half a hamburger bun, English muffin, or bagel
- 1 small roll, biscuit, or muffin
- 1 ounce of ready-to-eat cereal
- ½ cup cooked cereal, rice, or pasta
- 5–6 small or 2–3 large crackers

TERMS   cruciferous vegetables   Vegetables of the cabbage family, including cabbage, broccoli, brussels sprouts, kale, and cauliflower; the flower petals of these plants form the shape of a cross, hence the name.

If you are one of the many people who have trouble identifying an ounce of cereal or half a cup of rice, see the strategies in the box "Judging Serving Sizes." Choose foods that are typically made with little fat or sugars (bread, rice, pasta) over those that are high in fat and sugars (croissants, chips, cookies, doughnuts). For maximum nutrition, choose whole-grain breads, high-fiber cereals, whole-wheat pasta, and brown rice.

Vegetables (3–5 Servings)

Vegetables are rich in carbohydrates, dietary fiber, vitamin A, vitamin C, folate, iron, magnesium, and other nutrients. They are also naturally low in fat. A serving of vegetables is equivalent to the following:

- 1 cup raw leafy vegetables
- ½ cup raw or cooked vegetables
- ½ cup tomato sauce
- ¾ cup vegetable juice
- ½ cup cooked dry beans

Dry beans (legumes) such as pinto, navy, kidney, and black beans can be counted as servings of vegetables *or* as alternatives to meat. Other good choices from this group include dark-green leafy vegetables such as spinach, chard, and collards; deep-orange and red vegetables such as carrots, winter squash, red bell peppers, and tomatoes; broccoli, cauliflower, and other **cruciferous vegetables;** peas; green beans; potatoes; and corn.

Fruits (2–4 Servings)

Like vegetables, fruits are rich in carbohydrates, dietary fiber, and many vitamins, especially vitamin C. They are low in fat and sodium. The serving sizes used in the Pyramid are as follows:

Studies have shown that most people underestimate the size of their food portions, in many cases by as much as 50%. If you need to retrain your eye, try using measuring cups and spoons and an inexpensive kitchen scale when you eat at home. With a little practice, you'll learn the difference between 3 and 8 ounces of chicken or meat, and what a half-cup of rice really looks like. For quick estimates, use these equivalents:

- 1 teaspoon of margarine = the tip of your thumb.
- 1 ounce of cheese = your thumb or four dice stacked together.

- 3 ounces of chicken or meat = a deck of cards or an audio-cassette tape.
- ½ cup of rice or cooked vegetables = an ice cream scoop or one-third of a soda can.
- 2 tablespoons of peanut butter = a Ping-Pong ball.
- 1 cup of pasta = a woman's fist or a tennis ball.
- 1 medium potato = a computer mouse.

- 1 medium (apple, banana, peach, orange, pear) or 2 small (apricot, plum) whole fruit(s)
- 1 melon wedge
- ½ cup berries, cherries, or grapes
- ½ grapefruit
- ½ cup chopped, cooked, canned, or frozen fruit
- ¾ cup fruit juice (100% juice)
- ¼ cup dried fruit

Good choices from this group are citrus fruits and juices, melons, pears, apples, bananas, and berries. Choose whole fruits often—they are higher in fiber and often lower in calories than fruit juices. Fruit *juices* typically contain more nutrients than fruit *punches, ades,* and *drinks.* For canned fruits, choose those packed in their own juice rather than in syrup.

Milk, Yogurt, and Cheese (2–3 Servings)   Foods from this group are high in protein, carbohydrate, calcium, riboflavin, potassium, and zinc. To limit the fat in your diet, choose servings of low-fat or nonfat items from this group:

- 1 cup milk or yogurt
- 1½ ounces natural cheese
- 2 ounces processed cheese

Cottage cheese is lower in calcium than most other cheeses, and 1 cup of cottage cheese counts as only half a serving for this food group. Ice cream is also lower in calcium than many other dairy products (½ cup is equivalent to ⅓ serving); in addition, it is high in sugar and fat.

Meat, Poultry, Fish, Dry Beans, Eggs, and Nuts (2–3 Servings   This group of foods provides protein, niacin, iron, vitamin B-6, zinc, and thiamin, and vitamin B-12 (animal foods only). The Pyramid recommends 2–3 servings each day of foods from this group. The total amount of these servings should be the equivalent of 5–7 ounces of cooked lean meat, poultry, or fish per day. Many people misjudge what makes up a single serving for this food group:

- 2–3 ounces cooked lean meat, poultry, or fish (an average hamburger or a medium chicken breast half is about 3 ounces; 4 slices of bologna, 6 slices of hard salami, or ½ cup of drained canned tuna counts as about 2 ounces)
- The following portions of nonmeat foods are equivalent to 1 ounce of lean meat:

  ½ cup cooked dry beans (if not counted as a vegetable)

  1 egg

  2 tablespoons peanut butter

  ⅓ cup nuts

  ¼ cup seeds

  ½ cup tofu

To limit your intake of fat and saturated fat, choose lean cuts of meat and skinless poultry, and watch your serving sizes carefully. Nuts and seeds are high in fat, so eat them in moderation. Choose at least one serving of plant proteins every day.

Fats, Oils, and Sweets   The small tip of the Pyramid includes fats, oils, and sweets—foods such as salad dressings, oils, butter, margarine, gravy, mayonnaise, soft drinks, sugar, candy, jellies and jams, syrups, and sweet desserts. Foods from the tip of the Pyramid provide calories but few nutrients; they should not replace foods from the other groups. The total amount of fats, oils, and sweets you consume should be determined by your overall energy needs.

As indicated by the colored triangles and circles in the Pyramid, fats and added sugars are also found within the five major food groups (see Figure 8-5). ("Added sugars" refers to those sugars added to foods in processing or at the table, not the sugars found naturally in fruits and milk.) Foods that come from animals (the meat and milk groups) are naturally higher in fat than foods that come from plants. However, there are many lean meat and low-fat dairy choices available. Fruits, vegetables, and grain

TABLE 8-8 *Food Guide Pyramid Recommendations Compared with the Average American Diet*

	Recommended Diets at Three Calorie Levels[a]			Average American Diet	
	1600	2200	2800	Women (1600 calories)	Men (2400 calories)
Grain group (servings)	6	9	11	5.3	7.8
Vegetable group (servings)	3	4	5	3.0	4.2
Fruit group (servings)	2	3	4	1.5	1.6
Dairy group (servings)[b]	2–3	2–3	2–3	1.1	1.5
Meat group (ounces)[c]	5	6	7	4.0	6.5
Total fat (grams)[d]	53	73	93	58.0	90.8
Total added sugars (teaspoons)[d,e]	6	12	18	14.8	21.0

[a]The bottom of the recommended range of servings (1600 calories) is about right for many sedentary women and older adults. The middle range (2200 calories) is about right for most children, teenage girls, active women, and many sedentary men. The top of the range (2800 calories) is about right for teenage boys, many active men, and some very active women.
[b]Women who are pregnant or lactating, teenagers, and young adults to age 24 need 3 servings.
[c]The Pyramid recommends 2–3 servings per day, the equivalent of 5–7 ounces of cooked lean meat, poultry, or fish (see p. 203).
[d]Values for total fat and added sugars include fat and added sugars that are in food choices from the five major food groups as well as fat and added sugars from foods in the Fats, Oils, and Sweets group. The total for added sugars does not include sugars that occur naturally in foods such as fruit and milk. The recommended fat totals are based on a limit of 30% of total calories as fat.
[e]A teaspoon of sugar is equivalent to 4 grams (16 calories).

SOURCES: Shaw, A., et al. 1997. *Using the Food Guide Pyramid: A Resource for Nutrition Educators.* Center for Nutrition Policy and Promotion. U.S. Department of Agriculture (retrieved January 8, 1998; http://www.nal.usda.gov/fnic/Fpyr/guide.pdf). Cleveland, L. E., et al. 1997. *Pyramid Servings Data: Results from USDA's Continuing Survey of Food Intakes by Individuals.* Riverdale, Md.: Food Surveys Research Group. U.S. Department of Agriculture.

products are naturally low in fat, but they can be prepared in ways that make them higher-fat choices—for example, potatoes served as french fries and pasta served as fettucini alfredo. Added sugars in the food groups can be found in foods such as ice cream, sweetened yogurt, canned fruit packed in syrup, and baked goods such as cookies. Reduced-fat versions of foods such as cookies and ice cream are often *very* high in added sugars and just as high in calories as their full-fat versions.

The average American diet currently includes more fat and added sugars than recommended. The Pyramid suggests that Americans limit the fat in their diets to 30% of total calories. You will consume about half this amount if you eat the recommended number of servings from each food group, select the lowest-fat choices, and add no fat during cooking or at the table. Additional fat, up to 30% of total calories, is considered discretionary in that you can decide whether to get it from higher-fat food choices or additions to your foods.

Added sugars are less of a concern to health than fat, but consumption of large amounts of sugars adds empty calories to the diet and can make weight management more difficult. Analysis of the average diet of Americans has revealed that the number of servings from the fruit, dairy, and meat groups is below the recommended

ranges, and servings from the grain and vegetable groups are near the bottom of the recommended ranges (Table 8-8). Overconsumption of fat and added sugars leaves fewer calories available for healthier food choices from the five major food groups. For example, the average daily diet among American women includes about 9 teaspoons (36 grams) of added sugars and 5 grams of fat above recommended limits. The 200 calories in these extra sugars and fats could be better used to increase the number of servings from the food groups for which women typically fall short of Pyramid recommendations.

General strategies for controlling intake of fat and added sugars include choosing lower-fat foods within each food group, eating fewer foods that are high in sugar and low in other nutrients, and limiting the amount of fats and sugars added to foods during cooking or at the table.

The Food Guide Pyramid is a general guide to what you should eat every day. By eating a balanced variety of foods from each of the six food groups and including some plant proteins, you can ensure that your daily diet is adequate in all nutrients. A diet using low-fat food choices contains only about 1600 calories but meets all known nutritional needs, except possibly for iron in some women who have heavy menstrual periods. For these women, foods fortified in iron, such as breakfast cereals, can make up the deficit.

Dietary Guidelines for Americans

To provide further guidance for choosing a healthy diet, the U.S. Department of Agriculture and the Department of Health and Human Services have issued Dietary Guidelines for Americans, most recently in December 1995. What follows is a summary of the advice provided by the Dietary Guidelines, with additional comments from other health-related organizations, including the American Heart Association, the National Cancer Institute, the National Academy of Sciences, and the Surgeon General.

Eat a Variety of Foods　To obtain the nutrients and other substances needed for good health, vary the foods you eat. Focus on the Food Guide Pyramid, choosing an appropriate number of servings from each group. Use foods from the base of the Pyramid as the foundation for your meals, and choose a variety of foods from within each group. Everyone, especially adolescent girls and women, should take special care to consume adequate calcium and iron.

Balance the Food You Eat with Physical Activity: Maintain or Improve Your Weight　Emphasize balancing food intake with regular physical activity to avoid becoming overweight. Excess body fat increases the risk of diabetes, heart disease, cancer, and other diseases. People who are overweight and have one of these problems should try to lose weight or at least not gain weight.

Those who are overweight should not try to lose more than $1/2-1$ pound per week; avoid crash diets. Weight loss should be accomplished by increasing physical activity, eating less fat, and controlling portion sizes. If you are sedentary, try to become more active by accumulating 30 minutes or more of moderate physical activity on most or all days of the week. Choose low-fat, low-calorie, nutrient-dense foods—grains, vegetables, fruits, nonfat dairy products, and lean protein sources—rather than fatty foods, sugar and sweets, and alcoholic beverages.

Choose a Diet with Plenty of Grain Products, Vegetables, and Fruits　Foods from these food groups provide vitamins, minerals, complex carbohydrates, dietary fiber, and other substances important for good health. They also tend to be low in fat. Five or more servings of fruits and vegetables and six or more servings of grain products will help you reach a daily dietary fiber consumption of 20–35 grams. Emphasize complex, rather than simple, carbohydrates, and eat a variety of foods from each group. The availability of fresh fruits and vegetables varies by season and region of the country, but frozen and canned fruits and vegetables are readily available and are usually as high in nutrients. Fewer than 30% of Americans currently meet the Dietary Guidelines' goal for fruit and vegetable intake.

Choose a Diet Low in Fat, Saturated Fat, and Cholesterol　Some dietary fat is necessary for good health; good choices are monounsaturated and polyunsaturated fats found in vegetable oils, nuts, and fish. However, many Americans consume high-fat diets that increase their risk of heart disease, certain cancers, and obesity. Limit your overall intake of fat to 30% or less of daily calories, your saturated fat intake to less than one-third of your total daily fat intake (less than 10% of total daily calories), and your intake of cholesterol to 300 milligrams per day.

To control your intake of fat and saturated fat, choose lean meat, fish, poultry, and dry beans as protein sources; use nonfat or low-fat milk and milk products; and limit your consumption of high-fat foods. To reduce your intake of trans fats, avoid deep-fried fast foods and other products made with hydrogenated vegetable oils. Refer to the box "Reducing the Fat in Your Diet" for more suggestions.

Although less dangerous for heart health than saturated and trans fats, high cholesterol intake can be a problem for some people. Cholesterol is found only in animal foods. If you want to cut back on your cholesterol intake, follow the Food Guide Pyramid recommendations for consumption of animal foods; pay particular attention to serving sizes. In addition, limit your intake of foods that are particularly high in cholesterol content, including egg yolks and liver. Food labels provide the cholesterol content of prepared foods.

Choose a Diet Moderate in Sugars　Diets high in simple sugars do not cause hyperactivity or diabetes, but they do promote tooth decay. In addition, some foods that are high in sugar supply calories but few or no nutrients. For people who are very active and have high caloric needs, sugars can be an additional source of energy. However, because eating a nutritious diet and maintaining a healthy body weight are very important, most people should use sugars in moderation; people with low caloric needs should use sugars sparingly.

Moderation here means less than 15% of total calories—about 75 grams (15 teaspoons) per day from both naturally occurring simple sugars and added sugars. To reduce sugar consumption, cut back on items with added sugar, such as baked goods, candies, sweet desserts, sweetened beverages, canned fruits, and pre-sweetened breakfast cereals.

Choose a Diet Moderate in Salt and Sodium　Sodium is an essential nutrient, but it is required only in small

Your overall goal is to limit total fat intake to no more than 30% of total calories. Within that limit, favor unsaturated fats from vegetable oils, nuts, and fish over saturated and trans fats from animal products and foods made with hydrogenated vegetable oils. Limit saturated fat to less than 10% of total calories.

- Be moderate in your consumption of foods high in fat, especially those high in saturated and trans fat, including fast food, commercially prepared baked goods and desserts, meat, poultry, nuts and seeds, and regular dairy products (see Figure 8-4).

- When you do eat high-fat foods, limit your portion sizes, and balance your intake with foods low in fat.

- Choose lean cuts of meat, and trim any visible fat from meat before and after cooking. Remove skin from poultry before or after cooking.

- Replace whole milk with skim or low-fat milk in puddings, soups, and baked products. Substitute plain low-fat yogurt, blender-whipped cottage cheese, or buttermilk in recipes that call for sour cream.

- To reduce saturated and trans fat, use vegetable oil instead of butter or margarine. Use tub or squeeze margarine instead of stick margarine. Look for margarines that are free of trans fats.

- Season vegetables with herbs and spices rather than with sauces, butter, or margarine.

- Try lemon juice on salad, or use a yogurt-based salad dressing instead of mayonnaise or sour cream dressings.

- Steam, boil, or bake vegetables, or stir-fry them in a small amount of vegetable oil.

- Roast, bake, or broil meat, poultry, or fish so that fat drains away as the food cooks.

- Use a nonstick pan for cooking so that added fat will be unnecessary; use a vegetable spray for frying.

- Chill broths from meat or poultry until the fat becomes solid. Spoon off the fat before using the broth.

- Eat a low-fat vegetarian main dish at least once a week.

---

amounts—500 milligrams, or ¼ teaspoon, per day. Most Americans consume 8–12 times this amount. High sodium intake is linked to high blood pressure in some people and may also increase calcium loss, contributing to osteoporosis. It is recommended that you limit sodium intake to no more than 2400 milligrams per day, or about 1¼ teaspoons of salt per day.

Sodium is found primarily in processed and prepared foods; sodium content is provided on food labels. To lower your sodium intake, cut back on salty foods such as lunch meats, salted snack foods, canned soups, processed cheese, many tomato-based products, and many frozen dinners and baked goods. Add less salt during cooking and at the table; use lemon juice, herbs, and spices, rather than salt, to enhance the flavor of food. It usually takes only about a week or two to become accustomed to a lower-sodium diet.

If You Drink Alcoholic Beverages, Do So in Moderation Alcoholic beverages supply calories but few or no nutrients. Current evidence suggests that moderate drinking—no more than one drink daily for women and two drinks for men—is associated with a lower risk of cardiovascular disease in some people. However, higher levels of alcohol intake are associated with an increased risk for many diseases and with higher overall mortality rates. Adults who drink alcoholic beverages should do so in moderation, with meals, and when consumption does not put themselves or others at risk.

One further recommendation geared specifically for cancer prevention is to use moderation when consuming salt-cured, smoked, and nitrate-cured foods (such as ba-

con and sausage) because these may increase the risk of colon and other gastrointestinal cancers.

Reading Food Labels

Consumers can get help in applying the principles of the Food Guide Pyramid and the Dietary Guidelines for Americans from food labels. Beginning in 1994, all processed foods regulated by either the FDA or the USDA have included standardized nutrition information on their labels (see the box "Using Food Labels"). Every food label shows serving sizes and the amount of fat, saturated fat, cholesterol, protein, dietary fiber, and sodium in each serving. To make intelligent choices about food, learn to read and understand food labels. Lab 8-3 will give you the opportunity to compare foods using the information provided on their labels.

The Vegetarian Alternative

Some people choose a diet with one essential difference from the diets we've already described: Foods of animal origin (meat, poultry, fish, eggs, milk) are eliminated or restricted. Today, about 12 million Americans follow a vegetarian diet. Most do so because they think foods of plant origin are a more natural way to nourish the body. Some do so for religious, health, ethical, or philosophical reasons. If you choose to be a vegetarian, you can be confident of meeting your nutritional needs by following a few basic rules. (Vegetarian diets for children and pregnant women warrant individual professional guidance.)

Types of Vegetarian Diets There are a variety of vegetarian styles; the wider the variety of the diet eaten, the

Food labels are designed to help consumers make food choices based on the nutrients that are most important to good health. A food label states how much fat, saturated fat, cholesterol, protein, dietary fiber, and sodium the food contains. In addition to listing nutrient content by weight, the label puts the information in the context of a daily diet of 2000 calories that includes no more than 65 grams of fat (approximately 30% of total calories). For example, if a serving of a particular product has 13 grams of fat, the label will show that the serving represents 20% of the daily fat allowance. If your daily diet contains fewer or more than 2000 calories, you need to adjust these calculations accordingly. Refer to p. 189 for instructions on setting nutrient intake goals.

Food labels contain uniform serving sizes. This means that if you look at different brands of salad dressing, for example, you can compare calories based on the serving amount. Regulations also require that foods meet strict definitions if their packaging includes the terms "light," "low-fat," or "high-fiber" (see below). Health claims such as "good source of dietary fiber" or "low in saturated fat" on packages are signals that those products can wisely be included in your diet. Overall, the food label is an important tool to help you choose a diet that conforms to the Food Guide Pyramid and the Dietary Guidelines.

Beginning in 1999, dietary supplements will carry a similar "Supplement Facts" panel that specifies serving sizes and lists nutrients (with percent of Daily Value) and other ingredients.

Selected Nutrient Claims and What They Mean

Healthy A food that is low in fat, is low in saturated fat, has no more than 360–480 mg of sodium and 60 mg of cholesterol, *and* provides 10% or more of the Daily Value for vitamin A, vitamin C, protein, calcium, iron, or dietary fiber.

Light or lite One-third fewer calories or 50% less fat than a similar product.

Reduced or fewer At least 25% less of a nutrient than a similar product; can be applied to fat ("reduced fat"), saturated fat, cholesterol, sodium, and calories.

Extra or added 10% or more of the Daily Value per serving when compared to a similar product.

Good source 10–19% of the Daily Value for a particular nutrient.

High, rich in, or excellent source of 20% or more of the Daily Value for a particular nutrient.

Low calorie 40 calories or fewer per serving.

High fiber 5 g or more of fiber per serving.

Good source of fiber 2.5–4.9 g of fiber per serving.

Fat-free Less than 0.5 g of fat per serving.

Low-fat 3 g of fat or less per serving.

Saturated fat–free Less than 0.5 g of saturated fat and 0.5 g of trans fatty acids per serving.

Low saturated fat 1 g or less of saturated fat per serving and no more than 15% of total calories.

Cholesterol-free Less than 2 mg of cholesterol and 2 g or less of saturated fat per serving.

Low cholesterol 20 mg or less of cholesterol and 2 g or less of saturated fat per serving.

Low sodium 140 mg or less of sodium per serving.

Very low sodium 35 mg or less of sodium per serving.

Lean Cooked seafood, meat, or poultry with less than 10 g of fat, 4 g of saturated fat, and 95 mg of cholesterol per serving.

Extra lean Cooked seafood, meat, or poultry with less than 5 g of fat, 2 g of saturated fat, and 95 mg of cholesterol per serving.

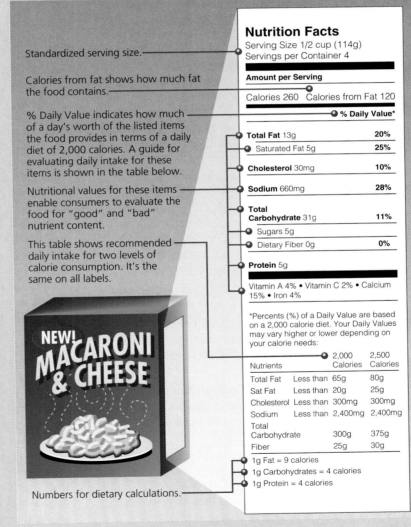

Standardized serving size.

Calories from fat shows how much fat the food contains.

% Daily Value indicates how much of a day's worth of the listed items the food provides in terms of a daily diet of 2,000 calories. A guide for evaluating daily intake for these items is shown in the table below.

Nutritional values for these items enable consumers to evaluate the food for "good" and "bad" nutrient content.

This table shows recommended daily intake for two levels of calorie consumption. It's the same on all labels.

Numbers for dietary calculations.

Nutrition Facts

Serving Size 1/2 cup (114g)
Servings per Container 4

Amount per Serving

Calories 260   Calories from Fat 120

	% Daily Value*
Total Fat 13g	20%
Saturated Fat 5g	25%
Cholesterol 30mg	10%
Sodium 660mg	28%
Total Carbohydrate 31g	11%
Sugars 5g	
Dietary Fiber 0g	0%
Protein 5g	

Vitamin A 4% • Vitamin C 2% • Calcium 15% • Iron 4%

*Percents (%) of a Daily Value are based on a 2,000 calorie diet. Your Daily Values may vary higher or lower depending on your calorie needs:

Nutrients		2,000 Calories	2,500 Calories
Total Fat	Less than	65g	80g
Sat Fat	Less than	20g	25g
Cholesterol	Less than	300mg	300mg
Sodium	Less than	2,400mg	2,400mg
Total Carbohydrate		300g	375g
Fiber		25g	30g

1g Fat = 9 calories
1g Carbohydrates = 4 calories
1g Protein = 4 calories

easier to meet nutritional needs. **Vegans** eat only plant foods. **Lacto-vegetarians** eat plant foods and dairy products. **Lacto-ovo-vegetarians** eat plant foods, dairy products, and eggs. Finally, **partial, semivegetarians,** or **pesco-vegetarians** eat plant foods, dairy products, eggs, and usually a small selection of poultry, fish, and other seafood. Including some animal protein in a diet makes planning much easier, but it is not necessary.

A Food-Group Plan for Vegetarians A food-group plan has been developed for lacto-vegetarians; it includes 6–11 servings from grains and 2–4 servings from legumes, nuts, and seeds. Add to this 3–5 servings from the vegetable group, 2–4 servings from the fruit group, and 2 or more servings from the milk, yogurt, and cheese group to complete the plan. By following this plan, lacto-vegetarians should have no problem obtaining an adequate diet. Consuming fruits with most meals is especially helpful, because any vitamin C present will improve iron absorption (the iron in plants is more difficult to absorb than the iron in animal sources).

In contrast to those who eat dairy products, vegans must do much more special diet planning to obtain all essential nutrients. A vegan must take special care to consume adequate amounts of protein, riboflavin, vitamin D, vitamin B-12, calcium, iron, and zinc; good strategies for obtaining these nutrients include the following:

- Eat proteins from a wide variety of sources, and include a couple of protein sources at each meal. A good rule of thumb is 11 servings of grains and 4 servings of legumes, nuts, and seeds. Soy milk, tofu (soybean curd), and tempeh (a cultured soy product) make important nutrient contributions to this diet plan.

- Eat green leafy vegetables, whole grains, yeast, and legumes to obtain riboflavin.

- Obtain vitamin D by spending 5–15 minutes a day out in the sun, by consuming vitamin D–fortified products like rice milk or soy milk, or by taking a supplement.

- Obtain vitamin B-12 (found only in animal foods) from a supplement or by consuming foods fortified with vitamin B-12, such as special yeast products, soy milk, and breakfast cereals.

- Consume fortified tofu, dark-green leafy vegetables, nuts, tortillas made from lime-processed corn, and fortified orange juice, bread, and soy milk to obtain calcium. Supplements may be necessary.

- Consume whole grains, fortified bread and breakfast cereals, dried fruits, dark-green leafy vegetables, nuts, and legumes to obtain iron.

- Obtain zinc from whole grains and legumes.

It takes a little planning and common sense to put together a good vegetarian diet. If you are a vegetarian or are considering becoming one, devote some extra time and thought to your diet. It's especially important that you eat as wide a variety of foods as possible to ensure that all of your nutritional needs are satisfied.

Dietary Challenges for Special Population Groups

The Food Guide Pyramid and Dietary Guidelines for Americans provide a basis that everyone can use to create a healthy diet. However, some population groups face special dietary challenges.

Women Women tend to be smaller and weigh less than men, meaning they have lower energy needs and therefore consume fewer calories. Because of this, women have more difficulty getting adequate amounts of all essential nutrients and need to focus on nutrient-dense foods. Two nutrients of special concern are calcium and iron, minerals for which many women fail to meet the RDAs. Low calcium intake may be linked to the development of osteoporosis in later life. Nonfat and low-fat dairy products and fortified cereal, bread, and orange juice are good choices. Iron is also a concern: Menstruating women have higher iron requirements than other groups, and a lack of iron in the diet can lead to iron-deficiency anemia. Studies indicate that about 10% of adolescent girls and women of childbearing age are iron deficient. Lean red meat, green leafy vegetables, and fortified breakfast cereals are good sources of iron. As discussed earlier, all women capable of becoming pregnant should consume adequate folate from fortified foods and/or supplements.

Men Men are seldom thought of as having nutritional deficiencies because they generally have high-calorie diets. However, many men have a diet that does not follow the Food Guide Pyramid but that includes more red meat and fewer fruits, vegetables, dairy products, and grains than recommended. This dietary pattern is linked to heart disease and some types of cancer. A high intake of calories can lead to weight gain in the long term if a man's activity level decreases as he ages. Men should use the Food Guide Pyramid as a basis for their overall diet and focus on increasing their consumption of fruits, vegetables, and grains to obtain vitamins, minerals, dietary fiber, and phytochemicals.

TERMS **vegan** A vegetarian who eats no animal products.

lacto-vegetarian A vegetarian who includes dairy products in the diet.

lacto-ovo-vegetarian A vegetarian who includes dairy products and eggs in the diet.

partial, semivegetarian, or **pesco-vegetarian** A person who includes plant foods, dairy products, eggs, and small amounts of poultry, fish, and seafood in the diet.

College Students Foods that are convenient for college students are not always the healthiest choices. It is easy for students who eat in buffet-style dining halls to overeat, and the foods offered are not necessarily high in essential nutrients and low in fat. The same is true of meals at fast-food restaurants, another convenient source of quick and inexpensive meals for busy students. Although no food is entirely "bad," consuming a wide variety of foods is critical for a healthy diet. See the box "Eating Strategies for College Students" for tips on making healthy eating convenient and affordable.

Older Adults As people age, they tend to become less active, so they require fewer calories to maintain their weight. At the same time, the absorption of nutrients tends to be lower in older adults because of age-related changes in the digestive tract. Thus, they must consume nutrient-dense foods in order to meet their nutritional requirements. As discussed earlier, foods fortified with vitamin B-12 and/or B-12 supplements are recommended for people over age 50. Because constipation is a common problem, consuming foods high in dietary fiber is another important goal.

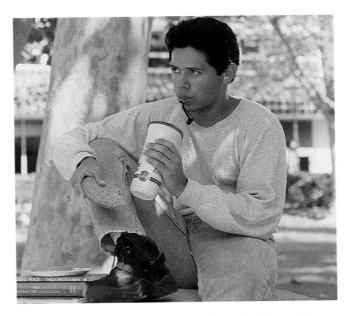

Eating on the run is a common—but not always healthy—habit among college students. After snacking on cookies, this young man should complete his day's diet with a low-fat, nutrient-dense dinner.

Athletes Key dietary concerns for athletes are meeting their increased energy requirements and drinking enough fluids during practice and throughout the day to remain fully hydrated. Individuals engaged in vigorous training programs expend more energy (calories) than sedentary and moderately active individuals and may have energy needs ranging from 2000 to more than 6000 calories per day. For athletes, the American Dietetic Association recommends a diet with 60–65% of calories coming from carbohydrate, 10–15% from protein, and no more than 30% from fat.

Endurance athletes involved in competitive events lasting longer than 90 minutes may benefit from increasing carbohydrate intake to 65–70% of total calories. High carbohydrate intake builds and maintains muscle glycogen stores, resulting in greater endurance and delayed fatigue during competitive events. Some endurance athletes engage in "carbohydrate loading"—a practice that involves increasing carbohydrate intake in the days prior to a competition.

Athletes for whom maintaining low body weight and body fat is important—such as skaters, gymnasts, and wrestlers—should consume adequate calories and nutrients and avoid falling into unhealthy patterns of eating. The combination of low levels of body fat, high physical activity, disordered eating habits, and, in women, amenorrhea, is associated with stress fractures and other injuries and with osteoporosis. Eating disorders are discussed in Chapter 9.

Strenuous exercise can lead to rapid loss of fluids. En-durance athletes should consume at least 16 ounces (2 cups) of fluid about 2 hours before a workout, followed by another 16 ounces about 20 minutes prior to exercise. In hot and humid conditions, an additional 4–6 ounces should be consumed every 15 minutes during a workout. Athletes should consume enough fluids during activity so that their body weight remains relatively constant before and after an exercise session. For workouts lasting less than 60–90 minutes, cool water is an appropriate fluid replacement; for longer workouts or for exercise in especially hot and humid conditions, a commercial sports beverage that contains carbohydrates may be beneficial.

There is no evidence that consuming supplements containing vitamins, minerals, protein, or specific amino acids will build muscle or improve sports performance. Strength and muscle are built with exercise, not extra protein, and carbohydrates provide the fuel needed for muscle-building exercise. Strenuous physical activity does increase the need for protein and some vitamins and minerals; however, the increased energy intake of athletes more than compensates for this increased need. (Indeed, the protein intake in the average American diet is already about 50% above the RDA, representing 16% of total calories.) For athletes, the American Dietetic Association recommends a daily protein intake of 1.0–1.5 grams per kilogram of body weight, up from the RDA of 0.8 gram per kilogram. A 160-pound athlete consuming 3500 calories per day needs to obtain only 12% of total calories from protein to achieve the upper end of the protein range for athletes. A balanced high-carbohydrate,

General Guidelines

- Eat slowly, and enjoy your food.

- Eat a colorful, varied diet. The more colorful your diet is, the more varied and rich in fruits and vegetables it will be. Many Americans eat few fruits and vegetables, despite the fact that these foods are typically inexpensive, delicious, rich in nutrients, and low in fat and calories.

- Eat breakfast. You'll have more energy in the morning and be less likely to grab an unhealthy snack later on.

- Choose healthy snacks—fruits, vegetables, grains, and cereals—as often as you can.

- Combine physical activity with healthy eating. You'll look and feel better and have a much lower risk of many chronic diseases. Even a little exercise is better than none.

Eating in the Dining Hall

- Choose a meal plan that includes breakfast, and don't skip it.

- If menus are posted or distributed, decide what you want to eat before getting in line, and stick to your choices. Consider what you plan to do and eat for the rest of the day before making your choices.

- Ask for large servings of vegetables and small servings of meat and other high-fat main dishes. Build your meals around grains and vegetables.

- Choose leaner poultry, fish, or bean dishes rather than high-fat meats and fried entrees.

- Ask that gravies and sauces be served on the side; limit your intake.

- Choose broth-based or vegetable soups rather than cream soups.

- Drink nonfat milk, water, mineral water, or fruit juice rather than heavily sweetened fruit drinks or whole milk.

- Choose fruit for dessert rather than pastries, cookies, or cakes.

- Do some research about the foods and preparation methods used in your dining hall or cafeteria. Discuss any food and nutrition suggestions you have with your food service manager.

Eating in Fast-Food Restaurants

- Most fast-food chains can provide a brochure with a nutritional breakdown of the foods on the menu. Ask for it. (See also the information in Appendix C.)

- Order small single burgers with no cheese instead of double burgers with many toppings. If possible, ask for them broiled instead of fried.

- Ask for items to be prepared without mayonnaise, tartar sauce, sour cream, or other high-fat sauces. Ketchup, mustard, and fat-free mayonnaise or sour cream are better choices and are available at many fast-food restaurants.

- Choose whole-grain buns or bread for burgers and sandwiches.

- Choose chicken items made from chicken breast, not processed chicken.

- Order vegetable pizzas.

- At the salad bar, choose a lowfat dressing. Put the dressing on the side and dip your fork into it—don't pour it over your salad. Avoid heavily dressed potato and pasta salads. Don't put croutons and bacon on vegetable salads.

- If you order french fries or onion rings, get the smallest size, and/or share them with a friend.

Eating on the Run

Are you chronically short of time? The following healthy and filling items can be packed for a quick snack or meal: fresh or dried fruit, fruit juices, raw fresh vegetables, plain bagels, bread sticks, fig bars, low-fat cheese sticks or cubes, low-fat crackers or granola bars, nonfat or low-fat yogurt, pretzels, rice or corn cakes, plain popcorn, soup (if you have access to a microwave), or water.

---

moderate-protein, low-fat diet can provide all needed nutrients for athletes.

People with Special Health Concerns   Many Americans have special health concerns that affect their dietary needs. For example, women who are pregnant or breastfeeding require extra calories, vitamins, and minerals. People with diabetes benefit from a well-balanced diet that is low in simple sugars, high in complex carbohydrates, and relatively rich in monounsaturated fats. And people with high blood pressure need to control their weight and may need to limit their sodium consumption. If you have a health problem or concern that may require

a special diet, discuss your situation with a physician or registered dietitian (R.D.).

A PERSONAL PLAN: APPLYING NUTRITIONAL PRINCIPLES

Now that you understand the basics of good nutrition, you can put together a diet that works for you. The basic principles of a healthy diet are simple—variety, balance, and moderation. But within this framework, no single diet is optimal for everyone. Many different diets can

There is no one ethnic diet that clearly surpasses all others in providing people with healthful foods. However, every diet has its advantages and disadvantages, and within each cuisine, some foods are better choices. It is in this area of personal choice that individuals can make a difference in their own health. The dietary guidelines described in this chapter can be applied to any ethnic cuisine. For additional guidance, refer to the table below, which lists some of the more and less healthful choices you can make when you eat out at various ethnic restaurants or cook ethnic meals at home.

	Choose Often	**Choose Seldom**
Chinese	Chinese greens Hunan or Szechuan dishes Rice, brown or white Steamed dishes Stir-fry dishes Wonton soup	Crispy duck or beef Egg rolls or fried wontons General Tso's chicken Kung pao dishes Rice, fried Sweet-and-sour dishes
Indian	Chapati (baked, tortilla-like bread) Dal (lentils) Karhi (chickpea soup) Khur (milk and rice dessert) Tandoori, chicken or fish Yogurt-based curry dishes	Bhatura, poori, or paratha (fried breads) Coconut milk–based dishes Ghee (clarified butter) Korma (rich meat dish) Pakoras (fried appetizer) Samosa (fried meat and vegetables in dough)
Italian	Cioppino (seafood stew) Minestrone soup, vegetarian Pasta with marinara sauce Pasta primavera Pasta with red or white clam sauce	Cannelloni, ravioli, or manicotti Fettucine alfredo Fried calamari Garlic bread Veal or eggplant parmigiana
Japanese	Kushiyaki (broiled foods on skewers) Nabemono (boiled dishes) Shabu-shabu (foods in boiling broth) Sushi	Agemono (deep-fried dishes) Sukiyaki Tempura (fried chicken, shrimp, or vegetables) Tonkatsu (fried pork)
Mexican	Beans and rice Burritos, bean or chicken Fajitas, chicken or vegetable Gazpacho Refried beans, nonfat or low-fat Tortillas, steamed	Chiles relleños Chimichangas, flautas, or quesadillas Enchiladas, beef or cheese Nachos or fried tortillas Refried beans made with lard Taco salad
Thai	Forest salad Larb (chicken salad with mint) Po tak (seafood soup) Yum neua (broiled beef with onions)	Fried fish, duck, or chicken Curries with coconut milk Dishes with peanut sauce Yum koon chaing (sausage with peppers)

SOURCES: The sat fat switch. 1997. *Nutrition Action Healthletter,* January/February. University of Southern Florida Student Health Service. 1997. Ethnic food (http://www.shs.usf.edu/Health/ethnic.html). The best of Asian cuisines. 1993. *University of California at Berkeley Wellness Letter,* January. Eating in ethnic restaurants. 1990. *Runner's World,* January. Reprinted by permission of *Runner's World Magazine.* Copyright © 1990 Rodek Press, Inc. All rights reserved.

meet people's nutritional requirements (see the box "Ethnic Foods"). Every individual needs to customize a food plan based on age, gender, weight, activity level, medical risk factors—and, of course, personal tastes.

Assessing and Changing Your Diet

The first step in planning a healthy diet is to examine what you currently eat. Labs 8-1 and 8-2 are designed to help you analyze your current diet and compare it to optimal dietary goals. (This analysis can be completed using either Appendix B or a nutritional analysis software program.)

Next, experiment with additions and substitutions to your current diet to bring it closer to your goals. If you are consuming too much fat, for example, try substituting fruit for a calorie-rich dessert. If you aren't getting enough iron, try adding some raisins to your cereal or garbanzo beans to your salad. If you need to plan your diet from the ground up, use the Food Guide Pyramid and the Dietary Guidelines.

To put your plan into action, use the behavioral self-management techniques and tips described in Chapter 1. If you identify several changes you want to make, focus on one at a time. You might start, for example, by substituting nonfat or low-fat milk for whole milk. When you become used to that, you can try substituting whole-wheat bread for white bread. The information on eating behavior in Lab 8-1 will help you identify and change unhealthy patterns of eating.

Staying Committed to a Healthy Diet

Beyond knowledge and information, you also need support in difficult situations. Keeping to your plan is easiest when you choose and prepare your own food at home. For meals prepared at home, advance planning is the key: mapping out meals and shopping appropriately, cooking in advance when possible, and preparing enough food for leftovers later in the week. A tight budget does not necessarily make it more difficult to eat healthy meals. It makes good health sense and good budget sense to use only small amounts of meat and to have a few meatless meals each week.

In restaurants, keeping to food plan goals becomes somewhat more difficult. Portion sizes in restaurants tend to be larger than serving sizes of the Food Guide Pyramid, but by remaining focused on your goals, you can eat only part of your meal and take the rest home for a meal later in the week. Don't hesitate to ask questions when you're eating in a restaurant. Most restaurant personnel are glad to explain how menu selections are prepared and to make small adjustments, such as serving salad dressings and sauces on the side so they can be avoided or used sparingly. To limit your fat intake, order meat or fish broiled or grilled rather than fried or sauteed, choose rice or a plain baked potato over french fries, and select a clear soup rather than a creamy one. Desserts that are irresistible can, at least, be shared.

Strategies like these can be helpful, but small changes cannot change a fundamentally high-fat, high-calorie meal into a moderate, healthful one. Often, the best advice is to bypass a steak with potatoes au gratin for a flavorful but low-fat entree. Many of the selections offered in ethnic restaurants are healthy choices (refer to the box on ethnic foods on p. 211 for suggestions).

Fast-food restaurants offer the biggest challenge to a healthy diet. Surveys show that about 70% of 18- to 24-year-olds and 64% of 25- to 34-year-olds visit a fast-food restaurant at least once a week. Fast-food meals are often high in calories, total fat, saturated fat, sodium, and sugar; they may be low in fiber and in some vitamins and minerals (see Appendix C). If you do eat at a fast-food restaurant, make sure the rest of your meals that day are low-fat meals.

Knowledge of food and nutrition is essential to the success of your program. The information provided in this chapter should give you the tools you need to design and implement a diet that promotes long-term health and well-being. If you need additional information or have questions about nutrition, be sure the source you consult is reliable.

COMMON QUESTIONS ANSWERED

Which is the healthier choice—butter or margarine? Both butter and margarine are concentrated sources of fat, containing about 11 grams of fat and 100 calories per tablespoon. However, butter is richer in saturated fat, a type of fat closely associated with elevated levels of artery-clogging LDLs ("bad" cholesterol). Each tablespoon of butter has about 8 grams of saturated fat; margarine averages only 2 grams of saturated fat per tablespoon, regardless of the type of vegetable oil it contains. In addition, butter contains cholesterol; margarine does not.

Based on this information, margarine is clearly the best choice. However, recent research has turned up a potential health problem with margarine, too. As described earlier in the chapter, the process of hydrogenation produces trans fatty acids, which also raise blood cholesterol levels. A tablespoon of stick margarine contains about 2 grams of trans fat.

So what should you choose? Because the combined total of saturated and trans fats in butter is twice that of stick margarine, most nutritionists would recommend margarine over butter. However, there are better options. Tub and squeeze margarines contain less saturated and trans fat than stick margarines, and most vegetable oils are low in saturated fat and completely free of trans fats. Consumption of unhydrogenated, unsaturated fats is associated with a decreased risk of heart disease.

The Food Guide Pyramid seems to recommend such a large number of servings. How can I possibly follow its recommendations without gaining weight? First of all, consider how many servings from each food group are appropriate for you. The suggested number of servings is given as a range, 6–11 servings of grain products, 3–5 of vegetables, and so on. The smaller number of servings is for people who consume about 1600 calories per day, such as many sedentary women. The larger number is for those who consume about 2800 calories per day, such as active men. If the smaller number of servings is appropriate for you, concentrate on choosing nutrient-dense foods—those that are rich in nutrients but relatively low in calories, such as most grains, fruits, and vegetables.

Second, compare the serving sizes of the foods you eat with those used in the Food Guide Pyramid (see pp. 201–205). Some of the Pyramid's serving sizes are smaller than what you might typically eat. For example, many people eat a cup or more of pasta or rice in a meal, which would correspond to 2 or more servings from the grain products group. You'll probably find that your current diet already includes the minimum number of servings from most of the food groups. If not, you may find that you are eating too many servings from one group and not enough from another. Try to make small changes in your eating habits and food choices to bring your diet into line with the recommendations in the Pyramid, paying particular attention to your consumption of fat and added sugars. The Food Guide Pyramid is designed to help you balance your food choices to ensure good health.

Strategies for successful weight management are described in detail in the next chapter.

Do I have to give up meat in order to lower the fat content of my diet to recommended levels? No. The keys for including beef, pork, and poultry in a healthy diet are to select lower-fat choices and to limit the size of your servings to those given in the Food Guide Pyramid. The amount of fat in meat products varies considerably; see the box "Guidelines for Healthier Meat Choices" for more information. The recommended 2- to 3-ounce serving of meat is about the size of a deck of cards—far smaller than what many Americans eat, especially when they eat out. Think of meat as a side dish rather than as the center of a meal. Try stir-frying lean strips of lean steak with vegetables or adding a small portion of extra-lean ground beef to spaghetti sauce. Limit your intake of high-fat processed meats such as sausages, salami, and cold cuts. When you eat out, try sharing a steak with a friend or taking half of it home.

How common is food poisoning? Food poisoning—or foodborne illness, as scientists call it—is very common. Tens of millions of cases occur each year; it is likely that your last case of "stomach flu" was actually a case of foodborne illness. The most common symptoms are diarrhea, abdominal cramps, vomiting, fever, and weakness. Most cases clear up in a few days, as long as people consume enough fluids to prevent dehydration. Foodborne illness poses a greater risk for young children, the elderly, and people with underlying chronic illnesses. And in cases where a particularly dangerous organism is involved, even a healthy adult can become seriously ill. Foodborne illness is believed to kill 6000–9000 Americans each year.

Bacteria and the toxins they produce cause most cases of foodborne illness; parasites and viruses are less common causes. *Salmonella* bacteria are responsible for almost 60% of all cases of foodborne illness; they are most often found in eggs, poultry, meat, milk, and inadequately refrigerated and reheated leftovers. The bacteria *Staphylococcus aureus* is responsible for 20–40% of cases. It is usually transferred to food when people handle or sneeze or cough over food; it is most common on meat, prepared salads, cream sauces, and cream-filled pastries. Illness from *Clostridium botulinum* or *Escherichia coli* is rare, but it can be deadly. Botulism results primarily from improperly canned foods; *E. coli* is spread mainly by undercooked ground beef, unpasteurized juices, and poorly washed fruits and vegetables.

Several outbreaks of illness tied to a particularly dangerous strain of *E. coli* led to the passage of new federal food inspection regulations in 1996. However, the new microbiological tests will not eliminate all contamination. The key to protecting yourself from foodborne illness is to handle, cook, and store foods in ways that prevent the bacteria from spreading and multiplying. Keep these tips in mind:

- Don't buy food in containers that leak, bulge, or are severely dented. Refrigerated foods should be cold, and frozen foods should be solid.

- Use or freeze fresh meats within 3–5 days after purchase; use or freeze fresh poultry, fish, and ground meat within 1–2 days.

- Thaw frozen food in the refrigerator or in the microwave oven, not on the kitchen counter.

- Thoroughly wash your hands with hot soapy water before and after handling food, especially raw meat, fish, poultry, or eggs.

- Make sure counters, cutting boards, dishes, and other equipment are thoroughly cleaned before and after use. If possible, use separate cutting boards for meat and for foods that will be eaten raw, such as fruits or vegetables. Wash dishcloths and kitchen towels frequently.

- Thoroughly rinse and scrub fruits and vegetables, with a brush, if possible; or peel off the skin or outer layer.

- Cook foods thoroughly, especially beef, poultry, fish, pork, and eggs. Cooking kills most microbes. When eating out, order red meat prepared "well done."

- Cook stuffing separately from poultry; or wash poultry thoroughly, stuff immediately before cooking, and then transfer the stuffing to a clean bowl immediately after cooking.

- Store foods below 40°F. Do not leave cooked or refrigerated foods, such as meats or salads, at room temperature for more than 2 hours.

- Don't eat raw animal products. Use only pasteurized milk and juice.

- According to the USDA, "when in doubt, throw it out."

For a bout of foodborne illness, drink plenty of clear fluids to prevent dehydration, and rest to speed your recovery. See a physician for a fever higher than 102°F, blood in the stool, or dehydration, especially if symptoms persist for more than 2–3 days. In cases of suspected botulism—characterized by symptoms such as double vision, paralysis, dizziness, and vomiting—consult a physician immediately

Choose Often

Any unground meats labeled "extra lean."

Beef: Eye of round, top round.

Veal: All kinds not listed in next two columns.

Pork: Tenderloin, 95% lean ham.

Lamb: Foreshank.

Chicken: Skinless breast.

Turkey: Breast, drumstick, or wing without skin.

Choose Sometimes

Any unground meats labeled "lean."

Beef: Tip or bottom round, sirloin, chuck pot roast, top loin, tenderloin, flank, T-bone, ground sirloin, extra-lean ground.

Veal: Loin, loin chop, ground.

Pork: Sirloin chop, top or center loin chop, rib chop, ham, Canadian bacon.

Lamb: Shank, leg, loin chop, sirloin.

Chicken: Skinless drumstick, thigh, or wing; breast with skin.

Turkey: Any piece with skin; thigh without skin; extra-lean ground.

Reduced-fat lunch meats or hot dogs, with 4 to 5 grams of fat per serving.

Choose Seldom

Beef: All cuts not listed in first two columns (such as brisket, rib roast, chuck blade roast, lean and regular ground).

Veal: Rib roast.

Pork: All kinds not listed in first two columns (such as spareribs, sausage, ground).

Lamb: All kinds not listed in first two columns (such as rib chop, arm, blade, shoulder, ground).

Chicken: Drumstick, thigh, or wing with skin; liver.

Turkey: Lean or regular ground.

Duck, goose.

Regular lunch meats or hot dogs, with more than 5 grams of fat per serving.

SOURCE: Beyond the Pyramid: Healthy choices for a healthy diet. 1996. *Consumer Reports on Health,* September, p. 103. Copyright © 1996 by Consumers Union of U.S., Inc., Yonkers, NY 10703-1057. Reprinted by permission from Consumer Reports on Health, September 1996.

SUMMARY

- The six classes of nutrients are carbohydrates, proteins, fats, vitamins, minerals, and water.

- The 45 nutrients essential to humans are released into the body through digestion. Nutrients in foods provide energy, measured in kilocalories (commonly called calories); build and maintain body tissues; and regulate body functions.

- Protein, an important component of body tissue, is composed of amino acids, nine of which are essential to a diet. Foods from animal sources provide complete proteins; plants provide incomplete proteins.

- Fat, the major body fuel at times of rest and light activity, also insulates the body and cushions the organs; 1 tablespoon of vegetable oil per day supplies the essential fats. Dietary fat should be limited to 30% or less of total calories.

- Limiting saturated and trans fatty acids in the diet can reduce the risk of heart disease; unsaturated fats may promote cardiovascular health.

- Carbohydrates provide energy to the brain, nervous system, and blood and to muscles during high-intensity exercise. Naturally occurring simple carbohydrates and unrefined complex carbohydrates should be favored over added sugars and refined carbohydrates. Dietary fiber cannot be broken down by the body; it helps reduce cholesterol levels and promotes the passage of wastes through the intestines.

- The 13 essential vitamins are either water- or fat-soluble; they help unleash energy in food sources and act as antioxidants. The 17 known essential minerals regulate body functions, aid in growth and tissue maintenance, and act as catalysts to release energy. Deficiencies in vitamins and minerals can cause severe symptoms over time, but excess doses are also dangerous.

- Water, distributed in body tissues and fluids, aids in digestion and food absorption, allows chemical reactions to take place, serves as a lubricant or cushion, and helps regulate body temperature.

- Foods contain other substances, such as phytochemicals, which may not be essential nutrients but which may protect against chronic diseases.

- The Recommended Dietary Allowances, Dietary Reference Intakes, Food Guide Pyramid, and Dietary Guidelines for Americans provide standards and recommendations for getting all essential nutrients from a varied, balanced diet and for eating in ways that protect against chronic disease.

- Basic recommendations for a healthy diet include eating a variety of foods; reducing all fat, especially saturated fat; increasing complex carbohydrates; and limiting sugar, salt, alcohol, and smoked and nitrate-cured foods.

- A vegetarian diet requires special planning to meet all nutrient requirements; grains, legumes, and a variety of fruits and vegetables are central.
- Careful planning can help people of all ages, activity levels, and medical conditions meet special dietary challenges.

FOR MORE INFORMATION

For reliable nutrition advice, talk to a faculty member in the nutrition department on your campus, a registered dietitian (R.D.), or your physician. Many large communities have a telephone service called Dial a Dietitian. By calling this number, you can receive free nutrition information from an R.D.

Experts on quackery suggest that you steer clear of anyone who puts forth any of the following false statements:

- Most diseases are caused primarily by faulty nutrition.
- Large doses of vitamins are effective against many diseases.
- Hair analysis can be used to determine a person's nutritional state.
- A computer-scored nutritional deficiency test is a basis for prescribing vitamins.

Any practitioner—licensed or not—who sells vitamins in his or her office should be thoroughly scrutinized.

Books

Duyff, R. L. 1998. *The American Dietetic Association's Complete Food and Nutrition Guide*. Minneapolis, Minn.: Chronimed Publishing. *An excellent review of current nutrition information and issues.*

Coleman, E. 1997. *Eating for Endurance*. Rev. ed. Palo Alto, Calif.: Bull Publishing. *A concise, easy-to-understand guide to sports nutrition.*

Editors of Vegetarian Times Magazine. 1995. *Vegetarian Times Complete Cookbook*. New York: Macmillan. *Contains introductory chapters on the health benefits of vegetarianism and on meal planning, along with over 600 recipes.*

Finn, S. C. 1997. *The American Dietetic Association Guide to Women's Nutrition for Healthy Living*. New York: Perigee Books. *A complete guide to eating right for lifelong health.*

Nutrition and Your Health: Dietary Guidelines for Americans. 1995. U.S. Department of Health and Human Services and U.S. Department of Agriculture. Home and Garden Bulletin No. 232. *A 42-page booklet that describes the Guidelines and provides helpful tips for implementing them.*

Newsletters

Environmental Nutrition: P.O. Box 420235, Palm Coast, FL 32142; 800-829-5384.

Nutrition Action Health Letter: 1875 Connecticut Ave., N.W., Suite 300, Washington DC 20009; 202-332-9110 (http://www.cspinet.org).

Tufts University Health & Nutrition Letter: P.O. Box 57857, Boulder, CO 80322; 800-274-7581.

Organizations, Hotlines, and Web Sites

American Dietetic Association. Provides a wide variety of nutrition-related educational materials.
  800-366-1655 (For general nutrition information and referrals to registered dietitians.)
  900-CALL-AN-RD (For customized answers to nutrition questions.)
  http://www.eatright.org

Ask the Dietitian. Questions and answers on many topics relating to nutrition.
  http://www.dietitian.com

CyberDiet Nutritional Profile. Calculates calorie and nutrient needs based on your current or target body weight and creates a personalized nutrient profile.
  http://www.CyberDiet.com/profile/profile.html

FDA Center for Food Safety and Applied Nutrition. Offers information about topics such as food labeling, food additives, and foodborne illness.
  http://vm.cfsan.fda.gov

Meals Online. Includes over 10,000 healthful recipes.
  http://www.meals.com

National Osteoporosis Foundation. Provides up-to-date information on the causes, prevention, detection, and treatment of osteoporosis.
  202-223-2226
  http://www.nof.org

Tufts University Nutrition Navigator. Provides descriptions and ratings for many nutrition-related Web pages.
  http://www.navigator.tufts.edu

USDA Food and Nutrition Information Center. Provides a variety of materials relating to the Dietary Guidelines, food labels, and many other topics; Web site includes extensive links.
  301-504-5719
  http://www.nal.usda.gov/fnic

USDA Meat and Poultry Hotline. Information from USDA experts on topics such as the proper handling, preparation, storage, and cooking of food.
  800-535-4555

Vegetarian Resource Group. Information and links for vegetarians and people interested in learning more about vegetarian diets.
  http://www.vrg.org

You can obtain nutrient breakdowns of individual food items from the following sites:

Nutribase
  http://www.nutribase.com

Nutrition Analysis Tool, University of Illinois, Urbana/Champaign
  http://www.ag.uiuc.edu/~food-lab/nat

USDA Food and Nutrition Information Center
  http://www.nal.usda.gov/fnic/foodcomp

See also the resources listed in Chapters 9, 11, and 12.

SELECTED BIBLIOGRAPHY

The American Dietetic Association. 1996. Position Statement: Nutrition Education for the Public. *Journal of the American Dietetic Association* 96(11): 1183–1187.

The American Dietetic Association and the Canadian Dietetic Association. 1997. *Position Statement: Nutrition for Physical*

Fitness and Athletic Performance for Adults (retrieved September 20, 1997; http://www.eatright.org/afitperform.html).

American Society for Clinical Nutrition/American Institute of Nutrition Task Force. 1996. Position paper on *trans* fatty acids. *American Journal of Clinical Nutrition* 63:663–670.

Ascherio, A., et al. 1995. Dietary intake of marine *n-3* fatty acids, fish intake, and the risk of coronary disease among men. *New England Journal of Medicine* 332:977–982.

Bidlack, W. R. 1996. Interrelationships of food, nutrition, diet and health: The National Association of State Universities and Land Grant Colleges White Paper. *Journal of American College Nutrition* 15(5): 422–433.

Bowman, M. A., and J. G. Spangler. 1997. Osteoporosis in women. *Primary Care* 24(1): 27–36.

Burke, L. 1995. Practical issues in nutrition for athletes. *Journal of Sports Sciences* 13(Spec): S83–S80.

Clark, N. 1996. Nutrition knowledge: Answers to the top ten questions. *The Physician and Sportsmedicine* (retrieved September 20, 1997; http://www.physsportsmed.com/issues/oct_96/top_ten.htm).

Clark, N. 1997. Eating for vitamins: Do you need supplements? *The Physician and Sportsmedicine* (retrieved September 20, 1997; http://www.physsportsmed.com/issues/1997/07jul/vitamins.htm).

Coleman, E., and S. N. Steen. 1996. *The Ultimate Sports Nutrition Handbook.* Palo Alto, Calif.: Bull Publishing.

The facts about fats. 1997. *Consumer Reports on Health,* March.

Food and Nutrition Board. Institute of Medicine. National Academy of Sciences. 1998. *Dietary Reference Intakes for Thiamin, Riboflavin, Niacin, Vitamin B$_6$, Folate, Vitamin B$_{12}$, Pantothenic Acid, Biotin, and Choline.* Washington, D.C.: National Academy Press.

Georgiou, C., et al. 1996. Young adult exercisers and nonexercisers differ in food attitudes, perceived dietary changes, and food choices. *International Journal of Sport Nutrition* 6(4): 402–413.

Ghiselli, A., A. D'Amicis, and A. Giacosa. 1997. The antioxidant potential of the Mediterranean diet. *European Journal of Cancer Prevention* 6(Suppl 1): S15–S19.

Halliwell, B. 1996. Antioxidants in human health and disease. *Annual Review of Nutrition* 16:33–50.

Hu, F. B., et al. 1997. Dietary fat intake and the risk of coronary heart disease in women. *New England Journal of Medicine* 337(21): 1491–1499.

Kipp, D. E., J. D. Radel, and J. A. Hogue. 1996. The Internet and the nutritional scientist. *American Journal of Clinical Nutrition* 64(4): 659–662.

Kirwan, J. P., D. O'Gorman, and W. J. Evans. 1998. A moderate glycemic meal before endurance exercise can enhance performance. *Journal of Applied Physiology* 84(1): 53–59.

Kleiner, S. M. 1995. Nutrition on the run. *The Physician and Sportsmedicine* 23(2): 15–16.

Looker, A. C., et al. 1997. Prevalence of iron deficiency in the United States. *Journal of the American Medical Association* 277(12): 973–976.

Millen, B. E., et al. 1997. Population nutrient intake approaches dietary recommendations: 1991 to 1995 Farmingham Nutrition Studies. *Journal of the American Dietetic Association* 97(7): 742–749.

Monteleone, G. P., Jr., and D. G. Browning. 1997. Nutrition in women. Assessment and counseling. *Primary Care* 24(1): 37–51.

Muñoz, K. A., et al. 1997. Food intakes of U.S. children and adolescents compared with recommendations. *Pediatrics* 100(3 Pt 1): 323–329.

Neumark-Sztainer, D., et al. 1997. Adolescent vegetarians. A behavioral profile of a school-based population in Minnesota. *Archives of Pediatrics and Adolescent Medicine* 151(8): 833–838.

Nieman, D. C. 1999. *Exercise Testing and Prescription; A Health-Related Approach.* 4th ed. Mountain View, Calif.: Mayfield.

Schwartz, N. E., and S. T. Borra. 1997. What do consumers really think about dietary fat? *Journal of the American Dietetic Association* 97(7 Suppl): S73–S75.

Siega-Riz, A. M., T. Carson, and B. Popkin. 1998. Three squares or mostly snacks—what do teens really eat? A sociodemographic study of meal patterns. *Journal of Adolescent Health* 22(1): 29–36.

Slutsker, L., et al. 1997. *Escherichia coli* O157:H7 diarrhea in the United States: Clinical and epidemiologic features. *Annals of Internal Medicine* 126(7): 505–513.

Sundram, K., et al. 1997. Trans (elaidic) fatty acids adversely affect the lipoprotein profile relative to specific fatty acids in humans. *Journal of Nutrition* 127(3): 514S–520S.

U.S. Department of Agriculture. Center for Nutrition Policy and Promotion. 1996. *The Food Guide Pyramid.* Home and Garden Bulletin No. 252.

U.S. Food and Drug Administration. 1996. *Folic Acid Fortification.* Office of Public Affairs Fact Sheet (retrieved February 29, 1996; http://vm.cfsan.fda.gov/~dms/wh-folic.html).

Uusi-Rasi, K., et al. 1998. Associations of physical activity and calcium intake with bone mass and size in healthy women at different ages. *Journal of Bone Mineral Research* 13(1): 133–142.

Weber, J. L., et al. 1997. Multimethod training increases portion-size estimation accuracy. *Journal of the American Dietetic Association* 97(2): 176–179.

Wilson, J. W., et al. 1997. *Data Tables: Combined Results from USDA's 1994 and 1995 Continuing Survey of Food Intakes for Individuals and 1994 and 1995 Diet and Health Knowledge Survey.* ARS Food Surveys Research Group. U.S. Department of Agriculture (retrieved December 2, 1997; http://www.barc.usda.gov/bhnrc/foodsurvey/home.htm).

Name _____   Section _____   Date _____

LAB 8-1 *Your Daily Diet Versus the Food Guide Pyramid*

Keep a record of everything you eat for 3 consecutive days. Record all foods and beverages you consume, breaking each food item into its component parts (for example, a turkey sandwich would be listed as 2 slices of bread, 3 oz of turkey, 1 tsp of mayonnaise, and so on). Complete the first two columns of the chart during the course of the day; fill in the remaining information at the end of the day using Figure 8-5 and pp. 202–203 in your text.

DAY 1

Food	Portion Size	Food Group	Number of Servings*

Daily Total

Food Group	Number of Servings
Milk, yogurt, cheese	
Meat, poultry, fish, dry beans, eggs, nuts	
Fruits	
Vegetables	
Breads, cereals, rice, pasta	

*Your portion sizes may be smaller or larger than the serving sizes given in the Food Guide Pyramid; list the actual number of Food Guide Pyramid servings contained in the foods you eat.

DAY 2

Food	Portion Size	Food Group	Number of Servings*

Daily Total

Food Group	Number of Servings
Milk, yogurt, cheese	
Meat, poultry, fish, dry beans, eggs, nuts	
Fruits	
Vegetables	
Breads, cereals, rice, pasta	

*Your portion sizes may be smaller or larger than the serving sizes given in the Food Guide Pyramid; list the actual number of Food Guide Pyramid servings contained in the foods you eat.

DAY 3

Food	Portion Size	Food Group	Number of Servings*

Daily Total

Food Group	Number of Servings
Milk, yogurt, cheese	
Meat, poultry, fish, dry beans, eggs, nuts	
Fruits	
Vegetables	
Breads, cereals, rice, pasta	

*Your portion sizes may be smaller or larger than the serving sizes given in the Food Guide Pyramid; list the actual number of Food Guide Pyramid servings contained in the foods you eat.

Next, average your serving totals for the 3 days, and enter them in the chart below. Fill in the recommended serving totals that apply to you from Figure 8-5 and Table 8-8.

Food Group	Recommended Number of Servings	Actual Number of Servings
Milk, yogurt, cheese		
Meat, poultry, fish, dry beans, eggs, nuts		
Fruits		
Vegetables		
Breads, cereals, rice, pasta		

Are there any groups for which you need to increase your consumption? Decrease your consumption? List any areas of concern below, along with ideas for changing them. Think carefully about the reasons behind your food choices. For example, if you eat doughnuts for breakfast every morning because you feel rushed, make a list of ways to save time to allow for a more healthful breakfast.

Problem: _____

Possible solutions: _____

_____

_____

_____

_____

Problem: _____

Possible solutions: _____

_____

_____

_____

_____

Problem: _____

Possible solutions: _____

_____

_____

_____

_____

_____

To monitor your progress toward your goal, enter the results of this lab in the Preprogram Assessment column of Appendix D. After several weeks of dietary changes, do this lab again and enter the results in the Postprogram Assessment column of Appendix D. How do the results compare?

LAB 8-2 *Dietary Analysis*

You can complete this activity using either a nutrition analysis software program or the food composition data in Appendix B and the charts printed below. Information about the nutrient content of foods is also available online; see the For More Information section for recommended Web sites.

Part I. Analyze Your Diet for 3 Days

If you are using the software, follow the instructions to complete an analysis of your diet on 3 separate days; otherwise, complete the charts on the first three pages of this lab. Then go on to the second part of the lab.

Date_____   Day: M Tu W Th F Sa Su

Food	Amount	Calories	Protein (g)	Fat, total (g)	Saturated fat (g)	Carbohydrate[a] (g)	Dietary fiber (g)	Cholesterol (mg)	Sodium (mg)	Calcium (mg)	Iron (mg)
Recommended totals[b]			10–15%	≤30%	<10%	≥55%	20–35 g	≤300 mg	≤2400 mg	mg	mg
Actual totals[c]		cal	g / %	g / %	g / %	g / %	g	mg	mg	mg	mg

[a]To obtain a value for total grams of carbohydrate from Appendix B, add the values in the columns for carbohydrates ("Carbo.") and added sugars ("Sug.").
[b]Fill in the appropriate RDA or DRI values for calcium and iron from Tables 8-5 and 8-6.
[c]Total the values in each column. To calculate the percentage of total calories from protein, carbohydrate, fat, and saturated fat, use the formulas on p. 189. Protein and carbohydrate provide 4 calories per gram; fat provides 9 calories per gram. For example, if you consume a total of 270 grams of carbohydrate and 2000 calories, your percentage of total calories from carbohydrate would be (270 g × 4 cal/g) ÷ 2000 cal = 54%. Do not include data for alcoholic beverages in your calculations. Percentages may not total 100% due to rounding.

Date_____   Day: M Tu W Th F Sa Su

Food	Amount	Calories	Protein (g)	Fat, total (g)	Saturated fat (g)	Carbohydrate[a] (g)	Dietary fiber (g)	Cholesterol (mg)	Sodium (mg)	Calcium (mg)	Iron (mg)
Recommended totals[b]			10–15%	≤30%	<10%	≥55%	20–35 g	≤300 mg	≤2400 mg	mg	mg
Actual totals[c]		cal	g / %	g / %	g / %	g / %	g	mg	mg	mg	mg

Food	Amount	Calories	Protein (g)	Fat, total (g)	Saturated fat (g)	Carbohydrate[a] (g)	Dietary fiber (g)	Cholesterol (mg)	Sodium (mg)	Calcium (mg)	Iron (mg)
Recommended totals[b]			10–15%	≤30%	<10%	≥55%	20–35 g	≤300 mg	≤2400 mg	mg	mg
Actual totals[c]		cal	g / %	g / %	g / %	g / %	g	mg	mg	mg	mg

LABORATORY ACTIVITIES

To monitor your progress toward your goal, enter the results of one day's dietary analysis in the Preprogram Assessment column of Appendix D. After several weeks of dietary changes, do this lab again and enter the results in the Postprogram Assessment column of Appendix D. How do the results compare?

Part II. Making Changes in Your Diet to Meet the Dietary Guidelines

(*Note:* If your daily diet follows all the recommended intakes, you don't need to complete this section.) Choose one of your daily diet records. Make changes, additions, and deletions from it until it conforms to all or most of the Dietary Guidelines. Or, if you prefer, start from scratch to create a day's diet that meets all guidelines. Use the chart below to experiment and record your final, healthy sample diet for one day.

Date_____   Day: M Tu W Th F Sa Su

Food	Amount	Calories	Protein (g)	Fat, total (g)	Saturated fat (g)	Carbohydrate[a] (g)	Dietary fiber (g)	Cholesterol (mg)	Sodium (mg)	Calcium (mg)	Iron (mg)
Recommended totals[b]			10–15%	≤30%	<10%	≥55%	20–35 g	≤300 mg	≤2400 mg	mg	mg
Actual totals[c]		cal	g / g	g / g	g / mg	g / mg	mg	mg			

LAB 8-3 *Informed Food Choices*

Part I. Using Food Labels

Choose three food items to evaluate. You might want to select three similar items, such as regular, low-fat, and non-fat salad dressing, or three very different items. Record the information from their food labels in the table below. How do the items you chose compare?

Food Items			
Serving size			
Total calories	cal	cal	cal
Total fat—grams	g	g	g
—% Daily Value	%	%	%
Saturated fat—grams	g	g	g
—% Daily Value	%	%	%
Cholesterol—milligrams	mg	mg	mg
—% Daily Value	%	%	%
Sodium—milligrams	mg	mg	mg
—% Daily Value	%	%	%
Carbohydrates (total)—grams	g	g	g
—% Daily Value	%	%	%
Dietary fiber—grams	g	g	g
—% Daily Value	%	%	%
Sugars—grams	g	g	g
Protein—grams	g	g	g
Vitamin A—% Daily Value	%	%	%
Vitamin C—% Daily Value	%	%	%
Calcium—% Daily Value	%	%	%
Iron—% Daily Value	%	%	%

Part II. Evaluating Fast Food

Use the information from Appendix C, Nutritional Content of Popular Items from Fast-Food Restaurants, to complete the chart on the next page for the last fast-food meal you ate. Add up your totals for the meal. Compare the values for fat, protein, carbohydrate, cholesterol, and sodium content for each food item and for the meal as a whole with the levels suggested by the Dietary Guidelines for Americans. Calculate the percent of total calories derived from fat, saturated fat, protein, and carbohydrate using the formulas given.

If you haven't recently been to one of the restaurants included in the appendix, fill in the chart for any sample meal you might eat. If some of the food items you selected don't appear in Appendix C, ask for a nutrition information brochure when you visit the restaurant, or check out online fast-food information: Arby's (http://www.arbysrestaurant.com), Burger King (http://www.burgerking.com), Domino's Pizza (http://www.dominos.com), Jack in the Box (http://www.jackinthebox.com), KFC (http://www.kfc.com), McDonald's (http://www.mcdonalds.com), Taco Bell (http://www.tacobell.com), Wendy's (http://www.wendys.com).

Food Items

	Dietary Guidelines							Total[b]
Serving size (g)		g	g	g	g	g	g	g
Calories		cal	cal	cal	cal	cal	cal	cal
Total fat—grams		g	g	g	g	g	g	g
—% calories[a]	≤30%	%	%	%	%	%	%	%
Saturated fat—grams		g	g	g	g	g	g	g
—% calories[a]	<10%	%	%	%	%	%	%	%
Protein—grams		g	g	g	g	g	g	g
—% calories[a]	10–15%	%	%	%	%	%	%	%
Carbohydrate—grams		g	g	g	g	g	g	g
—% calories[a]	≥55%	%	%	%	%	%	%	%
Cholesterol[c]	100 mg	mg	mg	mg	mg	mg	mg	mg
Sodium[c]	800 mg	mg	mg	mg	mg	mg	mg	mg

[a]To calculate the percent of total calories from each food energy source (fat, carbohydrate, protein), use the following formula:

$$\frac{(\text{number of grams of energy source}) \times (\text{number of calories per gram of energy source})}{(\text{total calories in serving of food item})}$$

(*Note:* Fat and saturated fat provide 9 calories per gram; protein and carbohydrate provide 4 calories per gram.) For example, the percent of total calories from protein in a 150-calorie dish containing 10 grams of protein is

$$\frac{(10 \text{ grams of protein}) \times (4 \text{ calories per gram})}{(150 \text{ calories})} = \frac{40}{150} = 0.27, \text{ or } 27\% \text{ of total calories from protein}$$

[b]For the Total column, add up the total grams of fat, carbohydrate, and protein contained in your sample meal and calculate the percentages based on the total calories in the meal. (Percentages may not total 100% due to rounding.) For cholesterol and sodium values, add up the total number of milligrams.

[c]Recommended daily limits of cholesterol and sodium are divided by 3 here to give an approximate recommended limit for a single meal.

SOURCE: Insel, P. M., and W. T. Roth. 1998. Wellness Worksheet 48. *Core Concepts in Health.* 8th ed. Mountain View, Calif.: Mayfield.

Weight Management

9

LOOKING AHEAD

After reading this chapter, you should be able to answer these questions about weight management:

- How do overweight and obesity affect health?

- How do genetic factors and metabolic rate influence a person's weight?

- What are the components of a lifestyle that leads naturally to a healthy body weight?

- Why is dieting not a successful approach to weight loss?

- What are the most effective strategies for losing weight?

- What are the symptoms, effects, and treatments for eating disorders?

Controlling body weight is really a matter of controlling body fat. As explained in Chapter 6, the most important consideration for health is not total weight but body composition—the proportion of body fat to fat-free mass. Many people who are "overweight" are also overfat, and the health risks they face are due to the latter condition. Although this chapter uses the common terms *weight management* and *weight loss,* the goal of a wellness lifestyle is to achieve a healthy body composition, not to conform to rigid standards of total body weight.

Controlling body weight and body fat is not a mysterious process. The "secret" of weight management is simply balancing calories consumed with calories expended in daily activities—in other words, eating a moderate diet and exercising regularly. Unfortunately, this simple formula is not as exciting as the latest fad diet or "scientific breakthrough" that promises slimness without effort. The American public is assaulted year after year by a steady stream of diet books, dietary supplements, commercial weight-loss programs, and medical procedures for weight loss. However, dieting can undermine the development of a truly healthy lifestyle that will naturally allow a person to maintain an appropriate body weight. Dieting is not part of a wellness lifestyle. Weight management involves the adoption of healthy and sustainable eating and exercise habits that will maximize energy and well-being and reduce the risk of chronic diseases.

This chapter sorts out the factors that contribute to a weight problem, takes a closer look at weight management through lifestyle, and suggests specific strategies for permanent weight loss. This information is designed to provide all the tools necessary for integrating effective weight management into an overall wellness program.

HEALTH IMPLICATIONS OF OVERWEIGHT AND OBESITY

Excess body fat increases a person's risk of developing numerous diseases and unhealthy conditions, as discussed in Chapter 6. Obesity is one of five major controllable risk factors for heart disease; it increases risk for other forms of cardiovascular disease (CVD), hypertension, gallbladder disease, and diabetes. Obesity may also be associated with high levels of blood fats, and it is correlated with certain types of cancer, including cancer of the colon, prostate, ovary, breast, and cervix. Women who are obese are more likely to suffer from menstrual abnor-

VITAL STATISTICS

TABLE 9-1	The Prevalence of Overweight: Populations of Special Concern	
Group	Overweight and Obesity (BMI ≥25)	Obesity (BMI ≥30)
Adults (age ≥20)	54.9%	22.3%
Men	59.4	19.5
Women	50.7	25.0
Black women	66.0	36.7
Mexican American women	65.9	33.3
Men (age 50–59)	73.0	28.9
Women (age 50–59)	64.4	35.6

SOURCE: National Heart, Lung, and Blood Institute. 1998. *Clinical Guidelines on the Identification, Evaluation, and Treatment of Overweight and Obesity in Adults.* Bethesda, Md.: National Institutes of Health.

malities and complications during pregnancy; and in severely obese people of both sexes, the rates of respiratory problems and joint disease are higher than normal.

The overall health risks of obesity were illustrated in a study that followed over 120,000 women for more than 16 years. Among women who had never smoked, the slimmest—those with a body mass index (BMI) of 19 or less—had the lowest risk of death from all causes. The relative risk of death increased as BMI increased, and the risk doubled for women with a BMI over 29. Gaining pounds over the years was also shown to be hazardous: The women who reported gaining 22 or more pounds since they were 18 years old showed a sevenfold increase in their risk of coronary heart disease. The results of this study reinforce the compelling conclusion of many others: Obesity shortens lives.

Currently, about 55% of American adults are overweight and 22% are obese, making weight management one of the most serious and widespread challenges to health and wellness (Table 9-1).

FACTORS THAT CONTRIBUTE TO A WEIGHT PROBLEM

Why do some people become obese and others remain thin? A variety of factors—physical, psychological, cultural, and social—play significant roles in determining body weight. Research has linked genetic factors and metabolism, in particular, to body weight problems.

Genetic Factors Versus Environmental Factors

Both genetic and environmental factors influence the development of obesity. Genes influence body size and

TERMS **resting metabolic rate (RMR)** The energy required (in calories) to maintain vital body functions, including respiration, heart rate, body temperature, and blood pressure, while the body is at rest.

ENERGY IN
Food calories

ENERGY OUT
Physical activity 10–40%
Food digestion 5–15%
Resting metabolism 55–75%

Figure 9-1 The energy-balance equation. In order to maintain your current weight, you must burn up as many calories as you take in as food each day.

shape, body fat distribution, and metabolic rate. Genetic factors also affect the ease with which weight is gained as a result of overeating and where on the body extra weight is added. If both parents are overweight, their children are twice as likely to be overweight as children who have only one overweight parent. In studies that compared adoptees and their biological parents, the weights of the adoptees were found to be more like those of the biological parents than those of the adoptive parents, again indicating a strong genetic link. It's estimated that 25–70% of the BMI variance among people is due to genetics and associated biological factors.

In studies of mice, scientists located a gene (named *ob*) that appears to influence appetite and the development of obesity. The gene produces a hormonelike protein called leptin that is secreted by the body's fat cells and carried to the brain. Leptin seems to let the brain know how big or small the body's fat stores are, and the brain can regulate appetite and metabolic rate accordingly. Mice with a defective or missing *ob* gene overate and gained weight. But when injected with leptin, the obese mice ate less, had higher metabolic rates, and lost weight. Even mice of normal weight lost weight when injected with leptin.

Could leptin "cure" obesity in humans? As encouraging as this finding is, obesity in humans is likely to turn out to be more complicated than a one-gene phenomenon. Many obese people have been found to have normal or higher-than-normal levels of leptin in their bloodstream; researchers hypothesize that they may have faulty leptin receptors in their brains. Other chemicals that may also be significant in controlling appetite include orexin, cortisol, gluconlike peptide-1 (GLP-1), neuropeptide Y (NPY), and peptide YY. However, additional studies will be needed before a treatment can be developed based on any of these findings.

All this research points to a genetic component in the determination of body weight. However, hereditary influences must be balanced against the contribution of environmental factors. Not all children of obese parents become obese, and normal-weight parents also have overweight children. The incidence of obesity is rising in the United States, but not in most of the rest of the world. In a study comparing men born and raised in Ireland with their biological brothers who lived in the United States, the American men were found to weigh, on average, 6% more than their Irish brothers. Environmental factors like diet and exercise are probably responsible for this difference in weight. Thus, the *tendency* to develop obesity may be inherited, but the expression of this tendency is affected by environmental influences.

The message you should take from this research is that genes are not destiny. It is true that some people have a harder time losing weight and maintaining weight loss than others. However, with increased exercise and attention to diet, even those with a genetic tendency toward obesity can maintain a healthy body weight. And regardless of genetic factors, lifestyle choices remain the cornerstone of successful weight management.

Metabolism and Energy Balance

Metabolism is the sum of all the vital processes by which food energy and nutrients are made available to and used by the body. The largest component of metabolism, **resting metabolic rate (RMR),** is the energy required to maintain vital body functions, including respiration, heart rate, body temperature, and blood pressure, while the body is at rest. As shown in Figure 9-1, RMR accounts for 55–75% of daily energy expenditure. The energy required to digest food accounts for an additional 5–15% of daily energy expenditure. The remaining 10–40% is expended during physical activity.

Both heredity and behavior affect metabolic rate. Men, who have a higher proportion of muscle mass than women, have a higher RMR (muscle tissue is more metabolically active than fat). Also, some individuals inherit a higher or lower RMR than others. A higher RMR means that a person burns more calories while at rest and can therefore take in more calories without gaining weight.

Weight loss or gain also affects metabolic rate. When a person loses weight, both RMR and the energy required to perform physical tasks decrease. The body thus "defends" its original weight by conserving energy and making it easier to regain lost pounds. For example, a man who formerly weighed 165 pounds but who now weighs 150 pounds must eat about 15% fewer calories to maintain his new, lower weight than a man who has weighed 150 pounds throughout his adult life. The reverse occurs when weight is gained; RMR increases, pushing weight back down toward its original level. The message from this research is that although weight loss can be achieved and maintained, it requires ongoing commitment.

Exercise has a positive effect on metabolism. When people exercise, they increase their RMR—the number of calories their bodies burn at rest. They also increase their fat-free mass, which is associated with a higher metabolic rate. The exercise itself also burns calories, raising total energy expenditure. The higher the energy expenditure, the more the person can eat without gaining weight.

The two factors in the energy-balance equation illustrated in Figure 9-1 that fall under individual control are the amount of energy intake (in food) and the number of calories expended in physical activity. For these simple reasons alone, increased physical activity is a critical component of a long-term program of weight management. (To determine your own RMR, complete Lab 9-1.)

Other Explanations for Overweight

Researchers have proposed various other explanations for overweight besides heredity and metabolism. These explanations include weight cycling, binge eating, and psychological, social, and cultural factors.

Weight Cycling   It has been hypothesized that repeated dieting resulting in cycles of weight loss and weight gain ("yo-yo dieting") is harmful both to weight management and to overall health. Researchers proposed that cycling increases the body's efficiency at extracting and storing calories from food, making weight loss increasingly difficult with each successive diet. Although some studies have found support for this idea, most have not; and current thinking is that weight cycling probably does not result in increased efficiency. On balance, when the substantial health benefits of even modest weight loss are compared with the uncertain potential adverse health consequences of losing weight or weight cycling, the benefits of losing weight clearly exceed the potential risks.

The Restrained Eating Theory   According to the restrained eating theory, restrictive dieting can cause excessive hunger and feelings of deprivation, possibly leading to **binge eating.** Attempts to restrain food intake may contribute to confusion about internal hunger cues and increase susceptibility to external cues (the sight of food, for example). As hunger or fatigue increases, or if confronted with cues in the environment, a person's restraint may falter. For many restrained eaters, once they violate their self-imposed diet rules, they simply give up and overeat or even binge. This overeating is usually followed by feelings of guilt, shame, and self-blame. Binge eating may contribute to the development of obesity in some people.

Psychological, Social, and Cultural Factors   Many people have learned to use food as a means of coping with stress and negative emotions. Eating can provide a powerful distraction from difficult feelings—loneliness, anger, boredom, anxiety, shame, sadness, inadequacy. It can be used to combat low moods, low energy levels, and low self-esteem. When food and eating become the primary means of regulating emotions, binge eating or other disturbed eating patterns can develop.

Obesity is strongly associated with socioeconomic status. The prevalence of obesity goes down as income level goes up. More women are obese at lower income levels than men, but men are somewhat more obese at higher levels. These differences may reflect the greater sensitivity and concern for a slim physical appearance among upper-income women, as well as greater access to information about nutrition and to low-fat and low-calorie foods. It may also reflect the greater acceptance of obesity among certain ethnic groups, as well as different cultural values related to food choices.

In some families and cultures, food is used as a symbol of love and caring. It is an integral part of social gatherings and celebrations. In such cases, it may be difficult to change established eating patterns because they are linked to cultural and family values.

WEIGHT MANAGEMENT AND LIFESTYLE

When all the research has been assessed, it is clear that most weight problems are lifestyle problems. Looking at these problems in a historical context reveals why fad diets and other quick-fix approaches are not effective in reversing overweight.

TERMS   **binge eating**   A pattern of eating in which normal food consumption is interrupted by episodes of high consumption.

Foods that contain more calories than you might expect include the following:

- *Reduced-fat foods.* Manufacturers often replace fat with extra sugar, so many low-fat and fat-free foods have at least as many calories as their full-fat versions. Check food labels of reduced-fat foods for the appropriate serving size and total calories.

- *Regular sodas.* A 12-ounce serving of regular soda is high in added sugars and contains about 150–200 calories. Substitute plain water or, if you want something carbonated, mineral or sparkling water.

- *Alcoholic beverages.* As stated in Chapter 8, alcohol contains 7 calories per gram. A glass of wine contains about 100 calories, a beer or cocktail about 150 calories, and a wine cooler over 175 calories. Try light or nonalcoholic versions, or substitute a lower-calorie type of beverage.

- *Fruit juices, drinks, and ades.* A cup of juice contains the juice of many fruits and is therefore higher in calories than whole fruit (for example, a cup of orange juice has about 110 calories, an orange about 65 calories). Fruit drinks and ades are often low in nutrients and high in added sugar. Choose juices over drinks and ades, keep your juice servings small, and substitute whole fruits for juice often.

- *Muffins.* Many muffins are large, are high in fat, and contain more than 300–500 calories. Choose whole-grain breads, cereals, bagels, or English muffins instead.

- *Condiments.* Butter, margarine, mayonnaise, and salad dressing all contribute about 100 calories per tablespoon; jams and jellies have about 50 calories per tablespoon. Cream, sour cream, sugar, syrup, and honey are also packed with calories. Use these concentrated sources of fats and added sugars sparingly. Substitute low-fat and nonfat dairy products and dressings for the full-fat versions. Use herbs, spices, lemon juice, ketchup, mustard, or salsa to add flavor to foods.

SOURCES: Hidden calories. 1997. *Mayo Clinic Health Letter,* September. U.S. Department of Agriculture. Center for Nutrition Policy and Promotion. 1996. *The Food Guide Pyramid.* Home and Garden Bulletin No. 252.

About 100 years ago, Americans consumed a diet very different from today's diet and got much more exercise as well. Americans now eat more fat and refined sugars and fewer complex carbohydrates. And despite an increased interest in fitness, Americans today get far less exercise than their great-grandparents did. Walking, bicycling, and farm and manual labor have all declined, resulting in a decrease in daily energy expenditure of about 200 calories. This decline, coupled with dietary changes, is measurable in the number of overweight Americans: about 97 million, and rising.

Permanent weight loss is not something you start and stop. You need to adopt healthy behaviors that you can maintain throughout your life. Lifestyle factors that are critical for successful long-term weight management include diet and eating habits, physical activity and exercise, an ability to think positively and manage your emotions effectively, and the coping strategies you use to deal with the stresses and challenges in your life.

Diet and Eating Habits

In contrast to "dieting," which involves some form of food restriction, "diet" refers to your daily food choices. Everyone has a diet, but not everyone is dieting. You need to develop a diet that you enjoy and that enables you to maintain a healthy body composition.

Total Calories To maintain your current weight, the total number of calories you eat must equal the number you burn (refer to the energy-balance equation in Figure 9-1). To lose weight, you must decrease your calorie intake and/or increase the number of calories you burn. According to the Centers for Disease Control and Prevention, the average calorie intake by Americans has increased by 100–300 calories per day over the past decade (see the box "Avoiding Hidden Calories"). Levels of physical activity did not increase during this period, so the net result was a substantial increase in the number of Americans who are obese. To calculate your daily caloric needs, complete the calculations in Lab 9-1.

The best approach for weight loss is probably combining an increase in physical activity with moderate calorie restriction. Don't go on a "crash diet." You need to consume enough food to meet your need for essential nutrients. Also, to maintain weight loss, you will probably have to maintain some degree of the calorie restriction you used to lose the weight. Therefore, it is important that you adopt a level of food intake that you can live with over the long term.

Portion Sizes Overconsumption of total calories is closely tied with portion sizes. Most of us significantly underestimate the amount of food we eat. Limiting portion sizes to those recommended in the Food Guide Pyramid is critical for weight management. For many people, concentrating on portion sizes is also a much easier method of monitoring and managing total food intake than counting calories. (Refer to Chapter 8 for more on appropriate portion sizes.)

Fat Calories Although some fat is needed in the diet to provide essential nutrients, you should avoid overeating

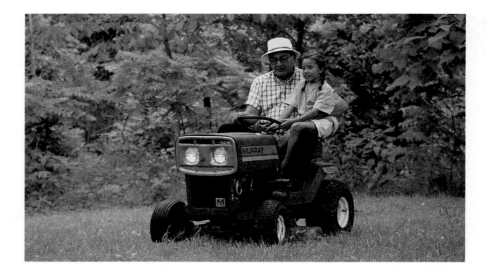

The typical American lifestyle does not lead naturally to healthy weight management. Labor-saving devices such as lawn mowers help reinforce our sedentary habits.

fatty foods for both chronic disease prevention and weight management. There is some evidence that fat calories are more easily converted to body fat than calories from protein or carbohydrate. Limiting fat in the diet can also help you limit your total calories. As described in Chapter 8, fat should supply no more than 30% of your average total daily calories, which translates into no more than 66 grams of fat in a 2000-calorie diet each day. Foods rich in fat include oils, margarine, butter, cream, and lard, which are almost pure fat; meat and processed foods, which contain a great deal of "hidden" fat; and nuts, seeds, and avocados, which are plant sources of fats.

Some people are better fat burners than others; that is, they burn more of the fat they take in as calories and therefore have less fat to store. Low fat burners convert more dietary fat to stored body fat. This tendency to hoard fat calories may be an important part of the genetic tendency toward obesity. For low fat burners, restricting fat calories to a level even below 30% may be helpful in weight control.

As Chapter 8 made clear, moving toward a diet strong in complex carbohydrates and fresh fruits and vegetables, and away from a reliance on meat and processed foods, is an effective approach to reducing fat consumption. Watch out for processed foods labeled "fat-free" or "reduced fat." Manufacturers often add sugar to improve the taste and texture lost when fat is removed, so such foods may contain as many calories as their fattier counterparts—or even more. Limiting fat is important, but so is limiting total calories. Researchers have found that many Americans compensate for a lower-fat diet by consuming more calories overall.

Complex Carbohydrates   It has long been the fashion among dieters to cut back on bread, pasta, and potatoes to control weight. But complex carbohydrates from these sources, as well as from vegetables, legumes, and whole grains, are precisely the nutrients that can help you

achieve and maintain a healthy body weight. They help provide a feeling of satiety, or fullness, that can keep you from overeating. Carbohydrates should make up about 55–65% of your total daily calories. Avoid high-fat toppings and sauces, however; try plain yogurt instead of sour cream on your baked potato and tomato-based sauces rather than cream sauces on your pasta.

Simple Sugars   Although there is no evidence to suggest that fat people consume more sugar than thin people, excess sugar can be a problem for some people. The average American consumes about 150 pounds of sugar per year. Simple sugars make up a large proportion of our "fun" foods, and, like fat, they are hidden in the convenience foods most of us rely on. Added sugars supply calories but few other nutrients. Substituting fresh fruits for sugar-rich desserts is the way to end a reliance on added sugars without giving up natural sweetness.

Protein   The typical American consumes more than an adequate amount of protein. Dietary supplements with extra protein are unnecessary for most people, and protein not needed by the body for growth and tissue repair will be stored as fat. Foods high in protein are often also high in fat, and diets high in fat and protein are linked to many serious health problems. Stick to the recommended protein intake of 10–15% of total daily calories.

Periodically, new diet books hit the market proclaiming a "scientific breakthrough" involving a high-protein, low-carbohydrate diet. Such diets usually cause an immediate and rather dramatic loss of body fluid, which may inaccurately be interpreted as fat loss. They typically involve significant calorie restriction, which is what actually causes any fat loss that does occur. A high-protein, low-carbohydrate diet does not conform to the Dietary Guidelines for Americans and is difficult to maintain. There is convincing evidence that diets rich in complex carbohydrates from grains, vegetables, and fruits lower the risk of

Studies of weight-loss programs have consistently shown that most people gain back lost weight within a fairly short period of time. But what about those people who *do* succeed in losing weight and keeping it off? Why are they successful? What can "yo-yo dieters" learn from their experiences? Researchers recently set out to answer these questions with the National Weight Control Registry (NWCR), a large-scale study of people who have dropped an average of 60 pounds and kept it off for 5 years. The average body mass index of NWCR participants fell from 35 to 24, bringing it into the healthy range (see Chapter 6). Findings from the NWCR study include the following:

- About half of the NWCR participants joined formal weight-loss programs; the remainder lost weight on their own. Fewer than 5% used any type of prescription medication.

- In order to maintain weight loss, participants made permanent changes in both their diet and their exercise habits. They incorporated the strategies they used to lose the weight into their daily routines.

- Common dietary strategies included restricting certain foods, cutting portion sizes, and monitoring calories or fat grams. (Other studies of successful weight managers have shown that increasing intake of vegetables, fruits, and

dietary fiber is also helpful.) Participants did not skip meals, and they ate out an average of three times per week.

- NWCR participants expended lots of energy in physical activity—an average of 2700 calories per week, the equivalent of walking 28 miles. This is well above the Surgeon General's minimum physical activity recommendation of 1000 calories per week. Popular activities among participants included walking, cycling, aerobic dance, and stair climbing.

- Nearly all participants reported improvements in energy level, mobility, mood, self-confidence, and physical health. They felt that the results of their lifestyle changes were well worth the effort.

People who have struggled with their weight should take heart from the NWCR. Most of the successful weight managers who participated in the study had tried unsuccessfully to lose weight in the past, and many of them had been overweight since childhood. The message from the NWCR is that weight management is possible but that it requires lifetime commitment and effort.

SOURCES: Weight loss: The secrets of success. 1998. *Harvard Women's Health Watch*, January. Klem, M. L., et al. 1997. A descriptive study of individuals successful at long-term maintenance of substantial weight loss. *American Journal of Clinical Nutrition* 66(2): 239–246.

heart disease, some types of cancer, and other chronic diseases. Most authorities recommend diets high in complex carbohydrates and moderate in protein consumption.

Eating Habits Equally important to weight management is eating small, frequent meals—three or more a day plus snacks—on a dependable, regular schedule. Skipping meals leads to excessive hunger, feelings of deprivation, and increased vulnerability to binge eating or snacking on high-calorie, high-fat, or sugary foods. A regular pattern of eating, along with some personal "decision rules" governing food choices, is a way of thinking about and then internalizing the many details that go into a healthy, low-fat diet. Decision rules governing breakfast might be these, for example: Choose a sugar-free, high-fiber cereal with nonfat milk most of the time; no more than once a week, have a hard-boiled egg; save pancakes and waffles for special occasions.

Decreeing some foods "off limits" generally sets up a rule to be broken. The better principle is "everything in moderation." If a particular food becomes troublesome, it might be placed off limits temporarily until control over it is regained. The ultimate goal for achieving a healthy diet that ensures successful weight management is to eat in moderation; no foods need to be entirely off limits, though some should be eaten judiciously. Making the healthier choice more often than not is the essence of moderation.

Physical Activity and Exercise

Regular physical activity is another important lifestyle factor in weight management (see the box "Strategies of Successful Weight Managers). In order to achieve long-term success, you must be able to stick with your weight-management program for a lifetime. Cutting food intake in order to lose weight is a difficult strategy to maintain; increasing your physical activity is a much better approach.

Physical activity and exercise burn calories and keep the metabolism geared to using food for energy instead of storing it as fat. Moderate-intensity endurance exercise, if performed frequently for a relatively long duration, can burn a significant number of calories. Endurance training also increases the rate at which your body uses calories after your exercise session is over—burning an additional 5–180 extra calories, depending on the intensity of exercise. Resistance training builds muscle mass, and more muscle translates into a higher metabolic rate. Resistance training can also help you maintain your muscle mass during a period of weight loss, helping you avoid the significant drop in RMR associated with weight loss.

The body's fuel-use patterns vary with exercise intensity and change during recovery. During exercise, a higher proportion of energy comes from fat during low-intensity exercise (50%) compared with high-intensity exercise (40%).

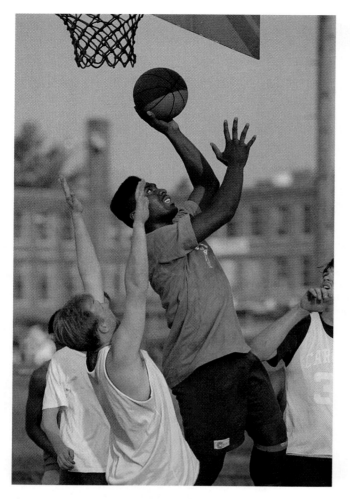

Physical activity is an essential component of any effective weight-management plan. Playing basketball is just one of innumerable activities that can help you keep in shape.

TABLE 9-2	Calorie Costs of Selected Physical Activities*		

To determine how many calories you burn when you engage in a particular activity, multiply the calorie multiplier given below by your body weight (in pounds) and then by the number of minutes you exercise.

Activity	Cal/lb/ min	× Body Weight	× Min =	Total Calories
Cycling (13 mph)	.071	_____	_____	_____
Digging	.062	_____	_____	_____
Driving a car	.020	_____	_____	_____
Housework	.029	_____	_____	_____
Painting a house	.034	_____	_____	_____
Shoveling snow	.052	_____	_____	_____
Sitting quietly	.009	_____	_____	_____
Sleeping and resting	.008	_____	_____	_____
Standing quietly	.012	_____	_____	_____
Typing or writing	.013	_____	_____	_____
Walking briskly (4.5 mph)	.048	_____	_____	_____

*See Chapter 7 for the energy costs of fitness activities.

SOURCE: Adapted from Kusinitz, I., and M. Fine. 1995. *Your Guide to Getting Fit,* 3d ed. Mountain View, Calif.: Mayfield.

However, high-intensity exercise burns more calories overall, so even though a lower proportion of those calories comes from fat, high-intensity exercise tends to burn more fat than low-intensity exercise. Intense exercise also causes your body to use more fat as fuel during the recovery period. However, high-intensity exercise is not necessarily the best strategy for controlling weight. All physical activity will help you manage your weight, and most people find that a program of moderate-intensity exercise is easier to maintain over the long term.

The first step in becoming more active is to incorporate more physical activity into your daily life. Follow the recommendations in the Surgeon General's report by accumulating 30 minutes or more of moderate-intensity physical activity—walking, gardening, housework, and so on—on most, or preferably all, days of the week. Take advantage of routine opportunities to be more active. Take the stairs instead of the elevator, walk or bike instead of driving. In the long term, even a small increase in activity level can help maintain your current weight or help you lose a moderate amount of weight (Table 9-2).

Once you become more active every day, begin a formal exercise program that includes cardiorespiratory endurance exercise, resistance training, and stretching exercises. (Consult Chapter 7 for advice on creating a complete, personalized exercise program.) Regular physical activity, maintained throughout life, makes weight management easier. The sooner you establish good habits, the better. The key to success is making exercise an integral part of the lifestyle you can enjoy now and will enjoy in the future.

Thoughts and Emotions

The third component of a lifestyle for weight management is thoughts and emotions. A healthy psychological adjustment can result from *and* encourage weight control for fitness. Psychological distress, on the other hand, can discourage and undermine a healthy program. Someone who is having difficulty making a commitment to weight management may be motivated by knowing that a moderate, low-fat diet based on solid nutritional principles can yield psychological as well as physical well-being.

Research on people who have a weight problem indicates that low self-esteem and the accompanying negative emotions are a significant part of the picture. These

- Develop realistic goals for yourself and your behavior.
- Eat a moderate number of calories every day. Watch portion sizes carefully.
- Limit your intake of dietary fat and added sugars.
- Increase your intake of complex carbohydrates.
- Limit your protein intake to recommended levels.
- Eat small, frequent meals.
- Maintain a structured pattern of eating.

- Engage in moderate cardiorespiratory endurance exercise of medium to long duration as part of a program of regular exercise.
- Include weight training as part of your exercise program.
- Think positively about yourself, and praise yourself for your accomplishments.
- Develop healthy ways of dealing with stress, boredom, fatigue, and loneliness that don't involve food.

emotions, interacting with beliefs and attitudes about the "ideal self," give rise to negative **self-talk**—self-deprecating or self-blaming internal comments—that can undermine weight control and contribute to anxiety and depression. Realistic self-talk, on the other hand—internal dialogue that leads step by step toward a goal and then offers praise for success—can be an important component in sustaining the commitment to a weight-management program over time. (Chapter 10 and Activity 11 in the Behavior Change Workbook at the end of the text include strategies for developing realistic self-talk.)

Coping Strategies

The fourth component of a healthy lifestyle for weight control is appropriate strategies for handling the stresses and challenges of life. Many people use eating as a means of coping, just as many use drugs, alcohol, smoking, spending, or gambling. They might use food to alleviate loneliness, as a pickup for fatigue, as an antidote to boredom, or as a distraction from problems. Some people even overeat as a means of punishing themselves for real or imagined transgressions.

Those who recognize that they are using food in these ways can analyze their eating habits with fresh eyes. At that point, they can consciously attempt to find new coping strategies and begin to use food appropriately—to fuel life's activities, to foster growth, and to bring pleasure, *not* to manage stress. For a summary of the components of weight management through healthy lifestyle choices, see the box "A Lifestyle for Weight Management."

STRATEGIES FOR LOSING WEIGHT

In cases in which weight loss is clearly desirable, the next step is assessing the various options and the available resources for support and guidance. No single weight-reduction approach is appropriate for all people. For example, most people who are less than 20% over their healthy goal weight can safely cut back on their fat intake and increase their exercise on their own. People who are 20–40% overweight, however, will be better served with some professional guidance and support—perhaps in a commercial weight-loss program (carefully researched to protect against dangerous or fraudulent claims) or a behavioral program supervised by a health professional. More serious degrees of overweight require a more aggressive approach under strict medical supervision.

Do-It-Yourself Approaches

People who aren't dangerously obese might find it most convenient to set up an individual program.

Doing It Alone   Research indicates that people are far more successful than was previously thought at losing weight and keeping it off. One study found that about 64% of the subjects achieved long-term success without joining a formal program or getting special help. Supporting these findings, a U.S. Public Health Service survey indicated that about 50% of the general public succeed with long-term weight management.

In developing a weight-management plan, it's important to remember that long-term success will depend on maintaining the lifestyle changes that help you lose the weight in the first place. Focus on adopting the healthy lifestyle described throughout this book. The "right" weight for you will naturally evolve, and you won't have to diet. However, if you must diet, do so in combination with exercise, and avoid very-low-calorie diets. Don't try to lose more than $1/2$–1 pound per week. Realize that most low-calorie diets cause a rapid loss of body water at first. When this phase passes, weight loss declines. As a result, dieters are often misled into believing that their efforts are not working. They then give up, not realizing that smaller losses later in the diet are better than the initial big losses, because later loss is mostly fat loss, whereas initial loss was primarily fluid.

self-talk   A person's internal comments and discussion; instrumental in shaping self-image.   **TERMS**

For more tips on losing weight on your own, refer to the section later in the chapter on creating an individual weight-management plan.

Using a Diet Book New diet books are published regularly, many of them making exciting but empty promises, and it can be dangerous or discouraging to rely on them too heavily. In assessing diet books, reject those that do the following:

- Advocate unbalanced meal plans—for example, those that advocate a high-carbohydrate–only diet or a low-carbohydrate, high-protein diet
- Claim to be based on a "scientific breakthrough" or a "secret"
- Use gimmicks, such as combining foods in certain ways or claiming that weight problems are due to food allergies, food sensitivities, or yeast infections
- Promise fast weight loss or limit the food selection

The most recent crop of popular diet books are those advocating high-protein regimens; these are often called 40/30/30 plans because they call for 40% of total calories from carbohydrates, 30% from protein, and 30% from fat. The American College of Sports Medicine, the American Dietetic Association, the Cooper Institute for Aerobics Research, and the Women's Sports Foundation recently released a joint statement saying that high-protein, low-carbohydrate diets are not a good weight-loss strategy, will not improve athletic performance, and can be harmful in some cases. The only reason such plans help people lose weight is that the diets they advocate provide so few calories. Remember, responsible diet books advocate a balanced, long-term approach to weight management that includes exercise and sound nutritional principles. (See the January 1998 issue of *Consumer Reports* magazine for reviews of many of the top-selling diet books.)

Using Diet Aids Diet aids are widely available without prescription, and many people are tempted to rely on them for quick-and-easy weight loss. However, the promises associated with these products are advertising gimmicks, and overreliance on them can be dangerous. Among the more common of these aids are dietary supplements for modified fasting. These supplements, in the forms of food bars and powder for shakes, provide far less than the daily nutritional and caloric requirements and should be used only under the guidance of a physician. They also teach dependence on products, not on sound, lifelong eating habits, and weight lost as a result of them is usually regained.

Diet pills are another common diet aid. The most common ingredient of diet pills sold in drugstores is phenylpropanolamine hydrochloride (PPA), which has been deemed a safe and effective mild appetite suppressant by the FDA. Nevertheless, studies on PPA's effectiveness are contradictory at best, and some reports suggest that it can cause dizziness, headaches, rapid pulse, palpitations,

sleeplessness, and hypertension. The use of PPA is approved by the FDA for periods of no more than 12 weeks.

Fiber is the second most common ingredient in diet aids sold in drugstores. However, the amount of fiber provided is usually small, and the FDA has found no data to suggest that fiber aids in weight control.

Although named for a formerly popular combination of prescription weight-loss drugs (fenfluramine and phentermine), the over-the-counter product "herbal fen-phen" does not contain either drug. Herbal fen-phen is usually a combination of ephedra (an herb containing the amphetamine-like stimulant ephedrine), caffeine, and other substances. Herbal fen-phen has not been shown to be safe or effective for weight loss.

Getting Help

Some people are helped by the support and experience of others as well as by professional guidance.

Commercial Weight-Loss Programs Some commercial weight-loss programs can be helpful for providing a food-and-exercise plan and reinforcing motivation. However, if you are considering enrolling in such a program, be sure to use your most acute consumer skills in assessing the available options (see the box "How to Evaluate Commercial Weight-Loss Programs"). Any weight-loss program should include medical supervision, counseling, nutrition education, and maintenance training.

Maintenance is an especially important feature of any program. Studies indicate that only about 10–15% of program participants maintain their weight loss—the rest gain back all or more than they had lost. One study of participants found that regular exercise was the best predictor of maintaining weight loss, while frequent television viewing was the best predictor of weight gain. This finding reinforces the idea that successful weight management requires long-term lifestyle changes.

Prescription Drugs A number of prescription drugs are designed to facilitate weight loss and treat obesity. Two drugs currently available are phentermine (Ionamin) and sibutramine (Meridia); both affect levels of serotonin, a neurotransmitter that controls appetite. Studies have generally found that these drugs produce modest weight loss—a 5–15% weight reduction. They do not eliminate the need to exercise and reduce food intake; they just help people do that by controlling appetite. Unfortunately, most people regain the weight they've lost if they stop taking the drugs.

As with all drugs, there are risks and side effects. In 1997, the FDA removed two other prescription weight-loss drugs, fenfluramine (Pondimin) and dexfenfluramine (Redux), from the market after their use was linked to potentially life-threatening heart valve problems. Such problems may not cause symptoms, so the FDA recommends that anyone who has taken either of these drugs be examined by a physician.

Almost 8 million Americans enroll in some kind of structured weight-loss program each year. Unfortunately, many people fail to lose weight permanently. Before you join a commercial program, evaluate it in terms of these criteria:

- *Proof that it works.* Most programs have data on quick weight loss, but ask for evidence of long-term results of all clients who have left the program.

- *A qualified staff.* A registered dietitian and specialists in behavior modification and exercise should design and supervise the program.

- *A nutritionally balanced diet.* You should be allowed reasonable portions from all the basic food groups and flexibility based on your needs and preferences. You should not be required to buy special products.

- *Exercise.* At minimum, you should receive instructions for starting a safe, moderate exercise program. Trained staff members should be available to customize a program for you and answer questions.

- *Lifestyle change.* Ask to see materials for helping you identify and change behaviors. Find out how the staff rewards and monitors your progress.

- *Follow-up and support.* After completing the formal part of the program, be sure you can obtain ongoing support easily and inexpensively.

SOURCE: Weight control: What works and why. 1994. *Supplement to Mayo Clinic Health Letter,* June. Reprinted with permission of Mayo Foundation for Medical Education and Research, Rochester, Minnesota 55905. For subscription information, call 1-800-333-9037.

Clearly, prescription weight-loss drugs are not for people who want to lose a few pounds to wear a smaller size of jeans. The latest federal guidelines advise people to try lifestyle modification for at least 6 months before trying drug therapy. Prescription drugs are recommended—in conjunction with lifestyle changes—only in certain cases: for people who have been unable to lose weight with nondrug options and who have a BMI over 30 (or over 27 if two or more additional risk factors such as diabetes and high blood pressure are present).

Surgery For people who are 100% or more overweight, obesity is considered a serious medical condition, and surgical intervention may be necessary as a treatment of last resort. Surgery may involve closing off or removing parts of the stomach, thereby limiting the amount of food the stomach can hold, or connecting the stomach to the lower portion of the small intestine, causing food to be poorly digested and absorbed. Both of these procedures can have serious side effects.

Psychotherapy If concern about body weight and shape develop into an eating disorder, the help of a professional is recommended. In choosing a therapist, be sure to ask about credentials and experience. The therapist should have experience working with body image issues and eating disorders (discussed later in the chapter); a physician may be able to provide a referral.

Hazards and Rewards in the Search for the "Perfect" Body

The American focus on attaining a perfect body has prompted a flood of weight-loss programs, fad diets, health clubs, exercise equipment, appetite-reducing drugs, and books on diet, and fitness. The mass media expose us to the single "right" look relentlessly, and the beauty and fitness industries promise to help us attain it. Presumably, with the right combination of programs and products, one can attain the promised rewards of a healthier, slimmer, fitter, more aesthetically appealing body.

During adolescence, both boys and girls become sensitive about their size and physical appearance. Studies have consistently shown a high prevalence of dissatisfaction with body weight or shape among teenagers. **Body image,** the collective picture of the body as seen through the mind's eye, consists of perceptions, images, thoughts, attitudes, and emotions. A negative body image is characterized by dissatisfaction with the body in general or some part of the body in particular. This dissatisfaction can cause significant psychological distress and is associated with restrictive dieting, binge eating, and other forms of disturbed eating.

Problems related to negative body image are much more common among girls and women than boys and men: Only 30% of eighth-grade girls are content with their bodies, while 70% of their male classmates express satisfaction with their bodies. The rate of dieting among adolescent girls is twice the rate among adolescent boys. And women are 20 times more likely than men to suffer from an eating disorder.

body image The mental representation a person holds about her or his body at any given moment in time, consisting of perceptions, images, thoughts, attitudes, and emotions about the body.   **TERMS**

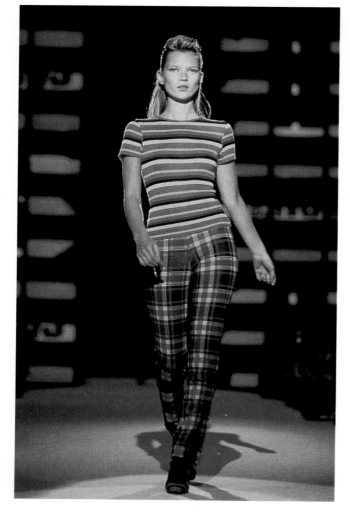

The image of the "ideal" female body promoted by the fashion and fitness industries doesn't reflect the wide range of body shapes and sizes that are associated with good health. An overconcern with body image can contribute to low self-esteem and the development of eating disorders.

It is important to remember that the thin, toned look as a feminine ideal is just a fashion and is not shared by all American women. The African American community is much more accepting of larger, more voluptuous body shapes than white Americans have been. In many traditional African societies, full-figured women's bodies are seen as symbols of health, prosperity, and fertility. African American teenage girls have a much more positive body image than white girls. Two-thirds of black teenage girls in one survey defined beauty as "the right attitude," whereas white teenage girls were much more preoccupied with weight and body shape. African American women are also less likely to suffer from eating disorders than their Latina, Native American, or white counterparts.

For women and men of any cultural background, a sensible approach to body image is focusing on good physical and psychological health, not a number on a scale. When you see idealized standards presented by the beauty and fitness industries, realize that one of their goals is to increase your dissatisfaction with yourself so you will buy their products. Remember, your worth as a human being is not a function of how you look.

Setting unrealistic weight-loss goals in response to cultural ideals can set people up for failure and psychological distress and may predispose them to abnormal eating patterns and eating disorders. Realistic weight-loss goals are much more achievable and can have very beneficial effects. For example, for an obese person, losing as few as 10 pounds can reduce blood pressure as much as antihypertensive medication.

Obesity *is* a serious health problem, but weight management needs to take place in a positive and realistic atmosphere. The hazards of excessive dieting and overconcern about body weight need to be countered by a change in attitude about what constitutes the "perfect" body and a reasonable body weight. Weight-loss goals should take into account a person's weight history, social circumstances, metabolic profile, and psychological well-being. Eating should be viewed as an enjoyable activity that can help the body function at its best rather than as a "bad" behavior that detracts from wellness.

EATING DISORDERS

Problems with body weight and weight control are not limited to excessive body fat. A growing number of people, especially adolescent girls and young women, experience **eating disorders**, characterized by severe disturbances in eating patterns and eating-related behavior. The major eating disorders are anorexia nervosa, bulimia nervosa, and binge-eating disorder. More than 8 million Americans, most of them women, suffer from eating disorders. Many more people have abnormal eating habits and attitudes about food that, although not meeting the criteria for a full-blown eating disorder, do disrupt their lives. (To assess your eating habits, complete the eating disorder checklist in Lab 9-3.)

Although many different explanations for the development of eating disorders have been proposed, they share one central feature: a dissatisfaction with body image and body weight. Such dissatisfaction is created by distorted thinking, including perfectionistic beliefs, unreasonable demands for self-control, and excessive self-criticism. Dissatisfaction with body weight leads to dysfunctional attitudes about eating, such as fear of fat, preoccupation with food, and problematic eating behaviors.

Anorexia Nervosa

A person suffering from **anorexia nervosa** does not eat enough food to maintain a reasonable body weight. Anorexia affects 1–3 million Americans, 90% of them female. Although it can occur later, anorexia typically develops between the ages of 12 and 18. People suffering from anorexia have an intense fear of gaining weight or becoming fat. Their body image is distorted so that even when emaciated, they think they are fat. (Distorted body image is also a hallmark of *muscle dysmorphia,* a disorder experienced by some body builders in which they see themselves as out of shape despite being very muscular.) People with anorexia may engage in compulsive behaviors or rituals that help keep them from eating; they also commonly use vigorous and prolonged physical activity to reduce body weight. Although they may express a great interest in food, their own diet becomes more and more extreme. Anorexic people are typically introverted, emotionally reserved, and socially insecure. Their entire sense of self-esteem may be tied up in their evaluation of their body shape and weight.

Anorexia nervosa has been linked to a variety of medical complications, including disorders of the cardiovascular, gastrointestinal, and endocrine systems. Because of extreme weight loss, females with anorexia often stop menstruating. When body fat is virtually gone and muscles are severely wasted, the body turns to its own organs in a desperate search for protein. Death can occur from heart failure caused by electrolyte imbalances. Depression and suicide are also serious risks. As many as 18% of people with anorexia die of disease-related complications.

Bulimia Nervosa

A person suffering from **bulimia nervosa** engages in recurrent episodes of binge eating followed by **purging.** During a binge, a bulimic person may consume anywhere from 1000 to 60,000 calories within a few hours. This is followed by an attempt to get rid of the food by purging, usually by vomiting or using laxatives or diuretics. During a binge, people with bulimia feel as though they have lost control and cannot stop or limit how much they eat. Some binge and purge only occasionally, while others do so many times every day. Binges may be triggered by a major life change or other stressful event. Binge eating and purging may become a way of dealing with difficult feelings such as anger and disappointment.

The binge-purge cycle of bulimia places a tremendous strain on the body and can have serious health effects, including tooth decay, esophageal damage and chronic hoarseness, menstrual irregularities, depression, liver and kidney damage, and cardiac arrhythmia. Bulimia is often difficult to recognize because sufferers conceal their eating habits and usually maintain a normal weight, although they may experience fluctuations of 10–15 pounds. About 3% of Americans suffer from bulimia.

Binge-Eating Disorder

Binge-eating disorder is characterized by uncontrollable eating without any compensatory purging behaviors. Common eating patterns are eating more rapidly than normal, eating until uncomfortably full, eating when not hungry, and preferring to eat alone. Uncontrolled eating is usually followed by weight gain and feelings of guilt, shame, and depression. Many people with binge-eating disorder mistakenly see rigid dieting as the only solution to their problem. However, rigid dieting usually causes feelings of deprivation and return to overeating. Compulsive overeaters rarely eat because of hunger. Instead, food is used as a means of coping with stress, conflict, and other difficult emotions. Binge eaters are almost always obese, so they face all the health risks associated with obesity. In addition, binge eaters may have higher-than-average rates of depression and anxiety. Binge-eating disorder may affect 25–50% of people who join formal weight-reduction programs.

Treating Eating Disorders

The treatment of eating disorders must address both problematic eating behaviors and the misuse of food to manage stress and emotions. Anorexia nervosa treatment first involves averting a medical crisis by restoring adequate body weight; then the psychological aspects of the disorder can be addressed. The treatment of bulimia nervosa or binge-eating disorder involves first stabilizing the eating patterns, then identifying and changing the patterns of thinking that lead to disordered eating. Treatment usually involves a combination of psychotherapy and medical management. Friends and family members often want to know what they can do to help someone with an eating disorder. For suggestions, see the box "If Someone You Know Has an Eating Disorder . . . ."

People with milder patterns of disordered eating may benefit from getting a nutrition checkup with a registered dietitian. A professional can help determine appropriate body weight and calorie intake and offer advice on how to budget calories into a balanced, healthy diet.

TERMS

eating disorder A serious disturbance in eating patterns or eating-related behavior, characterized by a negative body image and concerns about body weight or body fat.

anorexia nervosa An eating disorder characterized by a refusal to maintain body weight at a minimally healthy level and an intense fear of gaining weight or becoming fat; self-starvation.

bulimia nervosa An eating disorder characterized by recurrent episodes of binge eating and purging: overeating and then using compensatory behaviors such as vomiting and excessive exercise to prevent weight gain.

purging The use of vomiting, laxatives, excessive exercise, restrictive dieting, enemas, diuretics, or diet pills to compensate for food that has been eaten and that the person fears will produce weight gain.

binge-eating disorder An eating disorder characterized by binge eating and a lack of control over eating behavior in general.

- Educate yourself about eating disorders and their risks and about treatment resources in your community. (See the For More Information section at the end of this chapter for suggestions.)

- Write down specific ways the person's eating problem is affecting you or others in the household. Call a house meeting to talk about how others are affected by the problem and how to take action.

- Consider consulting a professional about the best way to approach the situation. Obtain information about how and where your friend can get help.

- Arrange to speak privately with the person, along with other friends or family members. Let one person lead the group and do most of the talking. Discuss specific incidents and the consequences of disordered eating.

- If you are going to speak with your friend, write down ahead of time what your concerns are and what you would like to say. Expect that the person you are concerned about will deny there is a problem, minimize it, or become angry

with you. Remain calm and nonjudgmental, and continue to express your concern.

- Avoid giving simplistic advice about eating habits. Gently encourage your friend to eat properly.

- Take time to listen to your friend, and express your support and understanding. Encourage honest communication. Emphasize your friend's good characteristics, and compliment all her or his successes.

- Help maintain the person's sense of dignity by encouraging personal responsibility and decision making. Be patient and realistic; recovery is a long process. Continue to love and support your friend.

- If the situation is an emergency—if the person has fainted or attempted suicide, for example—take immediate action. Call 911 for help.

- If you feel very upset about the situation, seek professional help. Remember, you are not to blame for another person's eating disorder.

CREATING AN INDIVIDUAL WEIGHT-MANAGEMENT PLAN

Would you like to lose weight on your own? Here are some strategies for creating a program of weight management that will last a lifetime.

Assess Your Motivation and Commitment

Before embarking on your chosen weight-management program, it's important that you take a fresh look within and assess your motivation and commitment. The point is not only to achieve success but also to guard against frustration, negative changes in self-esteem, and the sense of failure that attends broken resolves or "yo-yo dieting." Think about the reasons you want to lose weight. Self-focused reasons, such as to feel good about yourself or to have a greater sense of well-being, can often lead to success. Trying to lose weight for others or out of concern for how others view you is a poor foundation for a weight-management program. Make a list of your reasons for wanting to manage your weight, and post it in a prominent place.

Set Reasonable Goals

Choose a goal weight or body fat percentage that is both healthy and reasonable. Refer to the calculations you completed in Lab 6-2. Subdivide your long-term goal into a series of short-term goals. Be willing to renegotiate your final goal as your program moves along.

Assess Your Current Energy Balance

Your energy balance is the balance between calories consumed and calories used in physical activity. When your weight is constant, you are burning approximately the same number of calories as you are taking in. To tip your energy balance toward weight loss, you must either consume fewer calories or burn more through physical activity. To lose the recommended $1/2-1$ pound per week, you'll need to create a negative energy balance of between 1750 and 3500 calories a week, or 250–500 calories a day. Complete Labs 9-1 and 9-2 to assess your current daily expenditure and to develop strategies for achieving a negative energy balance that will lead to gradual, moderate weight loss. (See p. 242 for guidelines for altering your energy balance to *gain* weight.)

Increase Your Level of Physical Activity

To generate a negative energy balance, it's usually best to increase your activity level rather than decrease your calorie consumption. As discussed earlier, dieting reduces RMR; exercise raises it. Further, a diet with fewer than 1600 calories per day will probably not meet the RDAs for all essential nutrients. (No diet should reduce calorie intake below 1500 for men or 1200 for women.) Increasing energy output by adopting a program of regular exercise and by incorporating more physical activity into your daily routine is a better strategy. Table 9-2 lists the calorie costs of selected physical activities; refer to Table 7-1 for the calorie costs of different types of sports and fitness activities.

You need to adopt a weight-management plan that will last a lifetime. Look through the following list of strategies, and adopt those that will be most useful for you.

- When shopping for food, make a list and stick to it. Don't shop when you're hungry. Avoid aisles that contain problem foods.

- When serving food, use a small food scale to measure out portions before putting them on your plate.

- Serve meals on small plates and in small bowls to help you eat smaller portions without feeling deprived.

- Eat three meals a day; replace impulse snacking with planned, healthy snacks. Drink plenty of water to help fill you up.

- Eat only in specifically designated spots. Remove food from other areas of your house or apartment.

- When you eat, just eat—don't do anything else, such as read or watch TV.

- Eat slowly. Pay attention to every bite and enjoy your food. Try putting your fork or spoon down between bites.

- For problem foods, try eating small amounts under controlled conditions. Go out for a scoop of ice cream, for example, rather than buying half a gallon for your freezer.

- When you eat out, choose a restaurant where you can make healthy food choices. Ask the waiter not to put bread and butter on the table before the meal; request that sauces and salad dressings be served on the side.

- If you cook a large meal for friends, send leftovers home with your guests.

- If you're eating at a friend's, eat a little and leave the rest. Don't eat to be polite; if someone offers you food you don't want, thank the person and decline firmly. To turn down dessert or second helpings, try "No thank you, I've had enough" or "It's delicious, but I'm full."

- Develop strategies for handling stress—go for a walk or use a relaxation technique. Practice positive self-talk.

- Increase your level of daily physical activity. If you have been sedentary for a long time or are seriously overweight, increase your level of physical activity slowly. Start by walking 10 minutes at a time, and work toward 30 minutes of moderate physical activity per day.

- Begin a formal exercise program that includes cardiorespiratory endurance exercise, resistance training, and stretching.

- Tell family members and friends that you're making some changes in your eating and exercise habits. Ask them to be supportive.

SOURCES: Nash, J. D. 1997. *The New Maximize Your Body Potential.* Palo Alto, Calif.: Bull Publishing. Ferguson, J. M., and C. Ferguson. 1997. *Habits Not Diets: The Secret to Lifetime Weight Control.* 3d ed. Palo Alto, Calif.: Bull Publishing. Reprinted with permission from Bull Publishing Company.

Make Changes in Your Diet and Eating Habits

If you can't generate a large enough negative calorie balance solely by increasing physical activity, you may want to supplement exercise with small cuts in your calorie intake. Don't think of this as "going on a diet"; your goal is to make small changes in your diet that you can maintain for a lifetime. Focus on cutting your fat intake and on eating a variety of nutritious foods in moderation. Don't try skipping meals, fasting, or a very-low-calorie diet. These strategies seldom work, and they can have negative effects on your ability to manage your weight and on your overall health.

Making changes in eating habits is another important strategy for successful long-term weight management. If your program centers on conscious restriction of certain food items, you're likely to spend all your time thinking about the forbidden foods. It's better to focus on *how* you eat rather than on *what* you eat. Try adopting some of the behaviors listed in the box "Strategies for Managing Your Weight." You may find that your new eating habits make it much easier for you to achieve and maintain a healthy weight.

Put Your Plan into Action

Be systematic in your effort to change your behavior. Keeping written records of food intake and dietary changes seems to increase the likelihood of success, so devise a food journal similar to the one in Lab 8-1 or Figure 1-4. Write down what you plan to eat, in what quantity, before you eat it. Many people find that just having to record a food they know they should avoid helps stop them from eating it. Also, keep track of your daily activities and your formal exercise program so you can monitor increases in physical activity.

Other strategies for putting a successful plan into action include the following:

- Examine the environmental cues that trigger poor eating and exercise habits, and devise strategies for dealing with them. Anticipate problem situations, and plan ways to handle them more effectively. Create new cues that support healthy behaviors.

- Get others to help. Talk to friends and family members about what they can do to support your efforts. Find a buddy for your program.

- Give yourself lots of praise and rewards. Think about your accomplishments and congratulate yourself. Reward yourself often and for anything that counts toward success.

- If you do slip, get back on track immediately, and don't waste time on self-criticism. Think positively, and don't demand too much of yourself.

- Don't get discouraged. Be aware that although weight loss is bound to slow down after the first loss of body fluid, the weight loss at this slower rate is more permanent than earlier, more dramatic losses.

- Remember that weight management is a lifelong project. You need to adopt reasonable goals and strategies that you can maintain over the long term.

COMMON QUESTIONS ANSWERED

How can I safely gain weight? Although for most of us the focus of a weight-management program is losing weight, some people face the opposite challenge. Just as for losing weight, a program for weight gain should be gradual and should include both exercise and dietary changes. The foundation of a successful and healthy program for weight gain is a combination of strength training and a high-carbohydrate, high-calorie diet. Strength training is critical because it will help you add weight as muscle rather than fat.

Energy balance is also important in a program for gaining weight. You need to consume more calories than your body needs in order to gain weight, but you need to choose those extra calories wisely. Fatty, high-calorie foods may seem like an obvious choice, but consuming additional calories as fat can jeopardize your health and your weight-management program. A diet high in fat carries health risks, and your body is more likely to convert dietary fat into fat tissue than into muscle mass. A better strategy is to consume additional calories as complex carbohydrates—from grains, fruits, and vegetables. Experts recommend that a diet for weight gain should contain about 60–65% of total daily calories from carbohydrates. You do not need to be concerned with protein: Although protein requirements increase when you exercise, the protein consumption of most Americans is already well above the RDA for protein.

In order to gain primarily muscle weight instead of fat, a gradual program of weight gain is your best bet. Try these strategies for consuming extra calories:

- Don't skip any meals.

- Add two or three snacks to your daily eating routine.

- Try a sports drink or supplement that has at least 60% of calories from carbohydrates, as well as significant amounts of protein, vitamins, and minerals. (But don't use such supplements to replace meals, because they don't contain all food components.)

Can reduced-fat foods and snacks help me lose weight? Reduced-fat foods can be a part of a weight-management program, but they must be used carefully. Consider both what the food is and how much of it you eat. A reduced-fat food contains at least 25% less fat than the "regular" version of the food. But the total amount of fat depends on the type of food. For example, a serving of regular peanut butter has 17 grams of fat; the same serving of reduced-fat peanut butter has about 12—a lower amount, but still a substantial amount of fat. In addition, reduced-fat foods often contain the same number of calories as their regular versions. Studies indicate that many of us actually take in more calories when we consume low-fat foods by rationalizing that we can eat more if we decrease our fat intake. (The prevalence of obesity has increased significantly since the introduction of artificial sweeteners.) To be part of a successful weight-management program, reduced-fat foods cannot be considered as a license to eat more.

You also need to consider nutrients. Fruits and vegetables are still likely to be lower in fat and calories and higher in vitamins and minerals than reduced-fat cookies or muffins. Nutrients may also be a concern if you eat foods made with olestra (trade name, Olean), a fat substitute approved by the FDA in 1996 for use in deep-fried foods. Although olestra does significantly lower the fat content of popular foods like potato and tortilla chips, it also binds with certain nutrients, causing them to be carried through the digestive tract without being absorbed by the body. Foods made with olestra are fortified with some of these nutrients, including vitamins A and E, but not all of them. Some scientists are concerned that consumption of significant amounts of olestra could lead to nutrient deficiencies. (In addition, olestra can cause gastrointestinal problems.)

Overall, reduced-fat desserts and snacks should be considered as occasional treats rather than as a regular part of a healthy diet.

How can I achieve a "perfect" body? The current cultural ideal of an ultrathin, ultrafit body is impossible for most people to achieve. A reasonable goal for body weight and body shape must take into account an individual's heredity, weight history, social circumstances, metabolic rate, and psychological well-being. Don't set goals based on movie stars or fashion models. Modern photographic techniques can make people look much better on film or in magazines than they look in person. Many of these people are also genetically endowed with body shapes that are impossible for most of us to emulate. The best approach is to work with what you've got. Adopting a wellness lifestyle that includes regular exercise and a healthy diet will naturally result in the best possible body shape for you. Obsessively trying to achieve unreasonable goals can lead to problems such as eating disorders, overtraining, and injuries.

SUMMARY

- Excess body weight increases the risk of numerous diseases, particularly cardiovascular disease, cancer, gallbladder disease, and diabetes.

- Although genetic factors help determine a person's weight, the influence of heredity can be overcome.

- Resting metabolic rate, the amount of energy needed to maintain body functions, is partly determined by heredity; it can be increased through exercise and an increase in muscle mass.

- Energy-balance components that an individual can control are calories taken in and calories expended in physical activity.

- Nutritional guidelines for weight control and wellness include controlling consumption of total calories, fat, sugar, and protein; monitoring portion sizes; increasing consumption of complex carbohydrates; and developing an eating schedule based on decision rules.

- Activity guidelines for weight control emphasize regular, prolonged endurance exercise and weight training.

- The sense of well-being that results from a well-balanced, low-fat diet can reinforce commitment to weight control, improve self-esteem, and lead to realistic, as opposed to negative, self-talk. Successful weight-management results in not using food as a way to cope with stress.

- In cases of extreme obesity, weight loss requires medical supervision; otherwise, people can set up individual programs, perhaps getting guidance from reliable books, or they can get help by joining a commercial weight-loss program.

- Dissatisfaction with body image and body weight can lead to physical problems and serious eating disorders, including anorexia nervosa, bulimia nervosa, and binge-eating disorder.

- A successful personal plan assesses motivation, sets reasonable and healthy goals, and emphasizes increased activity rather than decreased calories.

FOR MORE INFORMATION

Books

Cash, T. F. 1995. *What Do You See When You Look in the Mirror? Helping Yourself to a Positive Body Image.* New York: Bantam. *An 8-step self-help program for overcoming a negative body image and developing more positive perceptions of one's body.*

Fairburn, C. 1995. *Overcoming Binge Eating.* New York: Guilford Press. *A self-help manual that sets forth a cognitive-behavioral treatment for bulimia nervosa and binge-eating disorder.*

Ferguson, J. M., and C. Ferguson. 1997. *Habits Not Diets: The Secret to Lifetime Weight Control,* 3d ed. Palo Alto, Calif.: Bull Publishing. *Focuses on changing behaviors that relate to weight in order to achieve permanent weight control.*

Fraser, L. 1997. *Losing It: America's Obsession with Weight and the Industry That Feeds on It.* New York: E. P. Dutton. *An exposé on the "diet" industry in America.*

Gaesser, G. A. 1996. *Big Fat Lies.* New York: Fawcett Columbine. *Advice from an exercise physiology researcher critical of general standards for determining "healthy" body weight; his program stresses a low-fat diet and exercise over weight loss.*

Nash, J. D. 1997. *The New Maximize Your Body Potential.* Palo Alto, Calif.: Bull Publishing. *Provides in-depth coverage of nutrition, exercise, and other key aspects of weight management.*

Organizations and Web Sites

Ask the Dietitian/Overweight. Provides questions and answers on many topics related to weight control, including tips for limiting fat intake and information about eating disorders. Site is also linked to the Healthy Body Calculator™, which calculates BMI, waist-to-hip ratio, and daily nutrient and calorie goals.
    http://www.dietitian.com/overweig.html

Eating Disorders Awareness and Prevention (EDAP). Provides educational resources on eating disorders.
    206-382-3587
    http://members.aol.com/edapinc/home.html

Eating Disorders Shared Awareness (EDSA). Provides information about eating disorders, including prevention, signs and symptoms, treatment options, tips for helping a friend, and links to many resources, including online support groups.
    http://www.something-fishy.com/ed.htm

Go Ask Alice. Sponsored by Columbia University Health Service, provides answers to a wide variety of students' questions, including many about weight management, diet, and exercise.
    http://www.goaskalice.columbia.edu

National Association of Anorexia Nervosa and Associated Disorders. Provides written materials, referrals, and telephone counseling.
    847-831-3438

National Heart, Lung, and Blood Institute (NHLBI). Provides information about the latest federal guidelines for the evaluation and treatment of overweight and obesity.
    http://www.nhlbi.nih.gov/nhlbi/nhlbi.htm

North American Association for the Study of Obesity (NAASO). Provides information and links about current research in obesity.
    http://www.naaso.org

National Institute of Diabetes and Digestive and Kidney Diseases (NIDDK). Health Information: Nutrition and Obesity. Provides information and referrals for problems related to obesity, weight control, and nutritional disorders.
    800-WIN-8098
    http://www.niddk.nih.gov/health/nutrit/nutrit.htm

Shape Up America! Founded by former Surgeon General C. Everett Koop, Shape Up America! provides written and on-line materials about safe dietary and physical fitness strategies for successful weight management. Web site includes an online BMI calculator and a physical activity IQ quiz.
    http://shapeup.org

See also the listings in Chapters 1, 6, and 8.

SELECTED BIBLIOGRAPHY

American Dietetic Association. 1996. *Position of the American Dietetic Association: Weight Management* (retrieved December 8, 1997; http://www.eatright.org/adap0197.html).

American Heart Association. 1998. *Press Release: Obesity Joins American Heart Association's List of Major Risk Factors for Heart Attack* (retrieved June 2, 1998; http://www.americanheart.org/Whats_News/AHA_News_Releases/obesity.html).

Brownell, K. D., and C. G. Fairburn, 1995. *Eating Disorders and Obesity: A Comprehensive Handbook.* New York: Guilford Press.

Carmichael, H. E., B. A. Swinburn, and M. R. Wilson. 1998. Lower fat intake as a predictor of initial and sustained weight loss in obese subjects consuming an otherwise ad libitum diet. *Journal of the American Dietetic Association* 98(1): 35–39.

Cash, T. F., and P. E. Henry. 1995. Women's body images: The results of a national survey in the U.S.A. *Sex Roles* 33:19–28.

Dietz, W. H. 1998. Childhood weight affects adult morbidity and mortality. *Journal of Nutrition* 128(2): 4118–4148.

Flynn, M. E. 1995. Fat-free food: A dieter's downfall? Studies show calories do count. *Environmental Nutrition* 18(4): 1, 6.

Foster, G. D., et al. 1996. Psychological effects of weight loss and regain: A prospective evaluation. *Journal of Consulting and Clinical Psychology* 64:752–757.

Grodstein, F., et al. 1996. Three-year follow-up of participants in a commercial weight loss program: Can you keep it off? *Archives of Internal Medicine* 156:1302–1306.

Halaas, J. L. 1995. Weight-reducing effects of the plasma protein encoded by the obese gene. *Science* 269:543–546.

Harvey-Berino, J. 1998. The efficacy of dietary fat vs. total energy restriction for weight loss. *Obesity Research* 6:202.

Kleiner, S. M. 1995. Healthy muscle gain. *The Physician and Sportsmedicine* 23(4): 21–22.

Kleiner, S. M. 1997. Fake sugars and fats: Net benefits or real risks? *The Physician and Sportsmedicine* (retrieved December 1, 1997; http://www.physsportsmed.com/issues/1997/04apr/lose.htm).

Kurtzwell, P. 1996. Taking the fat out of food. *FDA Consumer,* July/August.

Kushner, R. 1997. The treatment of obesity: A call for prudence and professionalism. *Archives of Internal Medicine* 157(6): 602–604.

Manson, J. E. 1995. Body weight and mortality among women. *New England Journal of Medicine* 333(11): 677–685.

Middleman, A. B., I. Vazquez, and R. H. Durant. 1998. Eating patterns, physical activity, and attempts to change weight among adolescents. *Journal of Adolescent Health* 22(1): 37–42.

Mussell, M. P., et al. 1995. Onset of binge eating, dieting, obesity, and mood disorders among subjects seeking treatment for binge eating disorder. *International Journal of Eating Disorders* 17:395–401.

National Heart, Lung, and Blood Institute. 1998. *Clinical Guidelines on the Identification, Evaluation, and Treatment of Overweight and Obesity in Adults: The Evidence Report.* Bethesda, Md.: National Institutes of Health.

Ogden, J., and C. Evans. 1996. The problem with weighing: Effects on mood, self-esteem and body image. *International Journal of Obesity* 20:272–277.

Parr, R. B. 1997. Exercising to lose 10 to 20 pounds. *The Physician and Sportsmedicine* 25(4).

Pelleymounter, M. A., et al. 1995. Effects of the *obese* gene product on body weight regulation in *ob/ob* mice. *Science* 269:540–543.

Pope, H. G., et al. 1997. Muscle dysmorphia: An underrecognized form of body dysmorphic disorder. *Psychosomatics* 38:548–557.

Racette, S. B., et al. 1995. Exercise enhances dietary compliance during moderate energy restriction in obese women. *American Journal of Clinical Nutrition* 62:345–349.

Thompson, J. K. (ed.). 1996. *Body Image, Eating Disorders, and Obesity.* Washington, D.C.: American Psychological Association.

U.S. Food and Drug Administration. 1997. *FDA Talk Paper: FDA Approves Sibutramine to Treat Obesity,* 24 November. FDA Press Office.

U.S. Food and Drug Administration. Center for Drug Evaluation and Research. 1997. *Questions and Answers About Withdrawal of Fenfluramine (Pondimin) and Dexfenfluramine (Redux)* (retrieved December 8, 1997; http://www.fda.gov/cder/news/fenphenqa2.htm).

U.S. Food and Drug Administration. Center for Drug Evaluation and Research. 1997. *Questions and Answers Concerning the Department of Health and Human Services (DHHS) Interim Recommendations for Patients Who Have Taken Either Fenfluramine or Dexfenfluramine* (retrieved December 8, 1997; http://www.fda.gov/cder/news/fenqa111397.htm).

Wadden, T. A., et al. 1996. Effects of weight cycling on the resting energy expenditure and body composition of obese women. *International Journal of Eating Disorders* 19:5–12.

Walsh, B. T., et al. 1997. Medication and psychotherapy in the treatment of bulimia nervosa. *American Journal of Psychiatry* 154(4): 523–531.

"Why Lost Weight Finds Its Way Back." 1995. *San Francisco Chronicle,* 9 March, A1, A13.

Wonderlich, S. A., et al. 1996. Childhood sexual abuse and bulimic behavior in a nationally representative sample. *American Journal of Public Health* 86:1082–1086.

LAB 9-1 *Calculating Daily Energy Balance*

Part I. Resting Metabolic Rate

Resting metabolic rate varies depending on age, gender, and weight. Use the equations below to calculate your approximate RMR.

World Health Organization Equations

1. Convert body weight to kilograms:

   _____ lb ÷ 2.2 lb/kg = _____ kg

2. Find the appropriate formula in the table below, and calculate your RMR. (For example, a 19-year-old male weighing 80 kg would have an RMR of approximately $(15.3 \times 80) + 679 = 1224 + 679 = 1903$ calories per day.)

	Age Range (years)	Equation to Derive RMR in cal/day
Males	10–18	$(17.5 \times$ wt$) + 651$
	18–30	$(15.3 \times$ wt$) + 679$
	30–60	$(11.6 \times$ wt$) + 879$
	Over 60	$(13.5 \times$ wt$) + 487$
Females	10–18	$(12.2 \times$ wt$) + 746$
	18–30	$(14.7 \times$ wt$) + 496$
	30–60	$(8.7 \times$ wt$) + 829$
	Over 60	$(10.5 \times$ wt$) + 596$

RMR = (_____ × _____ kg) + _____ = _____ **cal/day**
　　　　(factor from table)　(body weight)　　　(factor from table)

Harris Benedict Equations

1. Convert body weight to kilograms:

   _____ lb ÷ 2.2 lb/kg = _____ kg

2. Convert height to centimeters:

   _____ in. × 2.54 cm/in. = _____ cm

3. Use the appropriate equation to calculate RMR. (For example, a 20-year-old female 160 cm tall, weighing 60 kg, would have an RMR of approximately $655 + (9.56 \times 60) + (1.85 \times 160) - (4.68 \times 20) = 1431$ calories per day.)

   Women: RMR = 655 + (9.56 × weight _____ kg) + (1.85 × height _____ cm) −
   　　　　(4.68 × age _____ yr) = _____ **cal/day**

   Men: RMR = 66.5 + (13.8 × weight _____ kg) + (5 × height _____ cm) −
   　　　　(6.76 × age _____ yr) = _____ **cal/day**

Approximate Resting Metabolic Rate

Average the values you obtained from these equations to determine your approximate RMR.

World Health Organization Equation: _____ cal/day

Harris Benedict Equation: _____ cal/day

Average value for RMR: _____ cal/day

Part II. Daily Energy Expenditures

List all of your activities for a 3-day period, and classify them according to the categories listed in the table below. (Representative values of the calorie costs of different types of activities are presented below as multiples of resting metabolic rate.) Table 7-1 provides general guidelines for how to classify the sports and fitness activities you participate in: Activities with high cardiorespiratory endurance ratings probably fall in the heavy category, those with medium CRE ratings in the moderate category, and those with low CRE ratings in the light category. Take your intensity into account when classifying fitness activities; basketball, for example, can be played at an easy pace or very intensely.

Your total daily energy expenditure can be estimated by calculating a daily activity factor based on the amount of time you engage in activities in each category of intensity. By adding up weighted activity factors and finding the average, you can calculate total daily energy requirements. Since your activity levels probably vary widely from day to day, it's more accurate to calculate energy output for several different days to come up with an average daily range of calorie output.

Activity Category	Representative Value for Activity Factor per Unit Time of Activity
Resting	
Sleeping, lying down	RMR × 1.0
Very light	
Seated and standing activities such as driving, lab work, writing, typing, cooking, playing cards or a musical instrument	RMR × 1.5
Light	
Walking on a level surface 2.5–3.0 mph, house cleaning, child care, carpentry, restaurant trades, and sports/activities with low fitness ratings such as golf, bowling, and sailing	RMR × 2.5
Moderate	
Walking 3.5–4.0 mph, gardening, carrying a load, and sports/activities with medium fitness ratings such as baseball and volleyball	RMR × 5.0
Heavy	
Walking with a load uphill, heavy manual labor, sports/activities with high fitness ratings such as aerobic dance and cross-country skiing	RMR × 7.0

For each day's activities, add up the total number of hours for each activity category. Then multiply the total duration for each category by the category's activity factor. Add the weighted activity factors, then divide the total weighted activity factor by 24 to get an average daily activity factor. A sample of completed calculations for one day is shown on the next page.

SAMPLE

Activity	Duration	Category
sleeping	8 hours	resting
eating in dorm	1-1/2	very light
class	5	very light
bicycling to class, lab...	1	moderate
job in library	2-1/2	very light
cleaning room/laundry	1	light
basketball	1	heavy
studying in library	4	very light

Category	Activity Factor	Duration	Weighted Activity Factor
Resting	1.0	8	8.0
Very light	1.5	13	19.5
Light	2.5	1	2.5
Moderate	5.0	1	5.0
Heavy	7.0	1	7.0
Total		24 hours	42.0
Average daily activity factor (Total of weighted factors ÷ 24)			1.75

RECORDS FOR 3 DAYS

Day 1

Activity	Duration	Category

Day 1

Category	Activity Factor	Duration	Weighted Activity Factor
Resting	1.0		
Very light	1.5		
Light	2.5		
Moderate	5.0		
Heavy	7.0		
Total		24 hours	
Average daily activity factor (Total of weighted factors ÷ 24)			

Day 2

Activity	Duration	Category

Day 2

Category	Activity Factor	Duration	Weighted Activity Factor
Resting	1.0		
Very light	1.5		
Light	2.5		
Moderate	5.0		
Heavy	7.0		
Total		24 hours	
Average daily activity factor (Total of weighted factors ÷ 24)			

Day 3

Activity	Duration	Category

Day 3

Category	Activity Factor	Duration	Weighted Activity Factor
Resting	1.0		
Very light	1.5		
Light	2.5		
Moderate	5.0		
Heavy	7.0		
Total		24 hours	
Average daily activity factor (Total of weighted factors ÷ 24)			

Day 1 average daily activity factor _____

Day 2 average daily activity factor _____

Day 3 average daily activity factor _____

Finally, use the middle or average of your three daily activity factors to calculate your average daily energy output. For RMR, use the value you calculated in the first part of this lab. (For example, a person with an average daily activity factor of 1.75 and an RMR of 1450 calories per day would have an approximate daily energy expenditure of $1.75 \times 1450 = 2540$ calories per day.)

Average of three daily activity factors _____ × RMR _____ cal/day =

approximate daily energy expenditure: _____ cal/day
(from Part I)

How does this value compare to the average number of calories you eat each day, as determined in Lab 8-2?

To monitor your progress toward your goal, enter the results of this lab in the Preprogram Assessment column of Appendix D. After several weeks of a program to increase daily energy expenditure, do this lab again and enter the results in the Postprogram Assessment column of Appendix D. How do th e results compare?

SOURCES: World Health Organization. 1985. *Energy and Protein Requirements: Report of a Joint FAO/WHO/UNO Expert Consultation.* Geneva: World Health Organization, Technical Report Series 724. National Research Council. 1989. *Recommended Dietary Allowances*, 10th ed. Washington, D.C.: National Academy Press.

LAB 9-2 *Identifying Weight-Loss Goals and Ways to Meet Them*

Negative Calorie Balance

Complete the following calculations to determine your weekly and daily negative calorie balance goals and the number of weeks to achieve your target weight.

Current weight _____ lb − target weight (from Lab 6-2) _____ lb =
total weight to lose _____ lb

Total weight to lose _____ lb ÷ weight to lose each week _____ lb =
time to achieve target weight _____ weeks

Weight to lose each week _____ lb × 3500 cal/lb = weekly negative calorie balance _____ cal/week

Weekly negative calorie balance _____ cal/week ÷ 7 days/week = daily negative calorie balance
_____ cal/day

To keep your weight-loss program on schedule, you must achieve the daily negative calorie balance by either decreasing your calorie consumption (eating less) or increasing your calorie expenditure (being more active). A combination of the two strategies will probably be most successful.

Changes in Activity Level

Adding a few minutes of exercise every day is a good way of expending calories. Use the calorie costs for different activities listed in Table 7-1 and Table 9-2 to plan ways for raising your calorie expenditure level.

Activity	Duration	Calories Used
_____	_____	_____
_____	_____	_____
_____	_____	_____
_____	_____	_____
	Total calories expended:	_____

Changes in Diet

Look closely at your diet from one day, as recorded in Lab 8-2. Identify ways to cut calorie consumption by eliminating certain items or substituting lower-calorie choices. Be realistic in your cuts and substitutions; you need to develop a plan you can live with.

Food Item	Substitute Food Item	Calorie Savings
_____	_____	_____
_____	_____	_____
_____	_____	_____
_____	_____	_____
	Total calories cut:	_____

Total calories expended _____ + total calories cut _____ = Total negative calorie balance _____

Have you met your required negative energy balance? If not, revise your dietary and activity changes to meet your goal.

Common Problem Eating Behaviors

For each of the groups of statements that appear below, check those that are true for you. If you check several statements for a given pattern or problem, it will probably be a significant factor in your weight-management program. One possible strategy for dealing with each type of problem is given. For those eating problems you identify as important, add your own ideas to the strategies listed.

1. _____ I often skip meals.

   _____ I often eat a number of snacks in place of a meal.

   _____ I don't have a regular schedule of meal and snack times.

   _____ I make up for missed meals and snacks by eating more at the next meal.

   Problem: Irregular eating habits

   Possible solutions:

   • Write out a plan for each day's meals in advance. Carry it with you, and stick to it.

   • _____

   • _____

2. _____ I eat more than one sweet dessert or snack each day.

   _____ I usually snack on foods high in calories and fat (chips, cookies, ice cream).

   _____ I drink regular (not sugar-free) soft drinks.

   _____ I choose types of meat that are high in fat.

   _____ I consume more than one alcoholic beverage per day.

   Problem: Poor food choices

   Possible solutions:

   • Keep a supply of raw vegetables handy for snacks.

   • _____

   • _____

3. _____ I always eat everything on my plate.

   _____ I often go back for seconds and thirds.

   _____ I take larger helpings than most people.

   _____ I eat up leftovers instead of putting them away.

   Problem: Portion sizes too large

   Possible solutions:

   • Measure all portions with a scale or measuring cup.

   • _____

   • _____

LAB 9-3 *Eating Disorder Checklist*

For each statement, put a check in the column that best describes how often the statement is true for you.

Section One

Always 0	Very Often 0	Often 0	Some-times 1	Rarely 2	Never 3	
						1. I like eating with other people.
						2. I like my clothes to fit tightly.
						3. I enjoy eating meat.
						4. I have regular menstrual periods.
						5. I enjoy eating at restaurants.
						6. I enjoy trying new rich foods.

Section Two

Always 3	Very Often 2	Often 1	Some-times 0	Rarely 0	Never 0	
						7. I prepare foods for others, but do not eat what I cook.
						8. I become anxious prior to eating.
						9. I am terrified about being overweight.
						10. I avoid eating when I am hungry.
						11. I find myself preoccupied with food.
						12. I have gone on eating binges where I feel that I may not be able to stop.
						13. I cut my food into small pieces.
						14. I am aware of the calorie content of foods that I eat.
						15. I particularly avoid foods with a high carbohydrate content (bread, potatoes, rice, etc.).
						16. I feel bloated after meals.
						17. I feel others would prefer if I ate more.
						18. I vomit after I have eaten.
						19. I feel extremely guilty after eating.

Always 3	Very Often 2	Often 1	Some- times 0	Rarely 0	Never 0	
						20. I am preoccupied with a desire to be thinner.
						21. I exercise strenuously to burn off calories.
						22. I weigh myself several times a day.
						23. I wake up early in the morning.
						24. I eat the same foods day after day.
						25. I think about burning up calories when I exercise.
						26. Other people think I am too thin.
						27. I am preoccupied with the thought of having fat on my body.
						28. I take longer than others to eat my meals.
						29. I take laxatives.
						30. I avoid foods with sugar in them.
						31. I eat diet foods.
						32. I feel that food controls my life.
						33. I display self-control around foods.
						34. I feel that others pressure me to eat.
						35. I give too much time and thought to food.
						36. I suffer from constipation.
						37. I feel uncomfortable after eating sweets.
						38. I engage in dieting behavior.
						39. I like my stomach to be empty.
						40. I have the impulse to vomit after meals.

Total your points (use the numbers given at the top of each column for the two sections) _____

Norms	Range (0–120 points)
Eating disorder	>50 points
Borderline eating disorder	30–50 points
Normal*	<30 points

*Average score among those with normal eating habits = 15.4

SOURCE: Nieman, D. 1999. *Exercise Testing and Prescription: A Health-Related Approach,* 4th ed. Mountain View, Calif.: Mayfield.

Stress

LOOKING AHEAD

After reading this chapter, you should be able to answer these questions about stress:

- What is stress, and how does it affect health and wellness?

- How does the body respond to stress?

- How do emotional and behavioral responses to stress affect the ability to manage stress?

- What is the relationship between stress and disease, and what are some possible mechanisms of this relationship?

- What are common sources of stress?

- What are some approaches to successful stress management?

Like the term *fitness*, *stress* is a word many people use without really understanding its precise meaning. Stress is popularly viewed as an uncomfortable response to a negative event, which probably describes *nervous tension* more than the cluster of physical and psychological responses that actually constitute stress. In fact, stress is not limited to negative situations; it is also a response to pleasurable physical challenges and the achievement of personal goals. Whether stress is experienced as pleasant or unpleasant depends largely on the situation and the individual. Because learning effective responses to whatever induces stress can enhance psychological health and help prevent a number of serious diseases, stress management is an important component in any wellness program.

This chapter explains the physiological and psychological reactions that make up the stress response and describes how these reactions can be risks to good health. The chapter also presents ways of managing stress with a personal program or with the help of others.

TERMS

stressor Any physical or psychological event or condition that produces stress.

stress response The physiological changes associated with stress.

stress The collective physiological and emotional responses to any stimulus that disturbs an individual's homeostasis.

autonomic nervous system The branch of the peripheral nervous system that, largely without conscious thought, controls basic body processes; consists of the sympathetic and parasympathetic nervous systems.

parasympathetic division A division of the autonomic nervous system that moderates the excitatory effect of the sympathetic nervous system, slowing metabolism and restoring energy supplies.

sympathetic division A division of the autonomic nervous system that reacts to danger or other challenges by almost instantly accelerating body processes.

endocrine system The system of glands, tissues, and cells that secrete hormones into the bloodstream to influence metabolism and other body processes.

hormone A chemical messenger produced in the body and transported in the bloodstream to target cells or organs for specific regulation of their activities.

cortisol A steroid hormone secreted by the cortex (outer layer) of the adrenal gland; also called *hydrocortisone*.

epinephrine A hormone secreted by the inner core of the adrenal gland; also called *adrenaline*, the "fear hormone."

norepinephrine A hormone secreted by the inner core of the adrenal gland; also called *noradrenaline*, the "anger hormone."

endorphins Brain secretions that have pain-inhibiting effects.

fight-or-flight reaction A defense reaction that prepares an individual for conflict or escape by triggering hormonal, cardiovascular, metabolic, and other changes.

In common usage, *stress* refers to two different things: situations that trigger physical and emotional reactions *and* the reactions themselves. In this text, we'll use the more precise term **stressor** for a situation that triggers physical and emotional reactions and the term **stress response** for those reactions. A final exam, then, is a stressor; sweaty palms and a pounding heart are symptoms of the stress response. We'll use the term **stress** to describe the general physical and emotional state that accompanies the stress response. A person taking a final exam experiences stress.

Physical Responses to Stressors

Imagine a near miss: as you step off the curb, a car careens toward you. With just a fraction of a second to spare, you leap safely out of harm's way. In that split second of danger, and in the moments following it, you have experienced a predictable series of physical reactions. Your body has gone from a relaxed state to one prepared for physical action to cope with a threat to your life. Two major control systems in your body are responsible for your physical response to stressors: the nervous system and the endocrine system.

Actions of the Nervous System The nervous system consists of the brain, spinal cord, and nerves. The part of the system that is not under conscious supervision, the **autonomic nervous system,** controls your heart rate, breathing, blood pressure, and hundreds of other functions you normally take for granted. The autonomic nervous system consists of two divisions. The **parasympathetic division** is in control when you are relaxed; it aids in digesting food, storing energy, and promoting growth. In contrast, the **sympathetic division** is activated when there is an emergency, such as severe pain, anger, or fear. Sympathetic nerves act on many targets—on nearly every organ, sweat gland, blood vessel, and muscle, in fact—to enable your body to handle an emergency. In general, the sympathetic division commands your body to stop storing energy and instead to mobilize all energy resources to respond to the crisis.

Actions of the Endocrine System One important target of the sympathetic nervous system is the activation of the **endocrine system.** This system of glands, tissues, and cells helps control body functions by releasing **hormones** and other chemical messengers into the bloodstream. These chemicals act on a variety of targets throughout the body. Along with the nervous system with which it closely interacts, the endocrine system helps prepare the body to respond to a stressor.

How do both systems work together in an emergency? Let's go back to your near car collision. As the car travels

Pupils dilate to admit extra light for more sensitive vision.

Mucous membranes of nose and throat shrink, while muscles force a wider opening of passages to allow easier air flow.

Secretion of saliva and mucus decreases; digestive activities have a low priority in an emergency.

Bronchi dilate to allow more air into lungs.

Perspiration increases, especially in armpits, groin, hands, and feet, to flush out waste and cool overheating system by evaporation.

Liver releases sugar into bloodstream to provide energy for muscles and brain.

Muscles of intestines stop contracting because digestion has halted.

Bladder relaxes. Emptying of bladder contents releases excess weight, making it easier to flee.

Blood vessels in skin and viscera contract; those in skeletal muscles dilate. This increases blood pressure and delivery of blood to where it is most needed.

Endorphins are released to block any distracting pain.

Hearing becomes more acute.

Heart accelerates rate of beating, increases strength of contraction to allow more blood flow where it is needed.

Digestion, an unnecessary activity during an emergency, halts.

Spleen releases more red blood cells to meet an increased demand for oxygen and to replace any blood lost from injuries.

Adrenal glands stimulate secretion of epinephrine and norepinephrine, increasing blood sugar, blood pressure, and heart rate; also spur increase in amount of fat in blood. These changes provide an energy boost.

Pancreas decreases secretions because digestion has halted.

Fat is removed from storage and broken down to supply extra energy.

Voluntary (skeletal) muscles contract throughout the body, readying them for action.

Figure 10-1   The fight-or-flight reaction.   In response to a stressor, the autonomic nervous system and the endocrine system cause physical changes that prepare the body to deal with an emergency.

toward you, you feel only fear, but outside your awareness, things happen to prepare you to meet the danger. Chemical messages cause the release of key hormones, including **cortisol, epinephrine,** and **norepinephrine.** These hormones trigger a series of profound physiological changes (Figure 10-1):

- Hearing and vision become more acute.
- The heart rate accelerates in order to pump more oxygen through the body.
- The liver releases extra sugar into the bloodstream to provide an energy boost to the muscles and the brain.
- Perspiration increases to cool the skin.

- **Endorphins** are released to relieve pain in case of injury.

Taken together, these almost instantaneous physical changes are called the **fight-or-flight reaction.** They give you the heightened reflexes and strength you need to dodge the car or deal with other stressors. Although these physical changes may vary in intensity, the same basic set of physical reactions occurs in response to any type of stressor, positive or negative.

The Return to Homeostasis   Once a stressful situation ends, the parasympathetic division of your autonomic nervous system takes command and halts the reaction. It initiates the adjustments necessary to restore homeostasis, a state in which blood pressure, heart rate, hormone levels, and other vital functions are maintained within a narrow range of normal. Your parasympathetic nervous system calms your body down, slowing a rapid heartbeat, drying sweaty palms, and returning breathing to normal. Gradually, your body resumes its normal "housekeeping" functions, such as digestion and temperature regulation. Damage that may have been sustained during the fight-or-flight reaction is repaired. The day after you narrowly dodge the car, you wake up feeling fine. In this way, your body can grow, repair itself, and acquire reserves of energy. When the next crisis comes, you'll be ready to respond—instantly—again.

The Fight-or-Flight Reaction in Modern Life

The fight-or-flight reaction is a part of our biological heritage, and it's a survival mechanism that has served humankind well. In modern life, however, it is often absurdly inappropriate. Many of the stressors we face in everyday life do not require a physical response—for example, an exam, a mess left by a roommate, or a red traffic light. The fight-or-flight reaction prepares the body for physical action regardless of whether such action is a necessary or appropriate response to a particular stressor.

Emotional and Behavioral Responses to Stressors

The physical response to a stressor may vary in intensity from person to person and situation to situation, but we all experience a similar set of physical changes—the fight-or-flight reaction. Emotionally and behaviorally, however, individuals respond in very different ways to stressors.

Effective and Ineffective Responses

Common emotional responses to stressors include anxiety, depression, and fear. Although emotional responses are determined in part by inborn personality or temperament, we often can moderate or learn to control them. Coping techniques are discussed later in the chapter.

Behavioral responses to stressors—controlled by the **somatic nervous system,** which manages our conscious actions—are entirely under our control. Effective behavioral responses such as talking, laughing, exercising,

meditating, learning time-management skills, and finding a more compatible roommate can promote wellness and enable us to function at our best. Ineffective behavioral responses to stressors such as overeating and using tobacco, alcohol, or other drugs can impair wellness and even become stressors themselves.

Consider the individual variations demonstrated by two students, David and Amelia, responding to the same stressor—the first exam of the semester. David enters the exam with a feeling of dread, and, as he reads the exam questions, responds to his initial anxiety with more anxiety. The more emotionally upset he gets, the less he can remember and the more anxious he becomes. Soon he's staring into space, imagining what will happen if he fails the course. Amelia, on the other hand, takes a deep breath to relax before she reads the questions, wills herself to focus on the answers she knows, and then goes back over the exam to deal with those questions she's not sure of. She leaves the room feeling calm, relaxed, and confident that she has done well.

It's not difficult to see that avoiding destructive responses to stress and adopting effective and appropriate ones can have a direct effect on emotional and physical well-being.

Factors Influencing Emotional and Behavioral Responses to Stressors

A complex set of factors—temperament, health, life experiences, values, and coping skills—can influence an individual's response to a stressful situation. Personality, the sum of emotional and behavioral tendencies, plays a role in enabling people to cope more or less successfully with stress. People who are ultracompetitive, controlling, impatient, aggressive, and hostile (so-called Type A personalities) tend to react more explosively to stressors and have more problems coping with stress. In contrast, people with "hardy" personalities—those who view potential stressors as challenges and opportunities for growth and learning, rather than as burdens—tend to perceive fewer situations as stressful and to react more mildly to the stressors in their lives.

Past experiences can profoundly influence the evaluation of a potential stressor. Consider an individual who has had a bad experience giving a speech in the past. He or she is much more likely to perceive an upcoming speech assignment as stressful than someone who has had positive public speaking experiences. Gender and cultural background also influence our response to stressors. For example, some behavioral responses to stressors, such as crying or openly expressing anger, may be deemed more appropriate for one gender than the other.

The Stress Experience as a Whole

Physical, emotional, and behavioral responses to stressors are intimately interrelated. The more intense the emotional response, the stronger the physical response. Effec-

The experience of stress depends on many factors, including the nature of the stressor. Although stress-producing events are commonly thought of as negative, exciting and fun experiences like this amusement park ride can also cause stress.

tive behavioral responses can lessen stress; ineffective ones only worsen it. Sometimes people have such intense responses to stressors or such ineffective coping techniques that they need professional help. (Lab 10-1 highlights some of the signals of excess stress.) More often, however, people can learn to handle stressors on their own.

STRESS AND DISEASE

The role of stress in health and disease is complex, and much remains to be learned about the exact mechanisms by which stress influences health. However, mounting evidence suggests that stress—interacting with a person's genetic predisposition, personality, social environment, and health-related behaviors—can increase vulnerability to numerous illnesses and ailments. Several theories have been proposed to explain the relationship between stress and disease.

The General Adaptation Syndrome

Biologist Hans Selye was one of the first scientists to develop a comprehensive theory of stress and disease. Based on his work in the 1930s and 1940s, Selye coined the term **general adaptation syndrome (GAS)** to describe what he believed is a universal and predictable response pattern to all stressors. He recognized that stressors could be pleasant, such as attending a party, or unpleasant, such as a bad grade. He called stress triggered by a pleasant stressor **eustress** and stress triggered by an unpleasant stressor **distress.** The sequence of physical responses associated with GAS is the same for both eustress and distress and occurs in three stages: alarm, resistance, and exhaustion.

Alarm The alarm stage includes the complex sequence of events brought on by the activation of the sympathetic nervous system and the endocrine system—the fight-or-flight reaction. During this stage, the body is more susceptible to disease or injury because it is geared up to deal with a crisis. A person in this phase may experience headaches, indigestion, anxiety, and disrupted sleeping and eating patterns.

Resistance Selye theorized that with continued stress, the body develops a new level of homeostasis in which it is more resistant to disease and injury than normal. During the resistance stage, a person can cope with normal life and added stress.

Exhaustion Both the mobilization of forces during the alarm reaction and the maintenance of homeostasis during the resistance stage require a considerable amount of energy. If a stressor persists, or if several stressors occur in succession, general exhaustion results. This is not the sort of exhaustion people complain of after a long, busy day. It's a life-threatening type of physiological exhaustion characterized by such symptoms as distorted perceptions and disorganized thinking.

While Selye's model of GAS is still viewed as an important contribution to modern stress theory, some of its key aspects are now discounted. For example, it is no longer believed that an increased susceptibility to disease after prolonged stress is due to a depletion of resources (Selye's exhaustion stage). Rather, the stress response itself is believed to cause illness and disease over time. In addition, the focus of research has changed to also include the emotional and behavioral responses to stressors—areas in which individuals vary significantly and where they may make positive changes to better manage stress.

Psychoneuroimmunology

One of the most fruitful areas of current research into the relationship between stress and disease is **psychoneuroimmunology (PNI)**. PNI is the study of the interactions among the nervous system, the endocrine system, and the immune system. The underlying premise of PNI is that stress, through the actions of the nervous and endocrine systems, impairs the immune system and thereby affects health.

Researchers have discovered a complex network of nerve and chemical connections between the nervous and endocrine systems and the immune system. We have already seen the profound physical effects of the hormones and other chemical messengers released during the stress response. These compounds also influence the immune system by affecting the number and efficiency of immune system cells, or lymphocytes.

The nervous, endocrine, and immune systems share other connections. Hormonelike substances called neuropeptides appear to translate emotions into physiological events. Neuropeptides are produced and received by both brain and immune cells, so that the brain and the immune system share a biochemical "language," which also happens to be the language of emotions. The biochemical changes accompanying particular emotions can strongly influence the functioning of the immune system.

Links Between Stress and Specific Conditions

Although much remains to be learned, it is clear that people who have unresolved chronic stress in their lives or who handle stressors poorly are at risk for a wide range of health problems. In the short term, the problem might just be a cold, a stiff neck, or a stomachache. Over the long term, the problems can be more severe—cardiovascular disease, high blood pressure, or impairment of the immune system.

Cardiovascular Disease   The stress response profoundly affects the cardiovascular system, and these changes have important implications for cardiovascular health, especially over the long term. During the stress response, heart rate increases and blood vessels constrict, causing blood pressure to rise. Chronic high blood pressure is a major cause of atherosclerosis, a disease in which the lining of the blood vessels becomes damaged and caked with fatty deposits. These deposits can block arteries, causing heart attacks and strokes (see Chapter 11).

Recent research suggests that certain types of emotional responses increase a person's risk of cardiovascular disease. So-called "hot reactors," people who exhibit extreme increases in heart rate and blood pressure in response to emotional stressors, may face an increased risk of cardiovascular problems.

Altered Functioning of the Immune System   Sometimes you seem to get sick when you can least afford it—during exam week, when you're going on vacation, or when you have a job interview. As described earlier regarding PNI, research suggests that this is more than mere coincidence. Some of the health problems linked to stress-related changes in immune function include vulnerability to colds and other infections, asthma and allergy attacks, susceptibility to cancer, and flare-ups of chronic diseases such as genital herpes and HIV infection.

Other Health Problems   Many other health problems may be caused or worsened by uncontrolled stress, including the following:

- Digestive problems such as stomachaches, diarrhea, constipation, irritable bowel syndrome, and ulcers
- Tension headaches and migraines
- Insomnia and fatigue (see the box "Overcoming Insomnia")
- Injuries, including on-the-job injuries caused by repetitive strain
- Menstrual irregularities, impotence, and pregnancy complications
- Psychological problems, including depression, anxiety, panic attacks, eating disorders, and posttraumatic stress disorder (PTSD), which afflicts people who have suffered or witnessed severe trauma

---

COMMON SOURCES OF STRESS

We are surrounded by stressors—at home, at school, on the job, and within ourselves. Being able to recognize potential sources of stress is an important step in successfully managing the stress in our lives.

Major Life Changes

Any major change in your life that requires adjustment and accommodation can be a source of stress. Early adulthood and the college years are typically associated with many significant changes, such as moving out of the family home, establishing new relationships, setting educational and career goals, and developing a sense of identity and purpose. Even changes typically thought of as positive—graduation, job promotion, marriage—can be stressful.

Researchers have hypothesized that clusters of life changes, particularly those that are perceived negatively, may be linked to health problems. (Lab 10-1 includes a

TERMS   **psychoneuroimmunology (PNI)**   The study of the interactions among the brain, the endocrine system, and the immune system.

burnout   A state of physical, mental, and emotional exhaustion.

Lack of sleep can be both a cause and an effect of excess stress. Without sufficient sleep, our mental and physical processes steadily deteriorate. We get headaches, feel irritable, are unable to concentrate, forget things, and may be more susceptible to illness. Adequate sleep, on the other hand, improves mood, fosters feelings of competence and self-worth, and supports optimal mental and emotional functioning.

At some time of life, most people have trouble falling asleep or staying asleep—a condition known as insomnia. Most people can overcome insomnia by discovering the cause of poor sleep and taking steps to remedy it. Insomnia that lasts for more than 6 months and interferes with daytime functioning requires consultation with a physician. Sleeping pills are not recommended for chronic insomnia because they can be habit-forming; they also lose their effectiveness over time.

If you're bothered by insomnia, here are some tips for getting a better night's sleep:

- Determine how much sleep you need to feel refreshed the next day, and don't sleep longer than that (but do make sure you get enough).

- Go to bed at the same time every night and, more important, get up at the same time every morning, 7 days a week. Don't nap during the day.

- Exercise every day, but not too close to bedtime. Your metabolism takes up to 6 hours to slow down after exercise.

- Avoid tobacco (nicotine is a stimulant), caffeine in the later part of the day, and alcohol before bedtime (it causes disturbed, fragmented sleep).

- Have a light snack before bedtime; you'll sleep better if you're not hungry.

- Deal with worries before bedtime. Try writing them down, along with some possible solutions, and then allow yourself to forget about them until the next day.

- Use your bed only for sleep. Don't eat, read, study, or watch television in bed.

- Relax before bedtime with a warm bath (again, not too close to bedtime—allow about 2 hours for your metabolism to slow down afterward), a book, music, or some relaxation exercises. Don't lie down in bed until you're sleepy.

- If you don't fall asleep in 15–20 minutes, or if you wake up and can't fall asleep again, get out of bed, leave the room if possible, and do something monotonous until you feel sleepy.

- Keep a perspective on your plight. Losing a night's sleep isn't the end of the world. Getting upset only makes it harder to fall asleep. Relax, and trust in your body's natural ability to drift off to sleep.

checklist of life events to help you determine if major life changes are a current source of stress in your life.) Personality and coping skills are important moderating influences, however. People with a strong support network and a stress-resistant personality are less likely to become ill in response to major life changes than people with fewer internal and external resources.

Daily Hassles

While major life changes are undoubtedly stressful, they seldom occur regularly. Researchers have proposed that minor problems—life's daily hassles—can be an even greater source of stress because they occur much more often. People who perceive hassles negatively are likely to experience a moderate stress response every time they are faced with one. Over time, this can take a significant toll on health. Studies indicate that for some people, daily hassles contribute to a general decrease in overall wellness.

College Stressors

College is a time of major life changes and abundant minor hassles. You are learning new information and skills and making major decisions about your future. You may be away from home for the first time, or you may be adding extra responsibilities to a life already filled with job and family. Some common sources of stress associated with college include academic responsibilities, social and interpersonal changes, time-related pressures, and financial concerns.

Job-Related Stressors

In recent surveys, Americans rate their jobs as one of the key sources of stress in their lives. Tight schedules and overtime leave less time to exercise, socialize, and engage in other stress-proofing activities. Worries about job performance, salary, and job security and interactions with bosses, coworkers, and customers can contribute to stress. High levels of job stress are also common for people who are left out of important decisions relating to their jobs. When workers are given the opportunity to shape how their jobs are performed, job satisfaction goes up and stress levels go down.

If job-related (or college-related) stress is severe or chronic, the result can be **burnout,** a state of physical, mental, and emotional exhaustion. Burnout occurs most often in highly motivated and driven individuals who come to feel that their work is not recognized or that they are not accomplishing their goals. People in the helping professions—teachers, social workers, caregivers, police officers, and so on—are also prone to burnout. For some

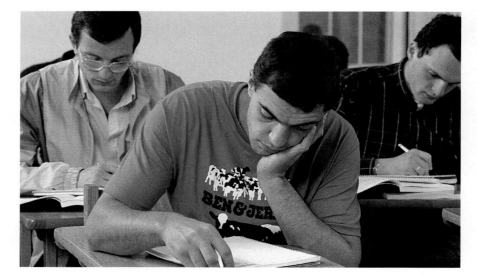

Taking exams is only one of many stressors associated with the college years. College can also be a time of major life events and numerous daily hassles.

people who suffer from burnout, a vacation or leave of absence may be appropriate. For others, a reduced work schedule, better communication with superiors, or a change in job goals may be necessary. Improving time-management skills can also help.

Interpersonal and Social Stressors

Although social support is a key buffer against stress, your interactions with others can themselves be a source of stress. Your relationships with family members and old friends may change during your college years as you develop new interests and a new course for your life. You will be meeting new people and establishing new relationships. All of these changes and experiences are potential stressors.

The community and society in which you live can also be major sources of stress. Social stressors include prejudice and discrimination. You may feel stress as you try to relate to people of other ethnic or socioeconomic groups. As a member of a particular ethnic group, you may feel pressure to assimilate into mainstream society. If English is not your first language, you face the added burden of conducting many daily activities in a language with which you may not be completely comfortable.

Other Stressors

Other stressors are found in the environment and in ourselves. Environmental stressors—external conditions or events that cause stress—include loud noises, unpleasant smells, industrial accidents, and natural disasters. Internal stressors can occur as we put pressure on ourselves to reach personal goals and evaluate our progress and performance. Physical and emotional states such as illness and exhaustion are other examples of internal stressors.

MANAGING STRESS

Stress is an inevitable part of life, and it's not going to go away. The issue is not how to avoid stress but rather how to manage it. While there are many approaches and specific techniques, in general the fundamental principles of physical and psychological fitness are themselves effective strategies for managing stress.

Social Support

People need people. Sharing fears, frustrations, and joys not only makes life richer but also seems to contribute—indirectly but significantly—to the well-being of body and mind. Research supports this conclusion: One study of college students living in overcrowded apartments, for example, found that those with a strong social support system were less distressed by their cramped quarters than were the "loners" who navigated life's challenges on their own. Other studies have shown that married people live longer than single people and have lower death rates from a wide range of conditions. And people infected with HIV remain symptom-free longer if they have a strong social support network. The crucial common denominator in all these findings is the meaningful connection with others. For more on developing and maintaining your social network, see the box "Building Social Support."

Exercise

One recent study found that taking a long walk can be effective at reducing anxiety and blood pressure. Another study showed that a brisk walk of as little as 10 minutes' duration can leave people feeling more relaxed and energetic for up to 2 hours. Regular exercise has even more

Meaningful connections with others can play a key role in stress management and overall wellness. A sense of isolation can lead to chronic stress, which in turn can increase one's susceptibility to temporary illnesses like colds and to chronic illnesses like heart disease. Although the mechanism isn't clear, social isolation can be as significant to mortality rates as factors like smoking, high blood pressure, and obesity.

There is no single best pattern of social support that works for everyone. You may need just one close friend and confidant, whereas your roommate may feel lonely without a large group of friends. To help determine whether your social network measures up, circle whether each of the following statements is true or false for you.

T   F   **1.** If I needed an emergency loan of $100, there is someone I could get it from.

T   F   **2.** There is someone who takes pride in my accomplishments.

T   F   **3.** I often meet or talk with family or friends.

T   F   **4.** Most people I know think highly of me.

T   F   **5.** If I needed an early morning ride to the airport, there's no one I would feel comfortable asking to take me.

T   F   **6.** I feel there is no one with whom I can share my most private worries and fears.

T   F   **7.** Most of my friends are more successful making changes in their lives than I am.

T   F   **8.** I would have a hard time finding someone to go with me on a day trip to the beach or country.

To calculate your score, add the number of true answers to questions 1–4 and the number of false answers to questions 5–8. If your score is 4 or more, you should have enough support to protect your health. If your score is 3 or less, you may need to reach out to strengthen your social ties. Some ways to do that include the following:

- *Foster friendships.* Keep in regular contact with your friends. Offer respect, trust, and acceptance, and provide help and support in times of need.

- *Keep your family ties strong.* Stay in touch with the family members you feel close to. Participate in family activities and celebrations.

- *Get involved with a group.* Do volunteer work, take a class, attend a lecture series, join a religious group. Choose activities that are meaningful to you and that include direct involvement with other people.

- *Build your communication skills.* The more you share your feelings with others, the closer the bonds between you will become. When others are speaking, be a considerate and attentive listener. (Chapter 15 includes more information on effective communication in intimate relationships.)

SOURCES: Social networks: The company you keep can keep you healthy. 1995. *Mayo Clinic Health Letter,* April. Ornish, D. 1991. The healing power of love. *Prevention,* February. QUIZ SOURCE: Japenga, A. 1995. A family of friends. *Health,* November/December, 94. Adapted with permission. Copyright © 1995 Health.

benefits. Researchers have found that people who exercise regularly react with milder physical stress responses before, during, and after exposure to stressors, and that their overall sense of well-being increases as well. Although even light exercise—a brisk walk, an easy bike outing—can have a beneficial effect, an integrated fitness program like the one recommended in this book can have a significant impact on stress.

One warning: For some people, exercise can become just one more stressor in a highly stressed life. People who exercise compulsively risk overtraining, a condition characterized by fatigue, irritability, depression, and diminished athletic performance. An overly strenuous exercise program can even make a person sick by compromising immune function. For the details of a safe and effective exercise program, refer to Chapter 7.

Nutrition

As discussed in Chapter 8, a healthy, balanced diet will supply the energy needed to cope with stress. Two additional nutrition tips for stress management are to limit or avoid caffeine and to avoid the high-potency vitamin compounds and amino acid supplements designated as "stress formulas." (These supplements are worthless for reducing tension or anxiety.)

Time Management

Learning to manage your time successfully can be crucial to coping with everyday stressors. Overcommitment, procrastination, and even boredom are significant stressors for many people. Along with gaining control of nutrition and exercise to maintain a healthy energy balance, time management is an important element in a wellness program. Try these strategies for improving your time-management skills:

- *Set priorities.* Divide your tasks into three groups: essential, important, and trivial. Focus on the first two. Ignore the third.

- *Schedule tasks for peak efficiency.* You've undoubtedly noticed you're most productive at certain times of the day (or night). Schedule as many of your tasks for those hours as you can, and stick to your schedule.

Exercise is a particularly effective antidote to stress. A lunchtime walk gives these coworkers a chance to both exercise and foster friendships.

- *Set realistic goals, and write them down.* Attainable goals spur you on. Impossible goals, by definition, cause frustration and failure. Fully commit yourself to achieving your goals by putting them in writing.

- *Budget enough time.* For each project you undertake, calculate how long it will take to complete. Then tack on another 10–15%, or even 25%, as a buffer.

- *Break up long-term goals into short-term ones.* Instead of waiting for or relying on large blocks of time, use short amounts of time to start a project or keep it moving.

- *Visualize the achievement of your goals.* By mentally rehearsing your performance of a task, you will be able to reach your goal more smoothly.

- *Keep track of the tasks you put off.* Analyze the reasons why you procrastinate. If the task is difficult or unpleasant, look for ways to make it easier or more fun. For example, if you find the readings for one of your classes particularly difficult, choose an especially nice setting for your reading and then reward yourself each time you complete a section or chapter.

- *Consider doing your least favorite tasks first.* Once you have the most unpleasant ones out of the way, you can work on the projects you enjoy more.

- *Consolidate tasks when possible.* For example, try walking to the store so that you run your errands and exercise in the same block of time.

- *Identify quick transitional tasks.* Keep a list of 5-minute tasks you can do while waiting or between other tasks, such as watering your plants, doing the dishes, or checking a homework assignment.

- *Delegate responsibility.* Asking for help when you have too much to do is no cop-out; it's good time management. Just don't delegate to others the jobs you know you should do yourself.

- *Say no when necessary.* If the demands made on you don't seem reasonable, say no—tactfully, but without guilt or apology.

- *Give yourself a break.* Allow time for play—free, unstructured time when you ignore the clock. Don't consider this a waste of time. Play renews you and enables you to work more efficiently.

- *Stop thinking or talking about what you're going to do, and just do it!* Sometimes the best solution for procrastination is to stop waiting for the right moment and just get started. You will probably find that things are not as bad as you feared, and your momentum will keep you going.

For more help with time management, complete Activity 10 in the Behavior Change Workbook at the end of the text.

Cognitive Techniques

Certain thought patterns and ways of thinking, including ideas, beliefs, and perceptions, can contribute to stress and have a negative impact on health. But other habits of mind, if practiced with patience and consistency, can help break unhealthy thought patterns. Below are some suggestions for changing destructive thinking.

- Modify expectations; they often restrict experience and lead to disappointment. Try to accept life as it comes.

Do your patterns of thinking make events seem worse than they truly are? Do negative beliefs about yourself become self-fulfilling prophecies? Substituting realistic self-talk for negative self-talk can help you build and maintain self-esteem and cope better with the challenges in your life. Here are some examples of common types of distorted negative self-talk, along with suggestions for more accurate and rational responses.

Cognitive Distortion	Negative Self-Talk	Realistic Self-Talk
Focusing on negatives	School is so discouraging—nothing but one hassle after another.	School is pretty challenging and has its difficulties, but there certainly are rewards. It's really a mixture of good and bad.
Expecting the worst	Why would my boss want to meet with me this afternoon if not to fire me?	I wonder why my boss wants to meet with me. I guess I'll just have to wait and see.
Overgeneralizing	(After getting a poor grade on a paper) Just as I thought—I'm incompetent at everything.	I'll start working on the next paper earlier. That way, if I run into problems, I'll have time to consult with the TA.
Minimizing	I won the speech contest, but none of the other speakers was very good. I wouldn't have done as well against stiffer competition.	It may not have been the best speech I'll ever give, but it was good enough to win the contest. I'm really improving as a speaker.
Blaming others	I wouldn't have eaten so much last night if my friends hadn't insisted on going to that restaurant.	I overdid it last night. Next time I'll make different choices.
Expecting perfection	I should have scored 100% on this test. I can't believe I missed that one problem through a careless mistake.	Too bad I missed one problem through carelessness, but overall I did very well on this test. Next time I'll be more careful.

SOURCE: Adapted from Schafer, W. 1996. *Stress Management for Wellness*, 3d ed. Copyright © 1996 by Holt, Rinehart, and Winston. Reprinted by permission of the publisher.

- Monitor your self-talk, and attempt to minimize hostile, critical, suspicious, and self-deprecating thoughts (see the box "Realistic Self-Talk").
- Live in the present; clear your mind of old debris and fears for the future in order to enjoy life as it is now.
- "Go with the flow." Accept what you can't change, forgive faults, be flexible.
- Laugh. Seek out therapeutic humor (not dark or offensive humor, which is an unconscious means of dealing with fears). Laughter can temporarily elevate the heart rate, aid digestion, relax muscles, ease pain, and trigger the release of endorphins.

Clear Communication

Clear, honest, open communication is a crucial component of healthy relationships. Poor communication can cause feelings of anger and frustration and significantly increase your levels of stress. The people who make up your social support system cannot respond to specific needs if they don't know what those needs are. See Chapter 15 for more information on effective communication.

Relaxation Techniques

According to Herbert Benson of Harvard Medical School, relaxation techniques can trigger the **relaxation response,** a physiological state characterized by a feeling of warmth and quiet mental alertness. This response is the opposite of the fight-or-flight reaction. When the relaxation response is triggered, heart rate, breathing, and metabolism slow down; blood flow to the brain and skin increases; and brain waves shift from an alert beta rhythm to a relaxed alpha rhythm.

The techniques described in this section, and in the box "Stress-Management Techniques from Around the World," are among the most popular techniques and the easiest to learn. Other techniques, such as massage, self-hypnosis, and biofeedback, require a partner or professional training or assistance. All these techniques take practice, and it may be several weeks before the benefits become noticeable in everyday life.

relaxation response A physiological state characterized by a feeling of warmth and quiet mental alertness. **TERMS**

The origins of techniques for relaxation span many continents and many centuries. Three techniques that originated outside Western culture but are growing in popularity in the United States are meditation, hatha yoga, and t'ai chi ch'uan. Although you may not choose to adopt the philosophical bases of these techniques, all of them can help you manage stress by promoting the relaxation response.

Meditation

At its most basic level, meditation, or self-reflective thought, involves quieting or emptying the mind in order to achieve deep relaxation. Some practitioners of meditation view it on a deeper level as a means of focusing concentration, increasing self-awareness, and bringing enlightenment to their lives. The origins of meditation can be traced back to the sixth century B.C. in Asia. Meditation has been integrated into the practices of several religions—Buddhism, Hinduism, Confucianism, and Taoism—but it is not a religion itself, nor does its practice require any special knowledge, belief, or background.

There are two general styles of meditation, centered around different ways of quieting the mind. In exclusive meditation, one focuses on a single word or thought, eliminating all others. In inclusive meditation, the mind is allowed to wander uncontrolled from thought to thought, but one must observe these thoughts in a detached way, without judgment or emotion. Exclusive meditation tends to be easier to learn. Several years ago, Herbert Benson developed a simple, practical technique for eliciting the relaxation response using exclusive meditation:

1. Pick a word, phrase, or object to focus on. You can choose a word or phrase that has a deep meaning for you, but any word or phrase will work. In Zen meditation, the word *mu* (literally, "absolutely nothing") is often used. Some meditators prefer to focus on their breathing.

2. Sit comfortably in a quiet place, and close your eyes if you're not focusing on an object.

3. Relax your muscles.

4. Breathe slowly and naturally. If you're using a focus word or phrase, silently repeat it each time you exhale. If you're using an object, focus on it as you breathe.

5. Keep your attitude passive. Disregard thoughts that drift in.

6. Continue for 10–20 minutes, once or twice a day.

7. After you've finished, sit quietly for a few minutes with your eyes closed, then open. Then stand up.

Allow relaxation to occur at its own pace; don't try to force it. Don't be surprised if you can't tune your mind out for more than a few seconds at a time. It's nothing to get angry about. The more you ignore the intrusions, the easier it will become. If you want to time your session, peek at a watch or clock occasionally, but don't set a jarring alarm.

The technique works best on an empty stomach, before a meal or about 2 hours after eating. Avoid times of day when you're tired, unless you want to fall asleep.

Although you'll feel refreshed even after the first session, it may take a month or more to get noticeable results. Be patient. Eventually the relaxation response will become so natural that it will occur spontaneously, or on demand, when you sit quietly for a few moments.

Progressive Relaxation   In this simple relaxation technique, you tense, then relax, the muscles of the body, one by one. Also known as deep muscle relaxation, this technique addresses the muscle tension that occurs when the body is experiencing stress. Consciously relaxing tensed muscles sends a message to other body systems to reduce the stress response.

To practice progressive relaxation, begin by inhaling as you contract your right fist. Then exhale as you release your fist. Repeat. Contract and relax your right bicep. Repeat. Do the same using your left arm. Then, working from forehead to feet, contract and relax other muscles. Repeat each contraction at least once, inhaling as you tense and exhaling as you relax. To speed up the process, tense and relax more muscles at one time—for example, both arms simultaneously. With practice you'll be able to relax quickly by simply clenching and releasing only your fists.

Visualization   Visualization, also known as using imagery, is so effective in enhancing sports performance that it has become a part of the curriculum at training camps for U.S. Olympic athletes. This same technique can be used to induce relaxation, to help change habits, or to improve performance on an exam, on stage, or on a playing field.

To practice visualization, imagine yourself floating on a cloud, sitting on a mountaintop, or lying in a meadow. Try to identify all the perceptible qualities of the environment—sight, sound, temperature, smell, and so on. Your body will respond as if your imagery were real.

An alternative is to close your eyes and imagine a deep purple light filling your body. Then change the color into a soothing gold. As the color lightens, so should your distress. Imagery can also enhance performance: Visualize yourself succeeding at a task that worries you.

Deep Breathing   Your breathing pattern is closely tied to your stress level. Deep, slow breathing is associated with relaxation. Rapid, shallow, often irregular breathing occurs during the stress response. With practice, you can learn to slow and quiet your breathing pattern, thereby

Hatha Yoga

Yoga is an ancient Sanskrit word meaning "union"; it refers specifically to the union of mind, body, and soul. The development and practice of yoga are rooted in the Hindu philosophy of spiritual enlightenment. The founders of yoga developed a system of physical postures, called *asanas,* designed to cleanse the body, unlock energy paths, and raise the level of consciousness.

Hatha yoga, the most common yoga style practiced in the United States, emphasizes physical balance and breathing control. It integrates components of flexibility, muscular strength and endurance, and muscle relaxation; it also sometimes serves as a preliminary to meditation.

A session of hatha yoga typically involves a series of *asanas,* held for a few seconds to several minutes, that stretch and relax different parts of the body. The emphasis is on breathing, stretching, and balance. There are hundreds of different *asanas,* and they must be performed correctly in order to be beneficial. For this reason, qualified instruction is recommended, particularly for beginners. Yoga classes are offered through many community recreation centers, YMCAs and YWCAs, and private clubs. Regardless of whether you accept the philosophy and symbolism of different *asanas,* the practice of yoga can induce the relaxation response as well as develop flexibility, muscular strength and endurance, and body awareness.

T'ai Chi Ch'uan

A martial art that developed in China, t'ai chi ch'uan is a system of self-defense that incorporates philosophical concepts from Taoism and Confucianism. An important part of this philosophy is *chi,* an energy force that surrounds and permeates all things. In addition to serving as a means of self-defense, the goal of t'ai chi ch'uan is to bring the body into balance and harmony with this universal energy, in order to promote health and spiritual growth. It teaches practitioners to remain calm and centered, to conserve and concentrate energy, and to harmonize with fear. T'ai chi ch'uan seeks to manipulate force by becoming part of it—"going with the flow," so to speak.

T'ai chi ch'uan is considered the gentlest of the martial arts. Instead of using quick and powerful movements, t'ai chi ch'uan consists of a series of slow, fluid, elegant movements, which reinforce the idea of moving *with* rather than *against* the stressors of everyday life. The practice of t'ai chi ch'uan promotes relaxation and concentration as well as the development of body awareness, balance, muscular strength, and flexibility. (An Emory University study found that a group of older adults who completed a t'ai chi ch'uan course reduced their risk of falling by nearly 50% compared with a control group.) It usually takes some time and practice to reap the stress-management benefits of t'ai chi ch'uan, and, as with yoga, it's best to begin with some qualified instruction.

SOURCES: Adapted from Can yoga make you fit? 1997. *UC Berkeley Wellness Letter,* May. A movement toward t'ai chi. 1997. *Harvard Health Letter,* July. Seaward, B. L. 1996. *Managing Stress: Principles and Strategies for Health and Wellbeing,* 2d ed. Boston: Jones and Bartlett. Benson, H., with W. Proctor. 1984. *Beyond the Relaxation Response.* New York: Times Books.

also quieting your mind and relaxing your body. Try one of the breathing techniques described in the box "Breathing for Relaxation" for on-the-spot tension relief, as well as for long-term stress reduction.

GETTING HELP

You can use the principles of behavioral self-management described in Chapter 1 to create a stress-management program tailored specifically to your needs. The starting point of a successful program is to listen to your body. When you learn to recognize the stress response and the emotions and thoughts that accompany it, you'll be in a position to take charge of how you handle stress. Labs 10-1 and 10-2 can guide you in identifying and finding ways to cope with stress-inducing situations.

If you have attempted to fashion a stress-management program to cope with the stressors in your life but still feel overwhelmed, you may want to seek outside help in the form of a self-help book, a peer counselor, a support group, or psychotherapy. Excellent self-help guides can be found in bookstores or in the library. Peer counseling, often available through the student health center or student affairs office, is usually staffed by volunteer students with special training that emphasizes maintaining confidentiality. Peer counselors can steer those seeking help to appropriate campus and community resources or just offer sympathetic listening.

Support groups are typically organized around a particular issue or problem; for example, all group members might be entering a new school, reentering school after a long interruption, struggling with single parenting, experiencing eating disorders, or coping with particular kinds of trauma. Simply voicing concerns that others share can relieve stress.

Psychotherapy, especially a short-term course of sessions, can also be tremendously helpful in dealing with stress-related problems. Not all therapists are right for all people, so it's a good idea to shop around for a compatible psychotherapist with reasonable fees.

Diaphragmatic Breathing

1. Lie on your back with your body relaxed.

2. Place one hand on your chest and one on your abdomen. (You will use your hands to monitor the depth and location of your breathing.)

3. Inhale slowly and deeply through your nose into your abdomen. Your abdomen should push up as far as is comfortable. Your chest should expand only a little and only in conjunction with the movement of your abdomen.

4. Exhale gently through your mouth.

5. Continue for about 5–10 minutes per session. Focus on the sound and feel of your breathing.

Breathing In Relaxation, Breathing Out Tension

1. Assume a comfortable position, lying on your back or sitting in a chair.

2. Inhale slowly and deeply into your abdomen. Imagine the inhaled, warm air flowing to all parts of your body. Say to yourself, "Breathe in relaxation."

3. Exhale from your abdomen. Imagine tension flowing out of your body. Say to yourself, "Breathe out tension."

4. Pause before you inhale.

5. Continue for 5–10 minutes or until no tension remains.

Chest Expansion

1. Sit in a comfortable chair, or stand.

2. Inhale slowly and deeply into your abdomen as you raise your arms out to the sides. Pull your shoulders and arms back and lift your chin slightly so that your chest opens up.

3. Exhale gradually as you lower your arms and chin, and return to the starting position.

4. Repeat five to ten times or until your breathing is deep and regular and your body feels relaxed and energized.

Quick Tension Release

1. Inhale into your abdomen slowly and deeply as you count slowly to 4.

2. Exhale slowly as you again count slowly to 4. As you exhale, concentrate on relaxing your face, neck, shoulders, and chest.

3. Repeat several times. With each exhalation, feel more tension leaving your body.

SOURCES: Stop stress with a deep breath. 1996. *Health*, October, 53. Breathing for health and relaxation. 1995. *Mental Medicine Update*, 4(2): 3–6. When you're stressed, catch your breath. 1995. *Mayo Clinic Health Letter*, December, 5.

SUMMARY

- Stress is the collective physiological and emotional response to any stressor. Physiological responses to stressors are the same for everyone.

- The autonomic nervous system and the endocrine system are responsible for the body's physical response to stressors. The sympathetic nervous system mobilizes the body and activates key hormones of the endocrine system, causing the fight-or-flight reaction. The parasympathetic system returns the body to homeostasis.

- Behavioral responses to stress are controlled by the somatic nervous system and fall under a person's conscious control.

- The general adaptation syndrome model and research in psychoneuroimmunology contribute to our understanding of the links between stress and disease. People who have many stressors in their lives or handle stress poorly are at risk for cardiovascular disease, impairment of the immune system, and many other problems.

- Potential sources of stress include major life changes, daily hassles, college and job-related stressors, and interpersonal and social stressors.

- Ways of managing stress include regular exercise, good nutrition, time management, support from other people, relaxation techniques, modified thought patterns, and clear communication.

- If a personal program for stress management doesn't work, peer counseling, support groups, and psychotherapy are available.

FOR MORE INFORMATION

You'll probably find courses and seminars on your campus or in your community that teach ways of dealing with stress. Some may be specifically devoted to such issues as time management, test taking, or public speaking. If you're experiencing severe symptoms of stress or if your symptoms last for several weeks, consult a physician or counselor. Most campuses provide student psychological services that are free and informal. Your student health center may also provide peer counseling.

Books

Ali, M. 1996. *What Do Lions Know About Stress?* Denville, N.J.: Life Span Press. *A provocative, often amusing look at the relationship between stress and health.*

COMMON QUESTIONS ANSWERED

Are there any relaxation techniques I can use in response to an immediate stressor? There are various strategies for dealing with stressors on the spot. In addition to the deep breathing techniques described in the chapter, try some of the following to see which ones work best for you:

- Do a full-body stretch while standing or sitting. Stretch your arms out to the sides and then reach them as far as possible over your head. Rotate your body from the waist. Bend over as far as is comfortable for you.

- Do a partial session of progressive muscle relaxation. Tense and then relax some of the muscles in your body. Focus on the muscles that are stiff or tense. Shake out your arms and legs.

- Take a short, brisk walk (3–5 minutes). Breathe deeply.

- Engage in realistic self-talk about the stressor. Mentally rehearse dealing successfully with the stressor. As an alternative, focus your mind on some other activity.

Can stress cause a person to become depressed? Although not often the sole factor in the development of depression, poor stress-management skills can contribute to depression, and depression can be a sign of excess stress. Depression is more than just having a bad day; it is a serious disorder characterized by a negative self-concept, meaning that a person feels unloved and ineffective. Poor stress-management skills can reinforce a negative self-concept by sabotaging personal relationships and academic and professional performance. In addition to a negative self-concept, severe depression can include the following:

- Pervasive feelings of sadness and hopelessness
- Loss of pleasure in usual activities
- Poor appetite and weight loss
- Insomnia, especially early morning awakening
- Restlessness or lethargy
- Thoughts of worthlessness and guilt
- An inability to concentrate
- Thoughts of suicide

Not all of these symptoms are present in everyone who is depressed, but most do experience a loss of interest or pleasure in their usual activities. In some cases, depression, like severe stress, is a clear-cut reaction to specific events, such as the loss of a loved one or failing in school or work. In other cases, no trigger event is obvious.

Suicide is a danger in cases of severe depression. Warning signs include expressing the wish to be dead; revealing contemplated suicide methods; increasing social withdrawal and isolation; and a sudden, inexplicable lightening of mood (which can indicate the person has finally decided to commit suicide). If you are severely depressed or know someone who is, expert help from a mental health professional is essential. Most communities have emergency help available, often in the form of a hotline telephone counseling service. Large colleges typically have health services and counseling centers that can provide help; professional therapists can also be located through the local telephone book.

Greenberg, J. S. 1996. *Comprehensive Stress Management.* Dubuque, Ia.: Brown and Benchmark. *An easy-to-understand guide to identifying and combatting stressors; includes a separate chapter on college stress.*

Sapadin, L., and J. Maguire. 1997. *It's About Time! The Six Styles of Procrastination and How to Overcome Them.* New York: Penguin. *Uses quizzes and case studies to trace procrastinating behavior to personality traits and early family dynamics.*

Sapolsky, R. M. 1994. *Why Zebras Don't Get Ulcers: A Guide to Stress-Related Diseases, and Coping.* New York: W. H. Freeman. *An entertaining look at the effects of stress on the body and the relationship between stress and disease.*

Smith, L. W. 1997. *Scientific American Focus: Of Mind and Body.* New York: Henry Holt. *An introduction to mind-body medicine, psychoneuroimmunology, and relaxation techniques.*

Organizations and Web Sites

American Psychological Association. Provides information on stress management and psychological disorders.
202-336-5500
http://www.apa.org

Association for Applied Psychophysiology and Biofeedback. Provides information and links about biofeedback.
800-477-8892
http://www.aapb.org

Center for Anxiety and Stress Treatment. A commercial site that includes an anxiety symptom checklist and stress-busting tips for work stress.
http://www.stressrelease.com

Duquesne University Stress Links. Provides links to sites with stress-management strategies, many designed especially for college students.
http://the-duke.duq-duke.duq.edu/special/stress.htm

The Humor Project. A clearinghouse for information and practical ideas related to humor.
518-587-8770
http://www.humorproject.com

National Institute of Mental Health (NIMH). Offers information about stress and stress management as well as other aspects of psychological health, including anxiety, depression, and eating disorders.
800-421-4211; 301-443-4536
http://www.nimh.nih.gov

Stress Free NET. A commercial Web site containing stress-related services and tools, including a directory of health and stress-management professionals.
http://www.stressfree.com

Yang Style Tai Chi. Provides an introduction to t'ai chi ch'uan, including its history and a discussion of various styles.
http://www.chebucto.ns.ca/Philosophy/Taichi

SELECTED BIBLIOGRAPHY

Andersen, B. L., et al. 1998. Stress and immune responses after surgical treatment for regional breast cancer. *Journal of the National Cancer Institute* 90(1): 30–36.

Anshel, M. 1996. Effect of chronic aerobic exercise and progressive relaxation on motor performance and affect following acute stress. *Behavioral Medicine* 21:186–196.

Arnetz, B., and C. Wilholm. 1997. Technological stress: Psychophysiological symptoms in modern offices. *Journal of Psychosomatic Research* 43(1): 35–42.

Ashton, C., Jr., et al. 1997. Self-hypnosis reduces anxiety following coronary artery bypass surgery. A prospective, randomized trial. *Journal of Cardiovascular Surgery* 38(1): 69–75.

Barnett, P. 1997. Psychological stress and the progression of carotid artery disease. *Journal of Hypertension* 15:49–55.

Birmaher, B., et al. 1994. Cellular immunity in depressed, conduct disorder, and normal adolescents: Role of adverse life events. *Journal of the American Academy of Child and Adolescent Psychiatry* 33(5): 671–678.

Brownley, K. 1996. Social support and hostility interact to influence clinic, work, and home blood pressure in black and white men and women. *Psychophysiology* 33:434–445.

Chicester, B., and P. Garfinkel. 1997. *Stress Blasters: Quick and Simple Steps to Take Control and Perform Under Pressure.* Emmaus, Pa.: Rodale Press.

Dill, P. L., and T. B. Henley. 1998. Stressors of college: A comparison of traditional and nontraditional students. *Journal of Psychology* 132(1): 25–32.

Domar, A. D., and H. Dreher. 1996. *Healing Mind, Healthy Woman: Using the Mind-Body Connection to Manage Stress and Take Control of Your Health.* New York: Henry Holt.

Flach, J., and L. Seachrist. 1994. Mind-body meld may boost immunity. *Journal of the National Cancer Institute* 86(4): 256–258.

Gillin, J. 1996. Race and sex differences in cardiovascular recovery from acute stress. *International Journal of Psychophysiology* 23:83–90.

Gramer, M. 1996. The availability of social support reduces cardiovascular reactivity to acute psychological stress. *Journal of Experimental Psychology* 43:256–278.

Hagihara, A., et al. 1997. Type A and Type B behaviors, work stressors, and social support at work. *Preventive Medicine* 26(4): 486–494.

Hansel, S. 1997. Appraisal and coping strategies in stressful situations: A comparison of individuals who binge eat and controls. *International Journal of Eating Disorders* 21:89–93.

How to get a good night's sleep. 1997. *Consumer Reports,* March.

Johansen, D. 1997. Psychological stress, cancer incidence and mortality from nonmalignant diseases. *British Journal of Cancer* 75:144–148.

Kamarck, T. W., et al. 1998. Effects of task strain, social conflict, and emotional activation on ambulatory cardiovascular activity: Daily life consequences of recurring stress in a multiethnic adult sample. *Health Psychology* 17(1): 17–29.

Kang, D. 1997. Immune responses to final exams in healthy and asthmatic adolescents. *Nurse Researcher* 46:12–19.

Krug, E. G., et al. 1998. Suicide after natural disasters. *New England Journal of Medicine* 338(6): 373–378.

Lester, D. 1996. Social stress, homicide, and suicide. *Psychological Reports* 79:922.

Pike, J. L., et al. 1997. Chronic life stress alters sympathetic, neuroendocrine, and immune responsivity to an acute psychological stressor in humans. *Psychosomatic Medicine* 59(4): 447–457.

Reinhold, B. B. 1996. *Toxic Work: How to Overcome Stress, Overload, and Burnout and Revitalize Your Career.* New York: Dutton.

Selye, H. 1976. *The Stress of Life,* rev. ed. New York: McGraw-Hill.

Spiegel, D., and R. Moore. 1997. Imagery and hypnosis in the treatment of cancer patients. *Oncology* 11(8): 1179–1189.

Strogatz, D. S., et al. 1997. Social support, stress, and blood pressure in black adults. *Epidemiology* 8(5): 482–487.

Toates, F. 1995. *Stress: Conceptual and Biological Aspects.* New York: Wiley.

Uchino, B. 1997. Cardiovascular effects of active coping behavior in mental and social stress situations during various incentive conditions. *Journal of Behavioral Medicine* 20:15–27.

Ystgaard, M. 1997. Life stress, social support, and psychological distress in late adolescence. *Social Psychiatry and Psychiatric Epidemiology* 32(5): 277–283.

LAB 10-1 *Identifying Your Stressors*

Signals of Excess Stress

To identify the sources of stress in your life, you must first be able to identify the signals of excess stress. Put a check mark next to any of the following signs you have experienced in the last month.

Emotional Signs

_____ Tendency to be irritable or aggressive
_____ Tendency to feel anxious, fearful, or edgy
_____ Hyperexcitability, impulsiveness, or emotional instability
_____ Depression
_____ Frequent feelings of boredom
_____ Inability to concentrate
_____ Fatigue

Behavioral Signs

_____ Increased use of tobacco, alcohol, or other drugs
_____ Excessive TV watching
_____ Sleep disturbances or excessive sleep
_____ Overeating or undereating
_____ Sexual problems
_____ Crying or yelling
_____ Job or school burnout

_____ Spouse or child abuse
_____ Panic attack

Physical Signs

_____ Pounding heart
_____ Trembling with nervous tics
_____ Grinding of teeth
_____ Dry mouth
_____ Excessive perspiration
_____ Gastrointestinal problems (diarrhea, constipation, indigestion, queasy stomach)
_____ Stiff neck or aching lower back
_____ Migraine or tension headaches
_____ Frequent colds or low-grade infections
_____ Cold hands and feet
_____ Allergy or asthma attacks
_____ Skin problems (e.g., hives, eczema, psoriasis)

Possible Stressful Life Changes

Listed below, in order of probable severity of effect, are 35 life events that cause stress. Put a check mark next to any item you have experienced recently or expect to experience soon. If you find you've checked several items, take time out from your daily routine to develop and cultivate your coping skills.

_____ Death of a close family member
_____ Divorce or separation from mate
_____ Detention in jail or other institution
_____ Major personal injury or illness
_____ Death of a close friend
_____ Divorce between parents
_____ Marriage
_____ Being fired from job or expelled from school
_____ Retirement
_____ Change in health of a family member
_____ Pregnancy
_____ Being a victim of crime
_____ Sexual difficulties
_____ Gaining new family members (through birth, adoption, older person moving in, etc.)
_____ New boyfriend or girlfriend
_____ Major business or academic readjustment (merger, change of job or major, failing course)
_____ Major change in financial state (a lot worse or a lot better off than before)
_____ Taking out a loan or mortgage for school or a major purchase

_____ Trouble with parents, spouse, or girlfriend or boyfriend
_____ Outstanding personal achievement
_____ Graduation
_____ First quarter/semester in college
_____ Denied admission to program or school
_____ Change in living conditions
_____ Serious argument with instructor, friend, or roommate
_____ Lower grades than expected
_____ Major change in working hours or conditions, or increased workload at school
_____ Major change in recreational, social, or church activities
_____ Major change in sleeping or eating habits
_____ Denied admission to required course
_____ Taking out a loan for a lesser purchase (e.g., a car, TV, or freezer)
_____ Chronic car trouble
_____ Change in number of family get-togethers
_____ Vacation
_____ Minor violation of the law (traffic tickets, etc.)

Weekly Stress Log

Now that you are familiar with the signals of stress, complete the weekly stress log to map patterns in your stress levels and identify sources of stress. Enter a score for each hour of each day according to the ratings listed below.

	A.M.							P.M.												Average
	6	7	8	9	10	11	12	1	2	3	4	5	6	7	8	9	10	11	12	
Monday																				
Tuesday																				
Wednesday																				
Thursday																				
Friday																				
Saturday																				
Sunday																				
Average																				

Ratings

1 = No anxiety; general feeling of well-being
2 = Mild anxiety; no interference with activity
3 = Moderate anxiety; specific signal(s) of stress present
4 = High anxiety; interference with activity
5 = Very high anxiety and panic reactions; general inability to engage in activity

To identify daily or weekly patterns in your stress level, average your stress rating for each hour and each day. For example, if your scores for 6:00 A.M. are 3, 3, 4, 3, and 4, with blanks for Saturday and Sunday, your 6:00 A.M. rating would be 17 ÷ 5, or 3.4 (moderate to high anxiety). Finally, calculate an average weekly stress score by averaging your daily average stress scores. Your weekly average will give you a sense of your overall level of stress.

Identifying Sources of Stress

External stressors: List several people, places, or events that caused you a significant amount of discomfort this week.

_____

_____

_____

Internal stressors: Make a list of any recurring thoughts or worries that produced feelings of discomfort this week.

_____

_____

_____

To monitor your progress toward your goal, enter the results of this lab in the Preprogram Assessment column of Appendix D. After several weeks of a stress-management program, do this lab again and enter the results in the Postprogram Assessment column of Appendix D. How do the results compare?

SOURCE: List of major life changes adapted with permission from Holmes, T. H., and R. H. Rahe. 1967. The social readjustment scale. *Journal of Psychosomatic Research* 11(2): 213–218. Elsevier Science, Inc.

LAB 10-2 *Stress-Management Techniques*

Part I. Lifestyle Stress Management

For each of the areas listed in the table below, describe your current lifestyle as it relates to stress management. For example, do you have enough social support? How are your exercise and nutrition habits? Is time management a problem for you? For each area, list two ways that you could change your current habits to help you manage your stress. Sample strategies might include calling a friend before a challenging class, taking a short walk before lunch, and buying and using a date book to track your time.

	Current lifestyle	Lifestyle change #1	Lifestyle change #2
Social support system			
Exercise habits			
Nutrition habits			
Time-management techniques			
Self-talk patterns			
Sleep habits			

Part II. Relaxation Techniques

Choose two relaxation techniques described in this chapter (progressive relaxation, visualization, deep breathing, meditation, yoga, t'ai chi ch'uan). If a taped recording is available for progressive relaxation or visualization, these techniques can be performed by your entire class as a group.

List the techniques you tried.

1. _____

2. _____

How did you feel before you tried these techniques?

_____

_____

_____

_____

What did you think, or how did you feel, as you performed each of the techniques you tried?

1. _____

_____

_____

2. _____

_____

_____

How did you feel after you tried these techniques?

_____

_____

_____

Cardiovascular Health

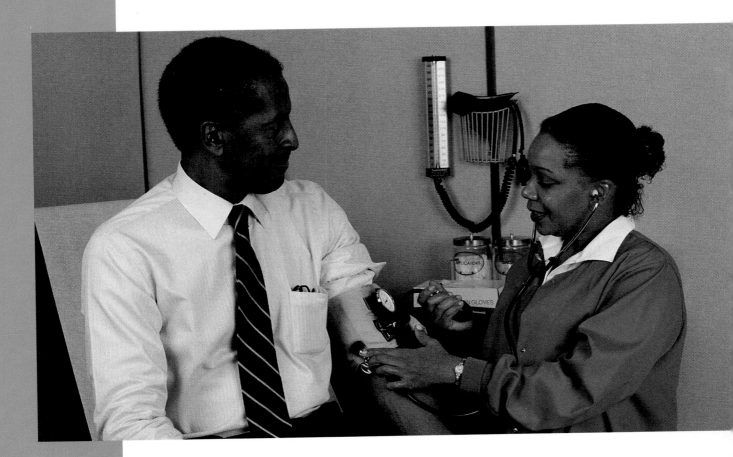

LOOKING AHEAD

After reading this chapter, you should be able to answer these questions about cardiovascular health and disease:

- What controllable and uncontrollable risk factors are associated with cardiovascular disease?

- What are the major forms of cardiovascular disease, and how do they develop?

- What steps can people take to keep their cardiovascular system healthy and avoid cardiovascular disease?

Cardiovascular disease (CVD) is the leading cause of death in the United States; nearly half of all Americans alive today will die from CVD. As discussed in Chapter 1, much of the incidence of CVD is attributable to the American way of life. Too many Americans eat a high-fat diet, are overweight and sedentary, smoke cigarettes, manage stress ineffectively, have uncontrolled high blood pressure or high cholesterol levels, and don't know the signs of CVD. Not all risk factors for CVD are controllable—some people have an inherited tendency toward high cholesterol levels, for example—but many are within the control of the individual.

This chapter explains the major forms of CVD, including hypertension, atherosclerosis, and stroke. It also considers the factors that put people at risk for CVD. Most important, it explains the steps individuals can take to protect their hearts and promote cardiovascular health throughout their lives.

RISK FACTORS FOR CARDIOVASCULAR DISEASE

Researchers have identified a variety of factors associated with an increased risk of developing cardiovascular disease. They are grouped into two categories: major risk factors and contributing risk factors. Some major risk factors, such as diet, exercise habits, and use of tobacco, are linked to controllable aspects of lifestyle and can therefore be changed. Others, such as age, sex, and heredity, are beyond an individual's control. (Part I of Lab 11-1 gives you the opportunity to evaluate your personal CVD risk factors.)

TERMS **cardiovascular disease (CVD)**   Disease of the heart and blood vessels.

high-density lipoproteins (HDLs)   Blood fats that help transport cholesterol out of the arteries, thereby protecting against heart disease.

platelets   Microscopic disk-shaped cell fragments in the blood that disintegrate on contact with foreign objects and release chemicals necessary for the formation of blood clots.

environmental tobacco smoke (ETS)   Smoke that enters the atmosphere from the burning end of a cigarette, cigar, or pipe, as well as smoke that is exhaled by smokers; also called *secondhand smoke.*

hypertension   Sustained abnormally high blood pressure.

atherosclerosis   Cardiovascular disease in which the inner layers of artery walls are made thick and irregular by deposits of a fatty substance; the internal channels of arteries become narrowed, and blood supply is reduced.

lipoproteins   Blood fats formed in the liver that carry cholesterol throughout the body.

Major Risk Factors That Can Be Changed

The American Heart Association (AHA) has identified five major risk factors for CVD that can be changed. These are tobacco use, high blood pressure, unhealthy blood cholesterol levels, physical inactivity, and obesity.

Tobacco Use   People who smoke a pack of cigarettes a day have twice the risk of heart attack that nonsmokers have; smoking two or more packs a day triples the risk. And when smokers do have heart attacks, they are two to four times more likely than nonsmokers to die from them. Women who smoke and use oral contraceptives are up to 39 times more likely to have a heart attack and up to 22 times more likely to have a stroke than women who don't smoke and take the pill.

Smoking harms the cardiovascular system in several ways. Smoking can reduce levels of **high-density lipoproteins (HDLs)**, "good cholesterol," in the bloodstream. The psychoactive drug in tobacco, nicotine, is a central nervous system stimulant, causing increased blood pressure and heart rate. The carbon monoxide in cigarette smoke displaces oxygen in the blood, reducing the amount of oxygen available to the heart and other parts of the body. Cigarette smoking also causes the **platelets** in blood to become sticky and cluster, compromises platelet survival rate, decreases clotting time, and thickens the blood. All these effects increase a person's risk of heart attack and other forms of CVD.

You don't have to smoke to be affected. **Environmental tobacco smoke (ETS)** in high concentrations has been linked to the development of cardiovascular disease. ETS and high cholesterol levels act together to damage the cells that line artery walls. Researchers estimate that 50,000 nonsmokers die from heart attacks each year as a result of exposure to ETS.

High Blood Pressure   High blood pressure, or **hypertension,** is a risk factor for many forms of CVD but is also considered a disease itself. High blood pressure occurs when too much force or pressure is exerted against the walls of the arteries. If your blood pressure is high, your heart has to work harder to push the blood forward. Over time, a strained heart weakens and tends to enlarge, which weakens it further. Increased blood pressure also scars and hardens arteries, making them less elastic. Heart attacks, strokes, **atherosclerosis,** and kidney failure can result.

Hypertension usually has no early warning signs, so it's important to have your blood pressure tested at least once every two years—more often if you have CVD risk factors. (High blood pressure and atherosclerosis are discussed later in the chapter.)

Unhealthy Cholesterol Levels   Cholesterol is a fatty, waxlike substance that circulates through the bloodstream and is an important component of cell mem-

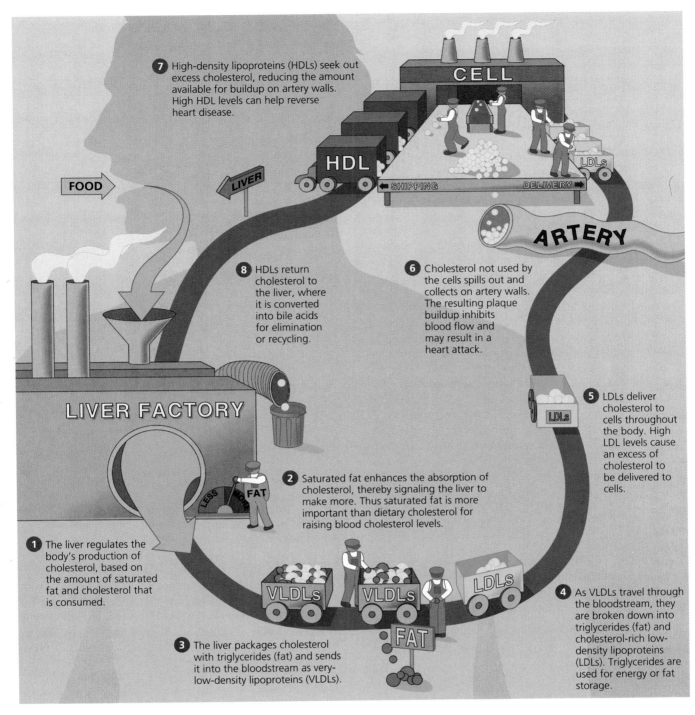

7 High-density lipoproteins (HDLs) seek out excess cholesterol, reducing the amount available for buildup on artery walls. High HDL levels can help reverse heart disease.

8 HDLs return cholesterol to the liver, where it is converted into bile acids for elimination or recycling.

6 Cholesterol not used by the cells spills out and collects on artery walls. The resulting plaque buildup inhibits blood flow and may result in a heart attack.

5 LDLs deliver cholesterol to cells throughout the body. High LDL levels cause an excess of cholesterol to be delivered to cells.

2 Saturated fat enhances the absorption of cholesterol, thereby signaling the liver to make more. Thus saturated fat is more important than dietary cholesterol for raising blood cholesterol levels.

1 The liver regulates the body's production of cholesterol, based on the amount of saturated fat and cholesterol that is consumed.

4 As VLDLs travel through the bloodstream, they are broken down into triglycerides (fat) and cholesterol-rich low-density lipoproteins (LDLs). Triglycerides are used for energy or fat storage.

3 The liver packages cholesterol with triglycerides (fat) and sends it into the bloodstream as very-low-density lipoproteins (VLDLs).

Figure 11-1   Travels with cholesterol.

branes, sex hormones, vitamin D, the fluid that coats the lungs, and the protective sheaths around nerves. Adequate cholesterol is essential for the proper functioning of the body. However, excess cholesterol can clog arteries and increase the risk of CVD (Figure 11-1).

Our bodies obtain cholesterol in two ways: from the liver, which manufactures it, and from the foods we eat.

Cholesterol levels vary depending on diet, age, sex, heredity, and other factors.

GOOD VERSUS BAD CHOLESTEROL   Cholesterol is carried in protein-lipid packages called **lipoproteins.** Lipoproteins can be thought of as shuttles that transport cholesterol to and from the liver through the circulatory system.

Low-density lipoproteins (LDLs) shuttle cholesterol from the liver to the organs and tissues that require it. LDL is known as "bad" cholesterol because if there is more than the body can use, the excess is deposited in the blood vessels. When it accumulates, it can block arteries and cause heart attacks and strokes. High-density lipoproteins (HDLs), or "good" cholesterol, shuttle unused cholesterol back to the liver for recycling.

RECOMMENDED BLOOD CHOLESTEROL LEVELS   The risk for CVD increases with increasing blood cholesterol levels. The first step in managing your cholesterol is to be tested. The National Cholesterol Education Program (NCEP) recommends testing at least once every 5 years for all adults, beginning at age 20, or at least every 3 years for people with a family history of heart disease. General cholesterol guidelines are given in Table 11-1. A total cholesterol level below 200 mg/dl (milligrams per deciliter) is considered desirable and indicates a relatively low risk of CVD; high levels, over 240 mg/dl, carry approximately double the CVD risk of desirable levels. An estimated 97 million American adults—over half the adult population—have total cholesterol levels of 200 mg/dl or higher.

Laboratory blood tests can measure your LDL and HDL levels. In general, high LDL levels and low HDL levels are associated with a high risk for CVD; low levels of LDL and high levels of HDL are associated with lower risk. HDL is especially important because a high HDL level seems to offer protection from CVD even in cases where total cholesterol is high. On the other hand, low total cholesterol may be associated with high CVD risk if HDL is also very low. For this reason, some experts use the ratio of total cholesterol to HDL to evaluate CVD risk.

IMPROVING CHOLESTEROL LEVELS   Important dietary changes that improve cholesterol levels include cutting total fat intake, substituting unsaturated for saturated and trans fats, and increasing soluble fiber intake. Decreasing your intake of saturated fat is particularly important because saturated fat promotes the production and excretion of cholesterol by the liver. You can raise your HDL levels by exercising regularly and, if you smoke, kicking the habit.

Physical Inactivity

An estimated 35–50 million Americans are so sedentary that they are at high risk for developing CVD. Exercise is thought to be the closest thing we have to a "magic bullet" against heart disease. It lowers CVD risk by helping decrease blood pressure, increase HDL levels, maintain desirable weight, improve the condition of the blood vessels, and prevent or control diabetes. One recent study found that women who accumulated at least 3 hours of brisk walking each week cut their

TABLE 11-1	*Cholesterol Guidelines*[a]
Total blood cholesterol	
Less than 200 mg/dl	Desirable[b]
200–239 mg/dl	Borderline high
240 mg/dl or more	High
LDL cholesterol	
Less than 130 mg/dl	Desirable[b]
130–159 mg/dl	Borderline high
160 mg/dl or more	High
HDL cholesterol	
More than 45 mg/dl	Desirable[b]
35–45 mg/dl	Borderline low
Less than 35 mg/dl	Low
Cholesterol ratio (total ÷ HDL)[c]	
4.5	Average
3.5	Optimal

[a]These guidelines are based on large-scale studies of middle-aged Americans; younger people should strive for somewhat lower levels. For example, for those age 19 and under, the desirable level for total blood cholesterol is below 170 mg/dl.
[b]For adults without known heart disease; for those with heart disease, an LDL level of 100 mg/dl or less is recommended.
[c]Higher ratios indicate higher risk.

SOURCES: American Heart Association. National Cholesterol Education Program.

risk of heart attack and stroke by more than half. (See Chapter 3 for more information on the physical and psychological effects of exercise.)

Obesity

In June 1998, the American Heart Association added obesity to its list of major controllable risk factors. A person whose body weight is more than 30% above the recommended level is at higher risk for heart disease and stroke, even if no other risk factors are present. Excess weight increases the strain on the heart by contributing to high blood pressure and high cholesterol. It can also lead to diabetes, another CVD risk factor (see below). As discussed in Chapter 6, distribution of body fat is also significant: Fat that collects in the torso is more dangerous than fat that collects around the hips. A sensible diet and regular exercise are the best ways to achieve and maintain a healthy body weight. For people who are obese, losing even a small amount of weight can have very beneficial effects on cardiovascular health.

Contributing Risk Factors That Can Be Changed

Various other factors that can be changed have been identified as contributing to CVD risk, including diabetes, triglyceride levels, and psychological and social factors.

TERMS   low-density lipoproteins (LDLs)   Blood fats that transport cholesterol to organs and tissues; excess amounts result in the accumulation of deposits on artery walls.

Diabetes   People with diabetes are at increased risk for CVD, partly because the disease affects the levels of cholesterol in the blood. Diabetes appears to have both a genetic component and a behavioral component. The best way to avoid diabetes is to exercise regularly and control body weight. (See Chapter 6 for more information on diabetes.)

Triglyceride Levels   Like cholesterol, triglycerides are blood fats that can be obtained from the diet and manufactured by the body. Studies have shown that high triglyceride levels are a reliable predictor of heart disease, especially if associated with other risk factors, such as low HDL levels, obesity, and diabetes. Elevated triglyceride levels may be of particular concern for women and for people who smoke.

Physicians often recommend that people with other risk factors for CVD have their total triglyceride level measured. A triglyceride level below 200 mg/dl is considered normal; a level of 400 mg/dl or above is considered high. The best ways to reduce triglycerides seem to be weight loss, regular exercise, and a diet that is high in fiber and low in simple sugars and refined carbohydrates and that favors unsaturated over saturated fats. Being moderate in the use of alcohol is also important because alcohol elevates triglyceride levels.

Psychological and Social Factors   Many of the psychological and social factors that influence other areas of wellness are also important risk factors for CVD.

• *Stress.* Excessive stress can strain the heart and blood vessels over time and contribute to CVD. A full-blown stress response causes blood vessels to constrict and blood pressure to rise. Blood platelets become more likely to cluster, possibly enhancing the formation of artery-clogging clots. People sometimes also adopt unhealthy habits such as smoking, overeating, or skipping meals as a means of dealing with severe stress.

• *Chronic hostility and anger.* Certain traits in the hard-driving "Type A" personality—hostility, cynicism, and anger—are associated with increased risk of heart disease. People who are prone to chronic hostility experience the stress response more intensely and frequently than more relaxed individuals. When they encounter the irritations of daily life, their blood pressure increases much more. They also seem to have trouble shutting down the stress response. Less hostile people tend to calm down much more quickly, taking the stress off their bodies—especially their hearts. (Part II of Lab 11-1 includes a hostility self-assessment and tips for managing anger.)

• *Suppressing psychological distress.* Consistently suppressing anger and other negative emotions may also be hazardous to a healthy heart. Several recent studies suggest that people who hide psychological distress—even

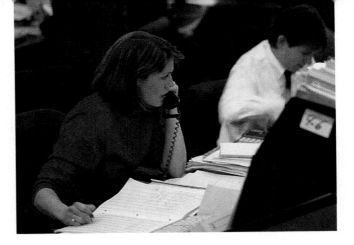

Before age 65, women are less susceptible to cardiovascular disease than men. Even though this woman has to cope with the same on-the-job stresses as men in her profession, she is less likely to have a heart attack in middle age than they are.

from themselves—have a higher rate of heart disease than people who experience similar distress but share it with others.

• *Depression and anxiety.* Both mild and severe depression are linked to an increased risk of fatal heart disease. Researchers have also found a strong association between anxiety disorders and an increased risk of death from heart disease, particularly sudden death from heart attack.

• *Social isolation.* People with little social support are at higher risk of dying from coronary heart disease (CHD) than people with close ties to others. A strong social support network is a major antidote to stress. Friends and family members can also promote and support healthy lifestyle behaviors (see the box "Religion and Wellness").

• *Socioeconomic status.* Low socioeconomic status and low educational attainment also increase risk for CVD. These associations are probably due to a variety of factors, including lifestyle and access to health care.

Major Risk Factors That Can't Be Changed

A number of major risk factors for CVD cannot be changed: heredity, aging, being male, and ethnicity.

Heredity   The tendency to develop CVD seems to be inherited. High cholesterol levels, abnormal blood-clotting problems, diabetes, and obesity are other CVD risk factors that have genetic links. People who inherit a tendency for CVD are not destined to develop it, but they may have to work harder than other people to prevent it.

Aging   The risk of heart attack increases dramatically after age 65. About 55% of all heart attack victims are age 65 or older, and almost four out of five who suffer fatal

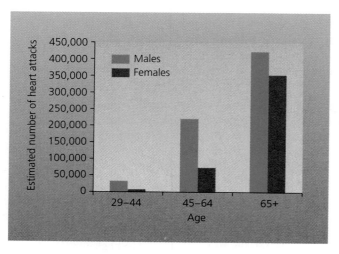
Of 212 clinical studies that evaluated the effect of religious commitment on Americans' health and well-being, 75% found a positive effect, according to research presented at the American Association for the Advancement of Science 1996 annual meeting. The report, sponsored by the National Institute for Health Care Research, found that religion was beneficial for both physical and psychological problems—including depression, hypertension, and heart disease—as well as overall quality of life.

The critical factor, says author Dale Matthews, M.D., of Georgetown University School of Medicine, seems to be the intensity of religious commitment: In general, those who had the greatest involvement with their church and the strongest devotion were the healthiest. For example, in one study of heart surgery patients, the death rate within 6 months of surgery was 5% for regular churchgoers—compared to a national average of 9%—and 0% for those who considered themselves "deeply religious." Overall, the report found these and other effects to be unrelated to a particular denomination.

The mechanism behind religion's apparent health benefits is still unclear, but Dr. Matthews speculates that the church provides a strong community that keeps people from becoming isolated and acts as a safety net when they are ill. Studies have consistently shown that social isolation contributes to poor health. In addition, people who are religious may follow a healthier lifestyle than the general population and be less inclined to smoke and drink excessive amounts of alcohol. Research has also found that the act of worship promotes relaxation, which itself confers other health benefits. And, of course, there is the possibility that all of this is outside the realm of medical science.

"I think religion *is* good for your health," Dr. Matthews says. "But we still need to do more research to understand how this works and whether there is a healing mechanism separate from

of hypertension than women. The incidence of stroke is about 19% higher for males than females. Estrogen production, which is highest during the childbearing years, may offer premenopausal women some protection against CVD.

Ethnicity   Death rates from heart disease vary among ethnic groups in the United States, with African Americans having much higher rates of hypertension, heart disease, and stroke than other groups (see the box "African Americans and CVD").

Puerto Rican Americans, Cuban Americans, and Mexican Americans are also more likely to suffer from high blood pressure and angina (a warning sign of heart disease) than non-Hispanic white Americans. These differences may be due in part to differences in education, income, and other socioeconomic factors.

Asian Americans historically have had far lower rates of CVD than white Americans. However, recent studies indicate that cholesterol levels among Asian Americans are rising, presumably because of the adoption of a high-fat American diet.

Possible Risk Factors Currently Being Studied

In recent years, several other possible risk factors for CVD have been identified. These include homocysteine, lipoprotein(a), and certain infectious agents.

Homocysteine is an amino acid circulating in the blood. High levels of homocysteine are associated with an increased risk of CVD, but researchers are not yet certain whether it is a direct cause or simply a marker for some

VITAL STATISTICS

Figure 11-2 Annual incidence of heart attack. Among heart attack victims under age 65, men significantly outnumber women; after age 65, women start to catch up. SOURCES: American Heart Association. 1998. *Heart and Stroke Statistical Update.*

heart attacks are over 65. For people over 55, the incidence of stroke more than doubles in each successive decade. However, many people in their thirties and forties, especially men, have heart attacks.

Being Male   Although CVD is the leading killer of both men and women in the United States, men face a greater risk of heart attack than women, especially earlier in life (Figure 11-2). Until age 55, men also have a greater risk

African American men are nearly 50% more likely to die from a heart attack than white men, and death from stroke is five times more common among African Americans than in other Americans. Hypertension is twice as common in blacks. What accounts for these higher rates of CVD among African Americans? Contributing factors can be grouped into three areas: biological/genetic factors, low income and discrimination, and lifestyle factors.

Biological/Genetic Factors

Researchers are investigating a number of genetic factors that may contribute to CVD in African Americans, including heightened sensitivities to lead and salt, which can lead to high blood pressure. Heredity may also play a role in higher cholesterol levels among blacks. And sickle-cell disease, a genetic disorder that occurs mainly in blacks, can lead to impaired blood flow and heart failure.

Low Income and Discrimination

Another factor in the high incidence of CVD among African Americans is low income. One-third live below the official poverty line. Economic deprivation usually means reduced access to adequate health care and health insurance. Associated with low income are poorer educational opportunities, which often mean less information about preventive health measures, such as diet and stress management.

Discrimination may also play a role in CVD among blacks. Research has shown that many physicians and hospitals treat the medical problems of African Americans differently than those of whites. Discrimination, along with low income and other forms of deprivation, may also increase stress, which is linked with hypertension and CVD.

Lifestyle Factors

Lifestyle factors may be the key in explaining high CVD rates among African Americans. A recent large-scale study determined that birthplace, not ethnicity, is the key indicator of CVD risk among African Americans. The study found that among New Yorkers born in the Northeast, blacks and whites have nearly identical risk for CVD. But black New Yorkers who were born in the South have a sharply higher risk, and black New Yorkers born in the Caribbean have a significantly lower risk. In fact, blacks who were born in the South and moved to New York City were twice as likely to die of heart disease as blacks or whites born in the Northeast.

Researchers speculate that some risk factors for CVD, including smoking and a high-fat diet, may be more common in the South. When combined with urban stress, these factors create a lifestyle that is far from heart-healthy. And people with low incomes, who are disproportionately African American, tend to smoke more, use more salt, and exercise less than those with higher incomes. In addition, half of African American women and one-third of African American men are significantly overweight.

Medical experts advise all Americans to have their blood pressure checked regularly, exercise, eat a healthy diet, manage stress, and avoid smoking. These preventive strategies may be particularly important for African Americans.

---

other risk factor. In laboratory studies, homocysteine appears to intensify blood clotting and damage the linings of blood vessels, both of which increase the risk of heart disease. Homocysteine levels tend to be higher among men than women and are particularly high among people who smoke; other risk factors include hypertension, high cholesterol levels, a sedentary lifestyle, and a diet deficient in vitamins B-12, B-6, and folic acid.

A specific type of LDL called lipoprotein(a), or Lp(a), has been identified as a possible independent risk factor for CHD. Lp(a) has a strong genetic component and is not influenced by diet or most cholesterol-lowering drugs. Preliminary research indicates that hormone replacement therapy and other treatments for lowering elevated LDL levels may also reduce the risk associated with high Lp(a).

Several infectious agents have also been identified as possible culprits in the development of heart disease. They are *Chlamydia pneumoniae, cytomegalovirus (CMV),* and *Helicobacter pylori,* a bacterium linked to ulcers and stomach cancer. Although the mechanism is not yet clear, it appears that some chronic infections may contribute to inflammation and the buildup of fatty deposits in arteries.

MAJOR FORMS OF CARDIOVASCULAR DISEASE

Collectively, the various forms of CVD kill more Americans than the next four leading causes of death combined. The financial burden of CVD, including the costs of medical treatments and lost productivity, exceeds $250 billion annually. Although the main forms of CVD are interrelated and have elements in common, we treat them separately here for the sake of clarity.

Hypertension

Blood pressure, the force exerted by the blood on blood vessel walls, is created by the pumping action of the heart. When the heart contracts (systole), blood pressure increases; when the heart relaxes (diastole), pressure decreases. Short periods of high blood pressure are normal, but blood pressure that is continually at an abnormally high level is known as hypertension.

Blood pressure is measured with a stethoscope and an instrument called a sphygmomanometer. It is expressed as two numbers—for example, 120 over 80—and

TABLE 11-2 — Blood Pressure Classification for Healthy Adults

Category[a]	Systolic (mm Hg)		Diastolic (mm Hg)	Recommended Follow-Up
Optimal[b]	below 120	and	below 80	Recheck in 2 years
Normal	below 130	and	below 85	Recheck in 2 years
High-normal	130–139	or	85–89	Recheck in 1 year
Hypertension[c]				
Stage 1	140–159	or	90–99	Confirm within 2 months
Stage 2	160–179	or	100–109	Physician evaluation within 1 month
Stage 3	180 and above	or	110 and above	Immediate physician evaluation

[a]When systolic and diastolic blood pressure fall into different categories, the higher category should be selected to classify an individual's blood pressure status.

[b]Optimal blood pressure with respect to cardiovascular risk is below 120/80 mm Hg; however, unusually low readings should be evaluated.

[c]Based on the average of two or more readings taken at different physician visits.

SOURCE: *The Sixth Report of the Joint National Committee on Prevention, Detection, Evaluation, and Treatment of High Blood Pressure.* 1997. Bethesda, Md.: National Heart, Lung, and Blood Institute. National Institutes of Health (NIH Publication No. 98-4080).

measured in millimeters of mercury. The first and larger number is the systolic blood pressure; the second is the diastolic blood pressure. Average blood pressure readings for young adults in good physical condition are 110–120 systolic over 70–80 diastolic. High blood pressure in adults is defined as equal to or greater than 140 over 90 (Table 11-2).

High blood pressure results from either an increased output of blood by the heart, often as a result of overweight, or because of increased resistance to blood flow in the arteries from narrowing and hardening. When a person has high blood pressure, the heart must work harder than normal to force blood through the arteries, and the arteries are under a greater strain than normal. Over time, high blood pressure causes the heart to enlarge and weaken, and the process of atherosclerosis speeds up.

High blood pressure is often called a "silent killer," because it usually has no symptoms or warning signs. In fact, it is possible to have high blood pressure for years without realizing it. Over that course of time, hypertension might be damaging vital organs (particularly the heart, brain, kidneys, and eyes) and increasing the risk of heart attack, congestive heart failure, stroke, kidney failure, and blindness. The key to avoiding the complications of hypertension is having your blood pressure measured regularly.

Hypertension cannot be cured, but it can be treated and controlled through diet, exercise, and medication. An estimated 50 million Americans, one in four adults, have hypertension; only about one-third of them have it under control. Cases of mild hypertension can frequently be treated by changes in diet alone, such as increased intake of fruits and vegetables and restricted salt intake in salt-sensitive people. Other lifestyle measures for preventing and treating hypertension include exercising regularly, maintaining a healthy weight, limiting alcohol intake, and not smoking. Treating more severe hypertension usually involves long-term drug therapy.

Atherosclerosis

Atherosclerosis is a slow, progressive hardening and narrowing of the arteries that can begin in childhood. Arteries become narrowed by deposits of fat, cholesterol, and other substances. As these deposits, called **plaques**, accumulate on artery walls, the arteries lose their elasticity and their ability to expand and contract, restricting blood flow. Once narrowed by a plaque, an artery is vulnerable to blockage by blood clots (Figure 11-3).

If the heart, brain, and/or other organs are deprived of blood, and thus the vital oxygen it carries, the effects of atherosclerosis can be deadly. **Coronary arteries**, which supply the heart with blood, are particularly susceptible to plaque buildup, a condition called **coronary heart disease (CHD)**, or coronary artery disease. The blockage of

TERMS

plaque A deposit of fatty (and other) substances on the inner wall of the arteries.

coronary arteries Two arteries branching from the aorta that provide blood to the heart muscle.

coronary heart disease (CHD) Heart disease caused by hardening of the arteries that supply oxygen to the heart muscle.

heart attack Damage to, or death of, heart muscle, sometimes resulting in a failure of the heart to deliver enough blood, carrying vital oxygen, to other organs of the body.

angina pectoris A condition in which the heart muscle does not receive enough blood, causing severe pain in the chest and often in the left arm and shoulder.

arrhythmia An irregularity in the force or rhythm of the heartbeat that often precedes a heart attack.

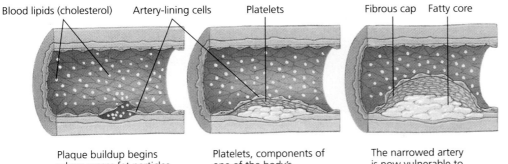

Blood lipids (cholesterol) Artery-lining cells Platelets Fibrous cap Fatty core

Figure 11-3 Stages of plaque development.

Plaque buildup begins when excess fat particles (lipids) collect beneath cells lining the artery that have been damaged by smoking, high blood pressure, or other causes.

Platelets, components of one of the body's protective mechanisms, collect at the damaged area and cause a cap of cells to form, isolating the plaque within the artery wall.

The narrowed artery is now vulnerable to blockage by clots that can form if the cap breaks and the fatty core of the plaque combines again with platelets and other clot-producing factors in the blood.

a coronary artery causes a heart attack. If a cerebral artery (leading to the brain) is blocked, the result is a stroke.

The main risk factors for atherosclerosis are cigarette smoking, physical inactivity, high levels of blood cholesterol, and high blood pressure. A 1998 study found that smoking and exposure to environmental tobacco smoke permanently accelerate the rate of plaque accumulation in the coronary arteries—50% for smokers, 25% for ex-smokers, and 20% for people regularly exposed to ETS.

Heart Disease and Heart Attacks

A **heart attack** is the end result of a long-term disease process. The heart requires a steady supply of oxygen-rich blood to function properly (Figure 11-4). If one of the coronary arteries that supplies blood to the heart becomes blocked by a blood clot, a heart attack results. A heart attack caused by a clot is called a coronary thrombosis, a coronary occlusion, or a myocardial infarction. In myocardial infarction, part of the heart muscle (myocardium) may die from lack of oxygen.

Although heart attacks often occur without warning, some people experience pain or an abnormal heartbeat first. Chest pain called **angina pectoris** is a signal that the heart isn't getting enough oxygen to supply its needs. Although not actually a heart attack, angina is a warning that the heart is overloaded. If the electrical impulses that control heartbeat are disrupted, the heart may beat too quickly, too slowly, or in an irregular fashion, a condition known as **arrhythmia**, another sign of impending heart attack.

If symptoms of heart trouble do occur, it is critical to go immediately to the nearest hospital or clinic with a 24-hour emergency cardiac facility (see the box "What to Do in the Event of a Heart Attack"). If a victim gets to the emergency room quickly enough, a clot-dissolving agent can be injected to dissolve a clot in the coronary artery, reducing the amount of damage to the heart muscle.

Physicians have a variety of diagnostic tools and treatments for heart disease. A patient may undergo a stress or

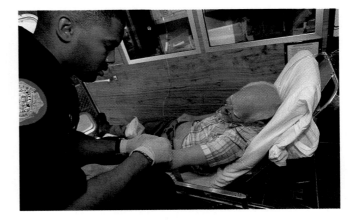

Many heart attack victims aren't sure they've had an attack and wait too long—2 hours or more— before getting help. Prompt attention from a paramedic greatly improves this man's chance of survival.

exercise test, in which he or she runs on a treadmill while being monitored with an electrocardiogram (ECG or EKG). Certain characteristic changes in the heart's electrical activity while under stress can reveal particular heart problems, such as restricted blood flow to the heart muscle. Tools that allow the physician to visualize a patient's heart and arteries include magnetic resonance imaging (MRI) and angiograms.

If tests indicate a problem or if a person has already had a heart attack, several treatments are possible. *Balloon angioplasty* involves threading a catheter with an inflatable balloon tip through a coronary artery until it reaches the area of blockage; the balloon is then inflated, flattening the plaque and widening the arterial opening. In *coronary bypass surgery,* healthy blood vessels are grafted to coronary arteries to bypass blockages. Along with a low-fat diet, regular exercise, and smoking cessation, many patients are also advised to take half an aspirin tablet daily to reduce clotting and inflammation.

Superior vena cava

Right atrium

Right coronary artery

Right ventricle

Inferior vena cava

Aorta

Pulmonary artery

Left atrium

Left coronary artery

Left ventricle

Figure 11-4 Blood supply to the heart. Blood is supplied to the heart from the right and left coronary arteries, which branch off the aorta. If a coronary artery becomes blocked by plaque buildup and a blood clot, a heart attack occurs; part of the heart muscle may die due to lack of oxygen.

Stroke

For brain cells to function as they should, they must have a continuous and ample supply of oxygen-rich blood. If brain cells are deprived of blood for more than a few minutes, they die. A **stroke,** also called a cerebrovascular accident (CVA), occurs when the blood supply to the brain is cut off. Strokes can be particularly serious because injured brain cells, unlike those of other organs, cannot regenerate.

A stroke may be caused by a blood clot that blocks an artery or by a burst blood vessel (cerebral hemorrhage).

TERMS **stroke** An impeded blood supply to some part of the brain resulting in the destruction of brain cells.

rheumatic fever A disease, mainly of children, characterized by fever, inflammation, and pain in the joints; often damages the heart muscle.

congestive heart failure A condition resulting from the heart's inability to pump out all the blood that returns to it. Blood backs up in the veins leading to the heart, causing an accumulation of fluid in various parts of the body.

High blood pressure and atherosclerosis (especially blockage of the cerebral arteries) greatly increase the risk of stroke. The interruption of the blood supply to any area of the brain prevents the nerve cells there from functioning—in some cases, causing death. Nerve cells control sensation and most body movements; depending on the area of the brain that is affected, a stroke may cause paralysis, walking disability, speech impairment, or memory loss. Of the 500,000 Americans who have strokes each year, approximately one-third die within a year; those who survive usually have some lasting disability.

Effective treatment requires the prompt recognition of symptoms—sudden numbness or weakness of the face, arm, and leg on one side of the body; loss of speech or difficulty speaking or understanding speech; dimming or loss of vision, especially in only one eye; and unexplained dizziness. Depending on the type of stroke, treatment may involve the use of clot-dissolving and antihypertensive drugs. If detection and treatment of stroke come too late, rehabilitation is the only treatment. Although damaged or destroyed brain tissue cannot regenerate, nerve cells in the brain can make new pathways, and some functions can be taken over by other parts of the brain.

Congestive Heart Failure

A number of conditions—high blood pressure, heart attack, atherosclerosis, **rheumatic fever**, birth defects—can damage the heart's pumping mechanism. When the heart cannot maintain its regular pumping rate and force, fluids begin to back up. When extra fluid seeps through capillary walls, edema (swelling) results, usually in the legs and ankles, but sometimes in other parts of the body as well. Fluid can collect in the lungs and interfere with breathing, particularly when a person is lying down. This condition is called *pulmonary edema,* and the entire process is known as **congestive heart failure.**

Congestive heart failure can be controlled. Treatment includes reducing the workload on the heart, modifying salt intake, and using drugs that help the body eliminate excess fluid.

PROTECTING YOURSELF AGAINST CARDIOVASCULAR DISEASE

There are several important steps you can take now to lower your risk of developing CVD in the future (see the box "A Heart-Healthy Lifestyle").

Eat Heart-Healthy

For most Americans, changing to a heart-healthy diet involves cutting total fat intake, substituting unsaturated fats for saturated fats, and increasing fiber. Such changes can lower a person's blood levels of total cholesterol, LDL cholesterol, and triglycerides.

Decreased Fat and Cholesterol Intake The NCEP recommends that all Americans over the age of 2 adopt a

A diet high in fiber and low in total fat and saturated fat can help lower levels of total cholesterol and LDL. This woman is enjoying a healthy dinner of baked chicken, broccoli, rice, fruit, and juice.

diet in which total fat consumption is no more than 30% of total daily calories. No more than one-third of those fat calories should come from saturated fat, which is found in animal products, palm and coconut oil, and hydrogenated vegetable oils. Most of the fat calories in your diet should come from unsaturated fats, which may raise HDL and lower total cholesterol. By controlling your intake of total fat and saturated fat, you'll also reduce your consumption of cholesterol-raising trans fatty acids (see Chapter 8 for more information on types of dietary fats and strategies for controlling fat intake).

Animal products contain cholesterol as well as saturated fat. The NCEP and AHA recommend that you limit dietary cholesterol intake to 300 mg per day or less.

Increased Fiber Intake Soluble fiber traps the bile acids the liver needs to manufacture cholesterol and carries them to the large intestine, where they are excreted. It also slows the production of proteins that promote blood clotting. Insoluble fiber may interfere with the absorption of dietary fat and may also help you cut total food intake because foods rich in insoluble fiber tend to be filling. To obtain the recommended 20–35 grams of dietary fiber per day, choose a diet rich in whole grains, fruits, and vegetables. Good sources of fiber include oatmeal, some breakfast cereals, barley, legumes, and most fruits and vegetables.

Alcohol A large-scale study released in 1997 found that people who average about one drink per day had a 30–40% lower risk of death from cardiovascular disease compared with nondrinkers. However, the mortality rate from breast cancer was 30% higher among women who had at least one drink daily. Other causes of death associated with drinking are alcoholism, cirrhosis of the liver, certain forms of cancer and cardiovascular disease, and injuries; overall death rates rise with the level of alcohol consumption. Because alcohol has both beneficial and adverse effects on health, you should consider your personal risk factors in making decisions about alcohol use. If you do drink, do so moderately (no more than one drink per day for women or two drinks per day for men), with food, and at times when drinking will not put you or others at risk.

DASH A study released in 1997 called "Dietary Approaches to Stop Hypertension," or DASH, suggests that many Americans can lower their blood pressure by adopting a diet that is low in fat and high in fruits, vegetables, and low-fat dairy products. In the study, the DASH diet caused a significant reduction in blood pressure for people with high and high-normal blood pressure. The DASH diet plan is as follows:

- 7–8 servings per day of grains and grain products
- 4–5 servings per day of vegetables
- 4–5 servings per day of fruits
- 2–3 servings per day of low-fat or nonfat dairy products
- 2 or fewer servings per day of meats, poultry, and fish
- 4–5 servings per *week* of nuts, seeds, and legumes
- 2–3 servings per day of added fats, oils, and salad dressings
- 5 servings per *week* of snacks and sweets

In the future, researchers hope to determine the effects of different levels of sodium intake (salt raises blood pressure in people who are salt-sensitive). The DASH diet also follows the dietary recommendations for lowering one's risk of cancer, osteoporosis, and heart disease.

Exercise Regularly

People who are sedentary develop heart disease an average of 5–6 years earlier than those who are active. You can significantly reduce your risk of CVD with a moderate amount of physical activity. Try to accumulate at least 30 minutes of moderate-intensity physical activity each day through such activities as brisk walking and stair climbing.

Avoid Tobacco

Remember: The number one risk factor for CVD that you can control is smoking. If you smoke, quit. If you don't, don't start. If you live or work with people who smoke, encourage them to quit—for their sake and yours. If you find yourself breathing in smoke, take steps to prevent or stop this exposure.

Know and Manage Your Blood Pressure

Currently, only about 30% of Americans with hypertension have their blood pressure under control. If you have no CVD risk factors, have your blood pressure measured at least once every 2 years; yearly tests are recommended if you have other risk factors. If your blood pressure is high, follow your physician's advice on how to lower it, and have it checked every 6 months.

Know and Manage Your Cholesterol Levels

Have your blood cholesterol levels measured if you've never had it done. When you know your "number," follow these guidelines from the NCEP:

- *Total cholesterol below 200 mg/dl.* If you HDL is 35 mg/dl or higher and you have no other risk factors for CVD, maintain a healthy lifestyle, including eating a low-fat diet, getting regular exercise, maintaining a healthy body weight, and not smoking. Get another test within 5 years. If your HDL level is less than 35 mg/dl, have your LDL level measured and evaluated, and follow your physician's advice.

- *Total cholesterol between 200 and 239 mg/dl.* If your HDL is 35 mg/dl or higher and you have fewer than two other risk factors for CVD, you may or may not be at increased risk. Work with your physician to control other CVD risk factors, and have your cholesterol levels rechecked in 1–2 years. If your HDL level is less than 35 mg/dl or you have two or more other risk factors for CVD, have your LDL level checked and evaluated, and follow your physician's advice.

- *Total cholesterol 240 mg/dl or more.* Your physician should order a more detailed cholesterol analysis and recommend therapy based on the results. Adopt a heart-healthy lifestyle immediately, including a cholesterol-improving diet and regular exercise. Follow your physician's advice for controlling other CVD risk factors, and have your cholesterol levels rechecked as recommended.

Develop Ways to Handle Stress and Anger and Manage Medical Conditions

To reduce the psychological and social risk factors for CVD, develop effective strategies for handling the stress in your life. Shore up your social support network, and try some of the techniques described in Chapter 10 for managing stress. If anger and hostility are problems for you, refer to Part II of Lab 11-1 for tips on diffusing your anger. If you have any medical problems such as diabetes, follow your physician's advice carefully.

COMMON QUESTIONS ANSWERED

Do women have a lower risk for cardiovascular disease than men, and, if so, why? Until about age 65, women have a significant advantage over men when it comes to CVD. Every year, more than 300,000 people under age 65 have a heart attack; of these, more than 75% are men. Women who develop CVD tend to be about 10 years older than men when they first have symptoms and about 20 years older when they have a heart attack.

What explains this difference? Research thus far has focused on the beneficial effects of estrogen, which, prior to menopause, circulates in high concentrations in a woman's body. Estrogen improves blood cholesterol levels by raising the concentration of HDL and lowering levels of LDL. Women, on average, have much better blood cholesterol profiles than men. Estrogen also seems to prevent blood clots from forming in the body and to dissolve clots that do form. This is significant because clots can lead to heart attacks and strokes. And estrogen may also lower blood concentrations of homocysteine, high levels of which may be linked with heart attacks and strokes.

But women should not be complacent about their risk for cardiovascular disease. CVD is the leading cause of death among women, killing five times as many women as breast cancer and significantly more women than all types of cancers combined. After menopause, estrogen levels fall and LDL levels begin to rise. By age 65, heart attack risk for women is almost equal to that of men. And women are even less likely to survive an attack, in part because they tend to suffer heart attacks at an older age and because CVD is less likely to be diagnosed in women.

As more studies of CVD among women are completed, scientists may learn more about how female biochemistry affects the development of CVD. In the meantime, it's important to note that the major risk factors for CVD are the same for both women and men. The general advice for preventing CVD presented in this chapter—exercising regularly, managing stress, eating a low-fat diet, and so on—is appropriate for everyone.

I know what foods to avoid to prevent CVD, but are there any foods I should eat to protect myself from CVD? The most important dietary change for CVD prevention is a negative one: cutting back on foods high in fat, particularly saturated and trans fat. However, research indicates that certain foods can be helpful. The positive effects of unsaturated fats, soluble fiber, and alcohol on heart health were discussed earlier in the chapter. Other potentially beneficial foods include those rich in the following:

- *Omega-3 fatty acids.* Found in fish, shellfish, and some nuts and seeds, omega-3 fatty acids may be helpful in lowering cholesterol and triglyceride levels.

(continued)

- *Folic acid, vitamin B-6, and vitamin B-12.* These three vitamins may affect CVD risk by lowering homocysteine levels; see Table 8-3 for a list of food sources.

- *Vitamin E.* Some recent studies indicate that vitamin E—found in nuts, vegetable oils, wheat germ, margarine, and avocados—may have a protective effect against heart disease.

- *Soy protein.* Some studies have shown that replacing some animal protein with soy protein can lower LDL cholesterol. Soy-based foods include tofu, tempeh, and baked goods made with soy flour.

More research is needed to clarify the effects of these compounds on CVD risk. Meanwhile, you can't go wrong by increasing your intake of fruits, grains, and vegetables.

The advice I hear from the news about protecting myself from CVD seems to be changing all the time. What am I supposed to believe? Health-related research is now described in popular newspapers and magazines rather than just medical journals, meaning that more and more people have access to the information. Researchers do not deliberately set out to mislead or confuse people. However, news reports may oversimplify the results of research studies, leaving out some of the qualifications and questions the researchers present with their findings. In addition, news reports may not differentiate between a preliminary finding and a result that has been verified by a large number of long-term studies. And researchers themselves must strike a balance between reporting promising preliminary findings to the public, thereby allowing people to act on them, and waiting 10–20 years until long-term studies confirm (or disprove) a particular theory.

This can leave you in a difficult position. You cannot become an expert on all subjects, able to effectively evaluate all the available health news. However, there are some general strategies you can use to better assess the health advice that appears in the media; see the box "Evaluating Health News."

SUMMARY

- The major controllable risk factors for CVD are smoking, hypertension, unhealthy cholesterol levels, a sedentary lifestyle, and obesity.

- Contributing factors for CVD that can be changed include diabetes, high triglyceride levels, inadequate stress management, a hostile personality, depression, anxiety, lack of social support, and poverty.

- Major risk factors that can't be changed are heredity, aging, being male, and ethnicity.

- Hypertension weakens the heart and scars and hardens arteries, causing resistance to blood flow. It is defined as blood pressure equal to or higher than 140 over 90.

- Atherosclerosis is a progressive hardening and narrowing of arteries that can lead to restricted blood flow and even complete blockage; high blood pressure and high levels of blood cholesterol are contributing factors.

- Heart attacks, strokes, and congestive heart failure are the results of a long-term disease process; hypertension and atherosclerosis are usually involved.

- Reducing heart disease risk involves eating heart-healthy, exercising regularly, avoiding tobacco, managing blood pressure and cholesterol levels, handling stress and anger, and managing medical conditions.

FOR MORE INFORMATION

Books

American Heart Association. 1998. *American Heart Association Guide to Heart Attack Treatment, Recovery, and Prevention.* New York: Times Books. *Provides information on a heart-healthy lifestyle.*

Fortmann, S., and P. Breitrose. 1996. *The Blood Pressure Book: How to Get It Down and Keep It Down.* Palo Alto, Calif.: Bull Publishing. *A step-by-step guide for making lifestyle changes to control blood pressure.*

Notelovitz, M., and D. Tonnessen. 1996. *The Essential Heart Book for Women.* New York: St. Martin's Press. *Explains how women can take action against their number one killer—heart disease—through prevention and treatment.*

Organizations and Web Sites

American Heart Association. Provides information on hundreds of topics relating to the prevention and control of CVD.
800-242-8721; 214-373-6300
http://www.americanheart.org

Cardiology Compass. An index and links to cardiovascular information on the Internet.
http://www.cardiologycompass.com

Dietary Approaches to Stop Hypertension (DASH). Provides information about the design, diets, and results of the DASH study, including tips on how to follow the DASH diet at home.
http://dash.bwh.harvard.edu

Franklin Institute Science Museum/The Heart: An On-Line Exploration. An online museum exhibit containing information on the structure and function of the heart, how to monitor your heart's health, and how to maintain a healthy heart.
http://www.fi.edu/biosci/heart.html

Americans face an avalanche of health information from newspapers, magazines, books, and television programs. It's not always easy to decide which news to believe and which news to ignore. The following questions can help you evaluate health news.

1. *Is the report based on research or on an anecdote?* Information or advice based on one or more carefully designed research studies has more validity than one person's experiences.

2. *What is the source of the information?* A study in a respected publication has been reviewed by editors and other researchers in the field—people who are in a position to evaluate the merits of a study and its results. Information put forth by government agencies and national research organizations is also usually considered fairly reliable.

3. *How big was the study?* A study that involves many subjects is more likely to yield reliable results than a study involving only a few people. Another indication that a finding is meaningful is if several different studies yield the same results.

4. *Who were the people involved in the study?* Research findings are more likely to apply to you if you share important characteristics with the subjects of the study. For example, the results of a study on men over age 50 who smoke may not be particularly meaningful for a 30-year-old nonsmoking woman.

5. *What kind of study was it?* Epidemiological studies involve observation or interviews in order to trace the relationships among lifestyle, physical characteristics, and diseases. While epidemiological studies can suggest links, they cannot establish cause-and-effect relationships. Experiments or interventional studies involve testing the effects of different treatments on groups of people who have similar lifestyles and characteristics. They are more likely to provide conclusive evidence of a cause-and-effect relationship. The best interventional studies share the following characteristics:

- *Controlled.* A group of people who receive the treatment is compared with a matched group who do not receive the treatment.
- *Randomized.* The treatment and control groups are selected randomly.
- *Double-blind.* Researchers and participants are unaware of who is receiving the treatment.

- *Multicenter.* The experiment is performed at more than one institution.

6. *What do the statistics really say?* First, are the results described as "statistically significant"? If a study is large and well designed, its results can be deemed statistically significant, meaning there is less than a 5% chance that the findings resulted from chance. Second, are the results stated in terms of relative or absolute risk? Many findings are reported in terms of relative risk—how a particular treatment or condition affects a person's disease risk. Consider the following examples of relative risk.

- According to some estimates, taking estrogen without progesterone can increase a postmenopausal woman's risk of dying from endometrial cancer by 233%.
- Giving AZT to HIV-infected pregnant women reduces prenatal transmission of HIV by 66%.

The first of these two findings seems far more dramatic than the second—until one also considers absolute risk, the actual risk of the illness in the population being considered. The absolute risk of endometrial cancer is 0.3%; a 233% increase based on the effects of estrogen raises it to 1%, a change of 0.7%. Without treatment, about 25% of infants born to HIV-infected women will be infected with HIV; with treatment, the absolute risk drops to about 8%, a change of 17%. Because the absolute risk of an HIV-infected mother passing the virus to her infant is so much greater than a woman's risk of developing endometrial cancer (25% compared with 0.3%), a smaller change in relative risk translates into a much greater change in absolute risk.

7. *Is new health advice being offered?* If the media report new guidelines for health behavior or medical treatment, examine the source. Government agencies and national research foundations usually consider a great deal of evidence before offering health advice. Above all, use common sense, and check with your physician before making a major change in your health habits based on news reports.

SOURCES: Medical news: How to assess the latest breakthrough. 1997. *Consumer Reports,* June. Why do those #&*?@! "experts" keep changing their minds? 1996. *University of California at Berkeley Wellness Letter,* February. Ten tips for judging the medical news. 1993. *Harvard Women's Health Watch,* October. Health headlines. 1994. *Mayo Clinic Health Letter,* December.

HeartInfo—Heart Information Network. Provides information for heart patients and others interested in learning how to identify and reduce their risk factors for heart disease; includes links to many related sites.

http://www.heartinfo.org

National Heart, Lung, and Blood Institute. Provides information on a variety of topics relating to cardiovascular health and disease, including cholesterol, smoking, obesity, and hypertension; Web site has special fact sheets covering women and CVD.

800-575-WELL; 301-251-1222

http://www.nhlbi.nih.gov/nhlbi/nhlbi.htm

National Stroke Association. Provides information and referrals for stroke victims and their families; the Web site has a stroke risk assessment.

800-787-6537

http://www.stroke.org

See also the listings for Chapters 9 and 10.

SELECTED BIBLIOGRAPHY

Alfthan, G. 1997. Plasma homocysteine and cardiovascular disease mortality. *Lancet* 349:397.

American Heart Association. 1998. *Heart and Stroke Statistical Update* (retrieved January 25, 1998; http://www.americanheart.org/Scientific/HSstats98/index.html).

Daviglus, M. L. 1997. Dietary vitamin C, beta-carotene and 30-year risk of stroke: Results from the Western Electric Study. *Neuroepidemiology* 16:69–77.

Daviglus, M. L., et al. 1997. Fish consumption and the 30-year risk of fatal myocardial infarction. *New England Journal of Medicine* 336(15): 1046.

Dietschy, J. M. 1998. Dietary fatty acids and the regulation of plasma low density lipoprotein cholesterol concentrations. *Journal of Nutrition* 128(2): 444S–448S.

Eckel, R. H., and R. M. Krauss. 1998. American Heart Association call to action: Obesity as a major risk factor for coronary heart disease. *Circulation* 97(21): 2099–2101.

Fang, J., S. Madhaven, and M. H. Alderman. 1996. The association between birthplace and mortality from cardiovascular causes among black and white residents of New York City. *New England Journal of Medicine* 335(21): 1545–1551.

Glassman, A. H., and P. A. Shapiro. 1998. Depression and the course of coronary artery disease. *American Journal of Psychiatry* 115(1): 4–11.

Goff, D. C., et al. 1997. Greater incidence of hospitalized myocardial infarction among Mexican Americans than non-Hispanic whites: The Corpus Christi Heart Project, 1988–1992. *Circulation* 95(6): 1433–1440.

Hennekens, C. H. 1997. Antioxidant vitamins and cardiovascular disease: Current perspectives and future directions. *European Heart Journal* 18:177–179.

Howard, G., et al. 1998. Cigarette smoking and progression of atherosclerosis: The Atherosclerosis Risk in Communities (ARIC) study. *Journal of the American Medical Association* 279(2): 119–124.

Hu, F. B., et al. 1997. Dietary fat intake and the risk of coronary heart disease in women. *New England Journal of Medicine* 337: 1491–1499.

Kelley, G. A. 1997. Cardiovascular disease risk factors in black college students. *Journal of American College Health* 45: 165–169.

Kris-Etherton, P. M. 1997. Efficacy of multiple dietary therapies in reducing cardiovascular disease risk factors. *American Journal of Clinical Nutrition* 65:560–561.

Lessmeier, T. J., et al. 1997. Unrecognized paroxysmal supraventricular tachycardia: Potential for misdiagnosis as panic disorder. *Archives of Internal Medicine* 157(5): 537–543.

McCarron, D. A. 1997. Nutritional management of cardiovascular risk factors. A randomized clinical trial. *Archives of Internal Medicine* 157:169–177.

Meade, T. W. 1997. Fibrinogen and cardiovascular disease. *Journal of Clinical Pathology* 50:13–15.

Nagata, C., et al. 1998. Decreased serum total cholesterol concentration is associated with high intake of soy products in Japanese men and women. *Journal of Nutrition* 128(2): 209–213.

Rejeski, W. J., L. R. Brawley, and S. A. Schumaker. 1996. Physical activity and health-related quality of life. *Exercise and Sport Sciences Reviews* 24:71–108.

Ridker, P. M., et al. 1997. Inflammation, aspirin, and the risk of cardiovascular disease in apparently healthy men. *New England Journal of Medicine* 336(14): 973.

Rimm, E. B., et al. 1998. Folate and vitamin B6 from diet and supplements in relation to risk of coronary heart disease among women. *Journal of the American Medical Association* 279(5): 359–364.

Thun, M. J., et al. 1997. Alcohol consumption and mortality among middle-aged and elderly U.S. adults. *New England Journal of Medicine* 337:1705–1714.

Tzonou, A., et al. 1998. Dietary iron and coronary heart disease risk. A study from Greece. *American Journal of Epidemiology* 147(2): 161–166.

U.S. Department of Health and Human Services. 1996. *Physical Activity and Health: A Report of the Surgeon General.* Atlanta, Ga.: U.S. Department of Health and Human Services.

Williams, M. J. 1997. Regional fat distribution in women and risk of cardiovascular disease. *American Journal of Clinical Nutrition* 65:855–860.

LAB 11-1 *Cardiovascular Health*

Part I. CVD Risk Assessment

Your chances of suffering a heart attack or stroke before age 55 depend on a variety of factors, many of which are under your control. To help identify your risk factors, circle the response for each risk category that best describes you.

1. Sex
   - 0 Female
   - 2 Male

2. Heredity
   - 0 Neither parent suffered a heart attack or stroke before age 60.
   - 3 One parent suffered a heart attack or stroke before age 60.
   - 7 Both parents suffered a heart attack or stroke before age 60.

3. Smoking
   - 0 Never smoked
   - 1 Quit more than 2 years ago
   - 2 Quit less than 2 years ago
   - 8 Smoke less than ½ pack per day
   - 13 Smoke more than ½ pack per day
   - 15 Smoke more than 1 pack per day

4. Environmental Tobacco Smoke
   - 0 Do not live or work with smokers
   - 2 Exposed to ETS at work
   - 3 Live with smoker
   - 4 Both live and work with smokers

5. Blood Pressure
   The average of the last three readings:
   - 0 130/80 or below
   - 1 131/81–140/85
   - 5 141/86–150/90
   - 9 151/91–170/100
   - 13 Above 170/100

6. Total Cholesterol
   The average of the last three readings:
   - 0 Lower than 190
   - 1 190–210
   - 2 Don't know
   - 3 211–240
   - 4 241–270
   - 5 271–300
   - 6 Over 300

7. HDL Cholesterol
   The average of the last three readings:
   - 0 Over 65 mg/dl
   - 1 55–65
   - 2 Don't know HDL
   - 3 45–54
   - 5 35–44
   - 7 25–34
   - 12 Lower than 25

8. Exercise
   - 0 Endurance exercise three times a week
   - 1 Endurance exercise once or twice a week
   - 2 Occasional exercise less than once a week
   - 7 Rarely exercise

9. Diabetes
   - 0 No personal or family history
   - 2 One parent with diabetes
   - 6 Two parents with diabetes
   - 9 Type 2 diabetes
   - 13 Type 1 diabetes

10. Weight
   - 0 Near ideal weight
   - 1 6 pounds or less above ideal weight
   - 3 7–19 pounds above ideal weight
   - 5 20–40 pounds above ideal weight
   - 7 More than 40 pounds above ideal weight

11. Stress
   - 0 Relaxed most of the time
   - 1 Occasionally stressed and angry
   - 2 Frequently stressed and angry
   - 3 Usually stressed and angry

Scoring

Total your risk-factor points. Refer to the list below to get an approximate rating of your risk of suffering a heart attack or stroke before age 55.

Score	Estimated Risk
Less than 20	Low risk
20–29	Moderate risk
30–45	High risk
Over 45	Extremely high risk

Part II. Hostility Assessment

Current research indicates that there are three aspects of hostility that are particularly harmful to health: cynicism (a mistrusting attitude regarding other people's motives), anger (an emotional response to other people's "unacceptable" behavior), and aggression (behaviors in response to negative emotions such as anger and irritation). To get an idea of how hostile you are, check any of the following statements that are true for you.

_____ 1. Stuck in a long line at the express checkout in the grocery store, I often count the number of items the people in front of me have to see if anyone is over the limit.

_____ 2. I am often irritated by other people's incompetence.

_____ 3. If a cashier gives me the wrong change, I assume he or she is probably trying to cheat me.

_____ 4. I've been so angry at someone that I've thrown things or slammed a door.

_____ 5. If someone is late, I plan the angry words I'm going to say.

_____ 6. I tend to remember irritating incidents and get mad all over again.

_____ 7. If someone cuts me off in traffic, I honk my horn, flash my lights, pound the steering wheel, or shout.

_____ 8. Little annoyances have a way of adding up during the day, leaving me frustrated and impatient.

_____ 9. If the person who cuts my hair trims off more than I want, I fume about it for days afterward.

_____ 10. When I get into an argument, I feel my jaw clench and my pulse and breathing rate climb.

_____ 11. If someone mistreats me, I look for an opportunity to pay them back, just for the principle of the thing.

_____ 12. I find myself getting annoyed at little things my spouse or significant other does that get under my skin.

Add up the number of items you checked. A score of 3 or less indicates a generally cool head. A score between 4 and 8 indicates that your level of hostility could be raising your risk of heart disease. A score of 9 or more indicates a hot head—a level of cynicism, anger, and aggression high enough to endanger both heart health and interpersonal relationships.

If you are a hot head, try keeping a log of your hostile responses to people and situations. Familiarize yourself with the patterns of thinking that lead to hostile feelings, and try to head them off before they develop into full-blown anger. If you feel your anger starting to build, ask yourself the following questions:

1. *Is this really important enough to get angry about?* For example, is having to wait an extra 5 minutes for a late bus so important that you should stew about it for half an hour?

2. *Am I really justified in getting angry?* Is the person in front of you really driving slowly, or are you trying to speed?

3. *Is getting angry going to make any real difference in this situation?* Will slamming the door really help your friend find the concert tickets he misplaced?

If you answered "yes" to all three questions, then you should calmly but assertively ask for what you want. A "no" to any question means that you should try to diffuse your anger. Reason with yourself, distract your mind with another activity, or try one of the techniques for meditation or deep breathing described in Chapter 10.

To monitor your progress toward your goal, enter the results of this lab in the Preprogram Assessment column of Appendix D. After several weeks of a program to reduce CVD risk, do this lab again and enter the results in the Postprogram Assessment column of Appendix D. How do the results compare?

SOURCE: CVD risk assessment from Insel, P. M., and W. T. Roth. 1998. *Core Concepts in Health.* 8th ed. Mountain View, Calif.: Mayfield. Hostility quiz from Williams, R. B., and V. Williams. 1993. *Anger Kills.* Copyright © 1993 by Redford B. Williams, M.D., and Virginia Williams, Ph.D. Adapted with permission of Times Books, a division of Random House, Inc.

Injury Prevention and Personal Safety

Injuries are the fifth leading cause of death among Americans overall and the leading killer of young people. Injuries affect all segments of the population, but they are particularly common among minorities and people with low income, primarily due to social, environmental, and economic factors. The economic cost of injuries in the United States last year alone was over $400 billion.

Injuries are generally classified into four categories, based on where they occur: motor vehicle injuries, home injuries, work injuries, and leisure injuries. The greatest number of deaths occur in motor vehicle crashes, but the greatest number of disabling injuries occur in the home.

MOTOR VEHICLE INJURIES

Incidents involving motor vehicles are the most common cause of death for people under age 45, the most common cause of paralysis due to spinal injury, and the leading cause of severe brain injury.

Nearly two-thirds of all motor vehicle injuries are caused by bad driving, especially speeding. As speed increases, momentum and force of impact increase and the time allowed for the driver to react (reaction time) decreases. Speed limits are posted to establish the safest *maximum* speed limit for a given area under *ideal* conditions. Anything that distracts a driver—sleepiness, bad mood, children or pets in the car, use of a cellular phone—can increase the risk of having a collision.

A second factor contributing to injury and death in motor vehicle collisions is failure to wear a safety belt. A person who doesn't wear a safety belt is twice as likely to be injured in a crash as a person who does wear a safety belt. Safety belts not only prevent the individual from being thrown from the car at the time of the crash but also provide protection from the "second collision," which occurs when the occupant of the car hits something inside the car, such as the steering column, dashboard, or windshield. The safety belt also spreads the stopping force of the collision over the body.

Since 1998, all new cars have been equipped with dual air bags—one for the driver and one for the front passenger seat. Although air bags provide some supplemental protection in the event of a collision, most are useful only in head-on collisions. They also deflate immediately after inflating and therefore do not provide protection in collisions involving multiple impacts. To ensure that air bags work as intended, always follow these basic guidelines: place infants in rear-facing infant seats in the back seat; transport children age 12 and under in the back seat; always use safety belts or appropriate safety seats; and keep 10 inches between the air bag cover and the breastbone of the driver or passenger. In the rare event that a person cannot comply with these guidelines, permission to install an on-off switch that temporarily disables the air bag can be applied for from the National Highway Traffic Safety Administration.

A third common factor in motor vehicle injuries is alcohol; it is involved in about half of all fatal crashes. Alcohol-impaired driving, defined by blood alcohol concentration (BAC), is illegal. The legal BAC limit varies from 0.08% to 0.10%, but driving ability is impaired at much lower BACs. All psychoactive drugs have the potential to impair driving ability.

About 75% of all motor vehicle collisions occur within 25 miles of home and at speeds lower than 40 mph. These crashes often occur because the driver believes safety measures are not necessary for short trips. Clearly, the statistics prove otherwise.

To prevent motor vehicle injuries:

- Obey the speed limit. If you have to speed to get to your destination on time, you're not allowing enough time. Try leaving 10–15 minutes earlier.

- Always wear a safety belt. Strap infants and toddlers into government-approved car seats in the back seat of the vehicle. Never hold a child in your lap while a car is moving.

- Never drive under the influence of alcohol or other drugs. Never ride with a driver who has been drinking or using drugs.

- Keep your car in good working order. Regularly inspect tires, oil and fluid levels, windshield wipers, spare tire, and so on.

- Always allow enough following distance. Follow the "3-second rule": When the vehicle ahead passes a reference point, count out 3 seconds. If you pass the reference point before you finish counting, drop back and allow more following distance.

- Always increase following distance and slow down if weather or road conditions are poor.
- Choose interstate highways rather than rural roads. Highways are much safer because of better visibility, wider lanes, fewer surprises, and other factors.
- Always signal when turning or changing lanes.
- Stop completely at stop signs. Follow all traffic laws.
- Take special care at intersections. Always look left, right, and then left again. Make sure you have plenty of time to complete your maneuver in the intersection.
- Don't pass on two-lane roads unless you're in a designated passing area and have a clear view ahead.

Motorcycle and Moped Injuries

About one out of every ten traffic fatalities among people age 15–34 involves someone riding a motorcycle. Injuries from motorcycle collisions are generally more severe than those involving automobiles because motorcycles provide little, if any, protection. Moped riders face additional challenges. Mopeds usually have a maximum speed of 30–35 mph and have less power for maneuverability.

To prevent motorcycle and moped injuries:

- Always wear a helmet.
- Wear eye protection in the form of goggles, a face shield, or a windshield.
- Maximize your visibility by wearing light-colored clothing, driving with your headlights on, and correctly positioning yourself in traffic.
- Develop the skills necessary to operate the vehicle; operator error is a contributing factor in 75% of fatal crashes involving motorcycles. Skidding from improper braking is the most common cause of loss of control.
- Drive defensively, and never assume that you've been seen by other drivers.

Pedestrian and Bicycle Injuries

Injuries to pedestrians and bicyclists are considered motor vehicle–related because they are usually caused by motor vehicles. About one-seventh of all motor vehicle deaths each year involve pedestrians; almost 90,000 pedestrians are injured each year. In most injuries, poor decision making is the crucial factor, not the traffic situation itself.

To prevent injuries when walking or jogging:

- Walk or jog in daylight.
- Maximize your visibility by wearing light-colored, reflective clothing.
- Face traffic when walking or jogging along a roadway, and follow traffic laws.

- Avoid busy roads or roads with poor visibility.
- Cross only at marked crosswalks and intersections.
- Don't listen to a radio or tape on headphones while walking.
- Don't hitchhike; it places you in a potentially dangerous situation.

Bicycle injuries result primarily from not knowing or understanding the rules of the road, failing to follow traffic laws, and not having sufficient skill or experience to handle traffic conditions. *Bicycles are considered vehicles; bicycle riders must obey all traffic laws that apply to automobile drivers, including stopping at traffic lights and stop signs.*

To prevent injuries when riding a bike:

- Wear a helmet. Three out of four cyclists killed in crashes die as a result of head injuries. The brain is very sensitive to any impact, even at low speeds. Since 1999, all bike helmets sold in the United States have met federal safety standards established by the U.S. Consumer Product Safety Commission. These standards ensure that helmets adequately protect the head and that chin straps are strong enough to prevent the helmet from coming off during a fall or crash.
- Wear other safety equipment, including eye protection, proper footwear, and gloves. Secure your pants with clips, and secure your shoelaces so they don't get tangled in the chain.
- Maximize your visibility by wearing light-colored, reflective clothing. Make sure your bicycle is equipped with reflectors. Use lights, especially at night or when riding in wooded or other dark areas.
- Ride with the flow of traffic, not against it, and follow traffic laws. Use bike paths when they are available.
- Ride defensively; never assume that drivers have seen you. Be especially careful when turning or crossing at corners and intersections. Watch for cars turning right.
- Know and use hand signals. Look around and signal before turning.
- Stop at all traffic lights and stop signs.
- Continue pedaling at all times to help keep the bike stable and to maintain your balance.
- Properly maintain the working condition of your bike.

HOME INJURIES

Contrary to popular belief, home is one of the most dangerous places to be. The most common fatal home injuries are caused by falls, fires, poisoning, and incidents involving firearms.

Falls

Falls are second only to motor vehicle injuries in terms of causing deaths. They are the fifth leading cause of unintentional death for people under age 25. Nearly two-thirds of the deaths occurring from falls are from falls at floor level (tripping, slipping, and so on) rather than from a height. Alcohol is a contributing factor in many falls.

To prevent injuries from falls:

- Place skidproof backing on rugs and carpets.
- Install handrails and nonslip applications in the shower and bathtub.
- Keep floors clear of objects or conditions that could cause slipping or tripping, such as heavy wax coating, electrical cords, and toys.
- Put a light switch by the door of every room so that no one has to walk across a room to turn on a light. Use night lights in bedrooms, halls, and bathrooms.
- Outside the house, clear dangerous surfaces created by ice, snow, fallen leaves, or rough ground.
- Install handrails on stairs. Keep stairs well lit and clear of objects.
- When climbing a ladder, use both hands. Never stand higher than the third step from the top. When using a stepladder, make sure the spreader brace is in the locked position.
- If there are small children in the home, place gates at the top and bottom of stairs. Never leave a baby unattended on a bed or table.

Fires

Each year about 80% of fire deaths and 65% of fire injuries occur in the home. Most home fires begin in the kitchen, living room, or bedroom. Many are caused by careless actions such as smoking in bed or leaving a cigarette burning in an ashtray.

To prevent fires:

- Dispose of all cigarettes in ashtrays. Never smoke in bed.
- Do not overload electrical outlets.
- Do not place extension cords under rugs or where people walk. Replace worn or frayed extension cords.
- Place a wire screen in front of fireplaces and wood stoves. Remove ashes carefully and store them in airtight metal containers, not paper bags.
- Properly maintain electrical appliances, kerosene heaters, and furnaces, and clean flues and chimneys annually.
- Keep portable heaters at least 3 feet away from curtains, bedding, towels, or anything that might catch fire. Never leave heaters on when you're out of the room or sleeping.

To be prepared for a fire:

- Plan at least two escape routes out of each room. Designate a location outside the home as a meeting place.
- Install a smoke-detection device on every level of your home. Clean the detectors and test batteries once a month, and replace the batteries at least once a year.
- Keep a fire extinguisher in your home, and know how to use it. Most fire extinguishers are operated by breaking the seal and pulling the pin on the handle, aiming the discharge at the base of the flames, and using a sweeping motion to cover the burning area.

To prevent injuries from fire:

- Get out as quickly as possible and go to the designated meeting place. Don't stop for a keepsake or a pet. Never hide in a closet or under a bed. Once outside, count heads to see if everyone is out. If you think someone is still inside the burning building, tell the firefighters. Never go back inside a burning building.
- If you're trapped in a room, feel the door. If it is hot, or if smoke is coming in through the cracks, don't open it; use the alternative escape route. If you can't get out of a room, go to the window and shout or wave for help.
- Smoke inhalation is the largest cause of death and injury in fires. To avoid inhaling smoke, crawl along the floor away from the heat and smoke. Cover your mouth and nose, ideally with a wet cloth, and take short, shallow breaths.
- If your clothes catch fire, don't run. Drop to the ground, cover your face, and roll back and forth to smother the flames. Remember: stop-drop-roll.

Poisoning

Over 2 million poisonings occur every year, a majority of them among children under age 5.

To prevent poisoning:

- Store all medicines out of the reach of children. Use medicines only as directed on the label or by a physician.
- Use cleaners, pesticides, and other dangerous substances only in areas with proper ventilation. Store them out of the reach of children.
- Never operate a vehicle in an enclosed space, have your furnace inspected yearly, and use caution with any substance that produces potentially toxic fumes, such as kerosene. If appropriate, install carbon monoxide detectors.
- Many common house and garden plants are poisonous if ingested, including azalea, oleander,

rhododendron, wild mushrooms, daffodil and hyacinth bulbs, mistletoe berries, apple seeds, morning glory seeds, wisteria seeds, and the leaves and stems of potato, rhubarb, and tomato plants. Keep these plants out of the reach of young children.

To be prepared in case of poisoning:

- Keep the number of the nearest Poison Control Center (or emergency room) in an accessible location.
- Keep a bottle of syrup of ipecac (this induces vomiting) on hand.

Emergency first aid for poisonings:

1. Remove the poison from contact with eyes, skin, or mouth, or remove the victim from contact with poisonous fumes or gases.

2. Do not follow emergency instructions on labels. Some may be out of date and carry incorrect treatment information.

3. Call the Poison Control Center immediately for instructions. You may be asked the name of the substance and its ingredients; the amount of substance involved; when exposure occurred and how long it lasted; whether any symptoms are present; and characteristics of the person exposed, including name, age, weight, and general health history.

4. If you are instructed to go to an emergency room, take the poisonous substance or container with you.

5. Administer syrup of ipecac to induce vomiting— *but only if advised by the Poison Control Center or a physician.*

Guidelines for specific types of poisonings:

- *Swallowed poisons:* If the person is awake and able to swallow, give water only; then call the Poison Control Center or a physician for advice.

- *Poisons on the skin:* Remove any affected clothing. Flood affected parts of the skin with warm water, wash with soap and water, and rinse. Then call for advice.

- *Poisons in the eye:* For children, flood the eye with lukewarm water poured from a pitcher held 3–4 inches above the eye for 15 minutes; alternatively, irrigate the eye under a faucet. For adults, get in the shower and flood the eye with a gentle stream of lukewarm water for 15 minutes. Then call for advice.

- *Inhaled poisons:* Immediately carry or drag the person to fresh air and, if necessary, give mouth-to-mouth resuscitation. If the victim is not breathing easily, call 9-1-1 for help. Ventilate the area. Then call for advice.

Unintentional Injury from Firearms

Firearms pose a significant threat, especially to people between ages 15 and 24, with most fatalities involving males who are cleaning or handling guns they thought were unloaded.

To prevent firearm injuries:

- Never point a loaded gun at something you do not intend to shoot.
- Store unloaded firearms under lock and key and separately from ammunition.
- Inspect firearms carefully before handling them.
- Follow the safety procedures advocated in firearms safety courses.

Other Home Injuries

Burns, choking, suffocation, and electrocution are other dangers in the home, particularly for small children. Burns are the third leading cause of death in young children (following motor vehicle collisions and drowning). House fires cause the most deaths, but hot water causes the most nonfatal burns. When a burn occurs, cold water should be poured on it immediately to cool the tissue and prevent the burn from going deeper.

To prevent burns in children:

- Place barriers around stoves and radiators, and keep children out of the kitchen where they might be burned by spills.
- Set your hot water heater no higher than 120°F.
- Always test the contents of a baby bottle on the wrist before feeding the baby. When bottles are heated in microwave ovens, the liquid can become scalding before the outside of the bottle gets very hot.
- Unplug and store extension cords when not in use.
- Apply sunscreen to children's skin when they are out in the sun.

To prevent other home injuries:

- Keep small objects out of the reach of children under age 3, and don't give them raw carrots, nuts, popcorn, or hard candy. Inspect toys for small parts that could be put in the mouth. Balloons also pose a serious choking hazard for young children.
- Keep infants away from plastic bags, which can suffocate them, and don't put infants to bed wearing jackets with drawstring hoods, which can strangle them.
- Keep electrical appliances away from a filled tub or sink. Use plastic covers over electrical outlets.

Leisure injuries are defined as those that occur in public places but do not involve a motor vehicle. Most leisure injuries involve recreational activities, such as swimming and boating, playground activities, and sports.

Drowning

Drowning is a special danger for children and for adolescents and adults who are using alcohol. Children under age 5 and people between ages 15 and 24 have the highest rates of death from drowning. Many drownings of children occur in residential pools, often when there is inadequate supervision. Many drownings also occur when people on boats fall overboard. Between one-third and two-thirds of these drownings involve alcohol.

To prevent drowning:

- Develop adequate swimming skills, and make sure children learn to swim.
- Make sure residential pools are fenced and adequately supervised.
- Use caution when swimming in unfamiliar surroundings (such as the ocean) or for an unusual length of time.
- Avoid being chilled by water colder than 70°F.
- Don't swim or boat under the influence of alcohol or other drugs.
- Don't swim alone.
- Check the depth of water before diving.
- When on a boat, use a personal flotation device. The U.S. Coast Guard recommends six different types, keyed to particular water conditions.

Playground Injuries

Over 200,000 injuries occur on school, park, and residential playground equipment every year. Most injuries are the result of falls from equipment to the ground; deaths are usually the result of head injuries.

To prevent playground injuries:

- Make sure equipment and surfaces under equipment comply with safety standards.
- Teach children to use equipment properly.

In-Line Skating Injuries

In-line skating has become a very popular recreational activity among people of all ages. Most injuries occur because users are not familiar with the equipment and do not wear appropriate safety gear. Injuries to the wrist and head are the most common. To reduce your risk of being injured while skating, wear a helmet, elbow and knee pads, wrist guards, a long-sleeved shirt, and long pants.

Sports Injuries

An increase in the number of people exercising to improve their health has brought with it an increase in sports-related injuries.

To prevent sports injuries:

- Develop the skills required for the activity.
- Recognize and guard against the hazards associated with the activity.
- Include appropriate exercises for warming up and cooling down.
- Make sure facilities are safe.
- Follow the rules, and practice good sportsmanship.
- Use proper safety equipment, including, where appropriate, helmets, eye protection, knee and elbow pads and wrist guards, and correct footwear.
- When it is excessively hot and humid, avoid heat stress by following the guidelines given in the box "Exercising in Hot Weather" in Chapter 3.

Many aspects of workplace safety are monitored by the Occupational Safety and Health Administration (OSHA), a federal agency. The highest rate of work-related injuries occurs among laborers, whose jobs usually involve extensive manual labor and lifting—two areas not addressed by OSHA safety standards. Back injuries are the most common work injury.

To protect your back when lifting:

- Don't try to lift beyond your strength. If you need it, get help.
- Get a firm footing, with your feet shoulder-width apart. Get a firm grip on the object.
- Keep your torso in a relatively upright position and crouch down, bending at the knees and hips. Avoid bending at the waist. To lift, stand up or push up with your leg muscles. Lift gradually, keeping your arms straight. Keep the object close to your body.
- Don't twist. If you have to turn with an object, change the position of your feet.
- Plan ahead. Make sure your pathway is clear before you pick up the object.

- Put the object down gently, reversing the rules for lifting.

A new type of work-related injury involves damage to the musculoskeletal system caused by repeated strain on the hand, arm, wrist, or other part of the body. Such injuries and disorders are referred to as repetitive-strain injuries. Carpal tunnel syndrome is one type. It is characterized by pain and swelling in the tendons of the wrists and sometimes numbness and weakness. Its growing incidence is associated with the use of computers.

To prevent carpal tunnel syndrome:

- Maintain good posture at the computer. Use a chair that provides back support, and place the feet flat on the floor or on a foot rest.
- Position the screen at eye level and the keyboard so the hands and wrists are straight.
- Take breaks periodically to lessen the cumulative effects of stress.

VIOLENCE AND INTENTIONAL INJURIES

Violence is emerging as a major public health concern. The United States ranks first among developed nations in the rate of violent death; the number of deaths caused by firearms (intentionally and unintentionally) exceeds the combined total of such deaths in the next 17 nations. Violence includes assault, homicide (murder), sexual assault, domestic violence, suicide, and various forms of abuse. About 2.2 million Americans are victims of violent injury every year.

Assault

Assault is the use of physical force to inflict injury or death on another person. Most assaults occur during arguments or in connection with another crime, such as robbery. Poverty, urban settings, and the use of alcohol and drugs are associated with higher rates of assault.

Homicide is the twelfth leading cause of death in the United States. Homicide victims are most likely to be male, between ages 19 and 24, and members of minority groups. Most homicides are committed with a firearm; the murderer and the victim usually know each other.

To protect yourself at home:

- Secure your home with good lighting and effective locks, preferably deadbolts.
- Make sure that all doors and windows are securely locked. Always lock windows and doors, including sliding glass doors, whenever you go out.
- Get a dog, or post "Beware of Dog" signs.
- Ensure that the landscaping around your home doesn't provide opportunities for concealment.
- Don't hide keys in obvious places. Don't give anyone the chance to duplicate your keys; for example, give only the car key, not your entire set of keys, to a parking attendant.
- Install a peephole in your front door. Don't open your door to people you don't know.
- Don't let strangers into your home or yard. When repair or delivery people or utility workers come to the door, ask to see identification, or call the company to verify that they've sent someone out.
- If you or a family member owns a weapon, store it securely. Store guns and ammunition in separate locations.
- If you are a woman living alone, use your initials rather than your full name in the phone directory. Don't use a greeting on your answering machine that implies you live alone or are not home.
- Teach everyone in the household how to obtain emergency assistance.
- Know your neighbors. Work out a system for alerting each other in case of an emergency.
- Establish a neighborhood watch program.

To protect yourself on the street:

- Avoid walking alone, especially at night. Stay where people can see and hear you.
- Dress sensibly, in clothing that allows you freedom of movement.
- Walk purposefully. Act alert and confident.
- Walk on the outside of the sidewalk, facing traffic.
- Know where you are going. Appearing to be lost increases your vulnerability.
- Don't hitchhike.
- Carry valuables in a fanny pack, pants pocket, or shoulder bag strapped diagonally across the chest. Conceal small purses inside a tote or shopping bag. Keep at least one hand free.
- Always have your keys ready as you approach your vehicle or home.
- Carry enough change so that you can make a telephone call or take public transportation. Carry a whistle to blow if you are attacked or harassed.
- Be aware of suspicious behavior. Listen to your own inner warning signals.
- If possible, allow at least two arm lengths between yourself and a stranger.
- If you feel threatened, run and/or yell. Go into a store or knock on the door of a home. If someone grabs you, yell "Help!" or "Fire!"

To protect yourself in your car:

- Keep your car in good working condition, carry emergency supplies, and keep the gas tank at least half full.
- When driving, keep doors locked and windows rolled up at least three-quarters of the way.
- Park your car in well-lighted areas or parking garages, preferably those with an attendant or a security guard.
- Lock your car when you leave it, and check the interior before opening the door when you return.
- Don't pick up strangers. Don't stop for vehicles in distress; drive on and call for help.
- Note the location of emergency call boxes along highways and in public facilities. If you travel alone frequently, consider investing in a cellular phone.
- If your car breaks down, raise the hood and tie a white cloth to the antenna or door handle. Wait in the car with the doors locked and windows rolled up. If someone approaches to offer help, open a window only a crack and ask the person to call the police or a towing service.
- When you stop at a light or stop sign, leave enough room to maneuver out if you need an escape route.
- If you are involved in a minor automobile crash and you think you have been bumped intentionally, don't leave your car. Motion to the other driver to follow you to the nearest police station. If confronted by a person with a weapon, give up your car.
- Don't get into disputes or arguments with drivers of other vehicles.

To protect yourself on public transportation:

- While waiting, stand in a populated, well-lighted area.
- Sit near the driver or conductor in a single seat or an outside seat.
- If traveling to an unfamiliar location, call the transit agency for the correct route and time. Make sure that the bus, subway, or train is bound for your destination before you board it.
- If you flag down a taxi, ensure that it's from a legitimate service. When you reach your destination, ask the driver to wait until you are safely inside the building.

To protect yourself on campus:

- Ensure that door and window locks are secure and that halls and stairwells have adequate lighting.
- Don't give dorm or residence keys to anybody.
- Don't leave your door unlocked or allow strangers into your room.

- Avoid solitary late-night trips to the library or laundry room. Take advantage of on-campus escort services.
- Don't jog or exercise outside alone at night. Don't take shortcuts across campus that are unfamiliar or seem unsafe.
- If security guards patrol the campus, know the areas they cover, and stay where they can see or hear you.

Sexual Assault, or Rape

Sexual assault, or rape, is sexual coercion that relies on the threat and use of physical force or takes advantage of circumstances that render a person incapable of giving consent (such as when drunk). If the victim is younger than the legally defined age of consent, the act constitutes statutory rape, regardless of whether consent is given. Coerced sexual activity in which the victim knows the rapist is often referred to as date rape or acquaintance rape. At least 3.5 million females are raped annually in the United States, and perhaps 10,000 males are raped each year by other males.

Rape victims suffer both physical and psychological injury. For most, the physical wounds are not severe, but the psychological pain can be substantial and long-lasting. Many victims experience shock, anxiety, depression, shame, and psychosomatic symptoms. These psychological reactions are called rape trauma syndrome; other symptoms include fear, nightmares, fatigue, crying spells, and digestive upset. Self-blame is common, a reaction reinforced by our society's tendency to blame the victim. Fortunately, this tendency is giving way to a more realistic view of the violent nature of rape.

To protect yourself against rape:

- Follow the guidelines listed earlier for protecting yourself against assault.
- Think out in advance what you would do if you were threatened with rape. However, no one knows what he or she will do when scared to death. Trust that you will make the best decision at the time—whether to scream, run, fight, or give in to avoid being injured or killed.

If you are raped:

- Tell what happened to the first friendly person you meet.
- Call the police. Tell them you were raped, and give your location.
- Try to remember everything you can about your attacker, and write it down.
- Don't wash or douche before the medical exam. Don't change your clothes, but bring a new set with you if you can.
- At the hospital you will have a complete exam. Show the physician any bruises or scratches.

- Tell the police exactly what happened. Be honest, and stick to your story.
- If you do not want to report the rape to the police, see a physician as soon as possible. Be sure you are checked for pregnancy and STDs.
- Contact an organization with skilled counselors so you can talk about the experience. Look in the telephone directory under "Rape" or "Rape Crisis Center" for a hotline number.

Date Rape

Most women are in much less danger of being raped by a stranger than of being sexually assaulted by a man they know or date. Surveys suggest that as many as one woman in four has had sex forced on her by a man she knew or was dating. Victims of date rape tend to shoulder much of the responsibility for the incident, questioning their own judgment rather than blaming the aggressor.

One factor in date rape appears to be the double standard about appropriate sexual behavior for men and women. It is still a cultural belief in our society that "nice" women don't say yes to sex, even when they want to, and that "real" men don't take no for an answer. There are also widespread differences between men and women in how romantic signals are perceived. Researchers in one study found that men tend to interpret women's actions on dates, such as smiling or talking in a low voice, as indicating an interest in having sex, while the women interpret the same actions as being "friendly." Men who rape their dates also tend to have certain characteristics, including hostility toward women and an acceptance of sexual violence. Both men and women must take responsibility for reducing the incidence of rape.

To protect yourself from date rape:

- Believe in your right to control what you do. Set limits and communicate them clearly, firmly, and early. Be assertive; men often interpret passivity as permission.
- Remember that some men think flirtatious behavior or sexy clothing indicates an interest in having sex.
- If you are unsure of a new acquaintance, go on a group date or double date. If possible, provide your own transportation.
- Remember that alcohol and drugs interfere with judgment, perception, and communication about sex.
- Use the statement that has proven most effective in stopping date rape: "This is rape and I'm calling the cops!"

Guidelines for men:

- Be aware of social pressure. It's OK not to "score."
- Understand that "No" means "No." Stop making advances when your date says to stop. Remember that she has the right to refuse sex.

- Don't assume that flirtatious behavior or sexy clothing means a woman is interested in having sex, that previous permission for sex applies to the current situation, or that your date's relationships with other men constitute sexual permission for you.
- Remember that alcohol and drugs interfere with judgment, perception, and communication about sex.

PROVIDING EMERGENCY CARE

You can improve someone else's chances of surviving if you are prepared to provide emergency help. A course in first aid, offered by the American Red Cross and on many college campuses, can teach you to respond appropriately when someone needs help.

Emergency rescue techniques can save the lives of people who have stopped breathing, who are choking, or whose hearts have stopped beating. Pulmonary resuscitation (also known as rescue breathing, artificial respiration, or mouth-to-mouth resuscitation) is used when a person is not breathing (Figure A-1). Cardiopulmonary resuscitation (CPR) is used when a pulse can't be found. Training is required before a person can perform CPR. Courses are offered by the American Red Cross and the American Heart Association.

Many choking victims can be saved with the Heimlich maneuver (also called abdominal thrusts). For instructions on performing this maneuver, see Figure A-1. Blows to the upper back in conjunction with chest thrusts are an acceptable way to dislodge an object from an infant's throat.

When you have to provide emergency care:

- Remain calm, and act sensibly. The basic pattern for providing emergency care is check-call-care.
- *Check the situation:* Make sure the scene is safe for both you and the injured person. Don't put yourself in danger; if you get hurt too, you will be of little help to the injured person.
- *Check the victim:* Conduct a quick head-to-toe examination. Assess the victim's signs and symptoms, such as level of responsiveness, pulse, and breathing rate. Look for bleeding and any indications of broken bones or paralysis.
- *Call for help:* Call 9-1-1 or a local emergency number. Identify yourself and give as much information as you can about the condition of the victim and what happened.
- *Care for the victim:* If the situation requires immediate action (no pulse, shock, etc.), provide first aid if you are trained to do so. Figure A-1 illustrates basic first aid for several types of emergency situations.

Figure A-1 Rescue breathing, first aid for choking, and ways to control bleeding; procedures recommended by the American Red Cross.

Books

American Red Cross. 1996. *First Aid: Responding to Emergencies,* 2nd ed. St. Louis, Mo.: Year Book Medical. *Provides current, straightforward information.*

Bever, D. L. 1996. *Safety: A Personal Focus,* 4th ed. New York: McGraw-Hill. *An overview of injury prevention, including automobile, fire, and recreational safety.*

Lipman, I. A. 1997. *How to Protect Yourself from Crime.* Pleasantville, N.Y.: Reader's Digest. *Provides advice to help you be safer at home, on the road, at work, and on vacation.*

Mufson, S., and R. Kranz. 1997. *Straight Talk About Date Rape.* New York: Facts on File. *Provides information about date rape, including strategies for prevention and suggestions for how victims can get help.*

Organizations, Hotlines, and Web Sites

American Automobile Association Foundation for Traffic Safety. Promotes research and provides consumer information, including brochures and videos about all aspects of traffic safety; Web site has links to many related sites.

    800-305-SAFE

    http://www.aaafts.org

CDC National Center for Injury Prevention and Control. Provides consumer-oriented information about preventing unintentional injuries and violence.

    770-488-1506 (automated information line)

    http://www.cdc.gov/ncipc/ncipchm.htm

National Highway Traffic Safety Administration. Supplies materials about reducing death, injuries, and economic losses from motor vehicle crashes, including safety test and recall information.

    800-424-9393

    http://www.nhtsa.dot.gov

National Safety Council. Provides information and statistics about preventing unintentional injuries.

    630-285-1121

    http://www.nsc.org

National Violence Hotlines. Provide information, referral services, and crisis intervention.

    800-222-2000 (family violence); 800-799-SAFE (domestic violence); 800-422-4453 (child abuse)

American Red Cross Staff. 1996. *Community First Aid and Safety.* St. Louis, Mo.: Mosby-Year Book.

Bayne, C. G. 1997. Falling: Why and what to do about it. *Nursing Management* 28:22–23.

Bicycle Helmet Safety Institute. 1998. *Bicycle Helmet Pamphlet* (retrieved March 10, 1998; http://www.helmets.org/webdocs/guide.htm).

Centers for Disease Control and Prevention. 1997. Rates of homicide, suicide, and firearm-related death among children—26 industrialized countries. *Morbidity and Mortality Weekly Report* 46:101–105.

Dobrin, A., et al., eds. 1996. *Statistical Handbook on Violence in America.* Phoenix, Ariz.: Oryx Press.

Jaffe, M. S., M. P. Dijkers, and M. Zametis. 1997. A population-based survey of in-line skaters' injuries and skating practices. *Archives of Physical Medicine and Rehabilitation* 78:1352–1357.

Mallonee, S., et al. 1996. Surveillance and prevention of residential-fire injuries. *New England Journal of Medicine* 335:27–31.

National Center for Injury Prevention and Control. 1998. *Fact Sheet: Pedestrian Deaths and Injuries* (retrieved March 10, 1998; http://www.cdc.gov/ncipc/duip/pedes.htm).

National Highway Traffic Safety Administration. 1997. *Air Bags and On-Off Switches: Information for an Informed Decision* (retrieved March 10, 1998; http://www.nhtsa.dot.gov/airbags/brochure).

National Safety Council. 1997. *Accident Facts, 1997 Edition.* Itasca, Ill.: National Safety Council.

Redelmeier, D. A., and R. J. Tibshirani. 1997. Association between cellular telephone calls and motor vehicle collisions. *New England Journal of Medicine* 336(7): 453–458.

Sinaver, N., J. L. Annest, and J. A. Mercy. 1996. Unintentional, nonfatal firearm-related injuries: A preventable public health burden. *Journal of the American Medical Association* 277(22): 1740–1743.

U.S. Consumer Product Safety Commission (CPSC). 1998. *Press Release: CPSC Issues New Safety Standards for Bike Helmets* (retrieved April 13, 1998; http://www.cpsc.gov/gophroot/pre%5Frel/pre%5Frel/98%5Fpre/98062.txt).

Nutritional Content of Common Foods

APPENDIX B

This food composition table has been prepared for Mayfield Publishing Company and is copyrighted by DINE Systems, Inc., the developer and publisher of the DINE System family of nutrition software for personal computers. The values in this food composition table were derived from the USDA Nutrient Data Base for Standard Reference Release 10 and nutrient composition information from over 300 food companies. Nutrient values used for each food were determined by collapsing similar foods into one food, using the median nutrient values. In the food composition table, foods are listed within the following eight groups: fruits, vegetables, beverages, alcoholic beverages, grains, dairy, fats/sweets/other, and protein foods. Further information can be obtained from DINE Systems, Inc., 586 N. French Road, Amherst, NY 14228, 716-688-2492, 716-688-2505 fax. SOURCE: © 1994 Dine Systems, Inc.

Order of fields: Name, Amount/Unit, Calories, Protein, Total Fat, Saturated Fat, Carbohydrates (minus added sugar), Added Sugar, Fiber, Cholesterol, Sodium, Calcium, Iron.

FRUITS

Name	Amount/Unit	Cal.	Pro. g	TFat g	SFat g	Carb. g	Sug. g	Fbr. g	Chol. mg	Sod. mg	Calc. mg	Iron mg
Apples, sweetened	½ cup	68	0	0.11	0	12.5	3.25	2	0	334	334	0.3
Apples, unsweetened	½ frt, ½ cup	41	0.25	0	0	9.5	0	2.1	0	0	4	0.2
Applesauce, sweetened	½ cup	97	0.25	0	0	12	11	1.8	0	4	4	0.4
Applesauce, unsweetened	½ cup	53	0.25	0	0	12.5	0	2.5	0	2	4	0.2
Apricots, sweetened	3 hlv, ¼ cup	65	0.5	0	0	3.75	10.75	1.1	0	3	8	0.4
Apricots, unsweetened	3 halves	27	0.5	0	0	5.5	0	1.1	0	3	8	0.3
Banana	1 fruit	105	1	0.33	0.22	24	0	2.3	0	1	7	0.4
Blueberries, sweetened	½ cup	103	0.5	0.11	0	8.5	16.25	2.3	0	3	7	0.4
Blueberries, unsweetened	½ cup	41	0.5	0.22	0	9	0	1.7	0	2	5	0.2
Cherries, sweetened	½ cup	106	0.75	0	0	12.25	13	0.9	0	4	13	0.4
Cherries, unsweetened	10 frt, ½ cup	44	0.75	0	0	10	0	0.9	0	2	12	0.4
Dates	5 frt, ¼ cup	118	0.75	0.22	0.11	28.5	0	3.7	0	1	14	0.5
Dried fruit	¼ cup	92	1	0	0	21.75	0	2.4	0	9	11	0.7
Figs, sweetened	2 fruit	45	0.25	0	0	7	3.75	1.3	0	1	15	0.2
Figs, unsweetened	2 frt, ¼ cup	74	0.75	0.33	0.11	17.5	0	4.2	0	3	39	0.6
Fruit cocktail, sweetened	½ cup	83	0.5	0	0	8.75	11	1.4	0	8	8	0.3
Fruit cocktail, unsweetened	½ cup	50	0.5	0	0	11.5	0	1.4	0	4	6	0.3
Grapefruit, sweetened	½ cup	76	0.5	0	0	10	8	0.5	0	2	18	0.5
Grapefruit, unsweetened	½ frt, ½ cup	39	0.5	0	0	9	0	0.7	0	0	14	0.2
Grapes, sweetened	½ cup	94	0.5	0	0	10.5	12	0.5	0	7	12	1.2
Grapes, unsweetened	20 frt, ½ cup	48	0.5	0	0	11.5	0	0.5	0	2	8	0.2
Guava	1 fruit	45	0.5	0.33	0.11	9.5	0	5	0	2	18	0.3
Juice, unsweetened	¾ cup	90	0.5	0	0	22.5	0	0.2	0	8	16	0.5
Kiwi fruit	1 fruit	46	0.75	0.33	0.11	10	0	2.1	0	4	20	0.3
Mango	½ frt, ½ cup	61	0.5	0.11	0	14.25	0	1.8	0	2	9	0.2
Melon	½ cup	30	0.5	0	0	7	0	0.7	0	9	8	0.2
Nectarines	1 fruit	68	1	0.56	0	14.5	0	3.3	0	0	6	0.2
Orange	1 frt, ¾ cup	63	1	0	0	14	0	3.9	0	1	53	0.2
Papaya	½ frt, ½ cup	56	0.75	0	0	12.75	0	1.8	0	4	35	0.2

continued

Fruits, *continued*

Name	Amount/Unit	Cal.	Pro. g	TFat g	SFat g	Carb. g	Sug. g	Fbr. g	Chol. mg	Sod. mg	Calc. mg	Iron mg
Peaches, sweetened	½ cup	94	0.5	0	0	5.25	17	1.2	0	8	3	0.4
Peaches, unsweetened	1 frt, ½ cup	44	0.5	0	0	10.75	0	1.3	0	3	5	0.1
Pears, sweetened	2 halves	103	0.5	0	0	6	18.5	3.2	0	8	8	0.4
Pears, unsweetened	2 hlv, ½ cup	60	0.5	0	0	15	0	3	0	4	10	0.2
Pineapple, sweetened	2 slices, ½ cup	93	0.5	0	0	7.5	15	0.9	0	2	15	0.4
Pineapple, unsweetened	2 slices, ½ cup	70	0.25	0	0	17.5	0	0.9	0	2	6	0.4
Plums, sweetened	2 fruit	67	0.5	0.11	0	8	7.75	0.7	0	17	9	0.7
Plums, unsweetened	1 raw, 2 canned	37	0.5	0	0	8.25	0	0.9	0	1	5	0.2
Prunes, cooked	½ cup	136	1.25	0.33	0	32	0	4.9	0	3	29	1.4
Prunes, dried	½ cup	209	2	0.44	0	49.25	0	6.8	0	4	45	2.1
Pumpkin, canned	½ cup	41	0.75	0.11	0.11	8.75	0	3.5	0	6	32	1.7
Raisins	¼ cup	109	1	0	0	26	0	2.5	0	5	19	0.8
Raspberries, sweetened	½ cup	117	0.75	0.11	0	12	18.25	4.2	0	0	19	0.5
Raspberries, unsweetened	½ cup	30	0.5	0.22	0	6.5	0	3	0	0	14	0.3
Strawberries, sweetened	½ cup	100	0.5	0.11	0	9	15	2	0	4	14	0.6
Strawberries, unsweetened	½ cup	24	0.5	0.22	0	5.5	0	1.6	0	2	11	0.5
Tangerines, sweetened	½ cup	76	0.5	0	0	10	8.5	0.9	0	8	9	0.4
Tangerines, unsweetened	1 frt, ½ cup	43	0.5	0	0	9.75	0	0.9	0	2	14	0.1
Watermelon	½ cup	25	0.5	0.22	0.22	5	0	0.3	0	2	6	0.2

VEGETABLES

Name	Amount/Unit	Cal.	Pro. g	TFat g	SFat g	Carb. g	Sug. g	Fbr. g	Chol. mg	Sod. mg	Calc. mg	Iron mg
Asparagus	6 spears, ½ cup	24	1.75	0.33	0.11	3.75	0	1.5	0	4	22	0.6
Asparagus, canned	½ cup	21	1.5	0.33	0.11	2.75	0	1.9	0	425	17	1.5
Avocados	½ frt, ½ cup	166	2	14.22	2.56	7.25	0	2.7	0	10	12	1
Bamboo shoots	¼ cup	4	0.25	0	0	0.5	0	0.3	0	1	4	0.1
Bamboo shoots, canned	¼ cup	6	0.5	0.11	0	1	0	0.6	0	2	1	0.1
Bean sprouts	½ cup	16	1.25	0	0	2.75	0	2.2	0	3	7	0.5
Bean sprouts, canned	½ cup	8	0.75	0	0	1.25	0	2.3	0	149	9	0.3
Beets, canned	½ cup	36	0.75	0	0	8	0	2.9	0	324	17	0.8
Beets, pickled	½ cup	82	0.75	0	0	8.5	11.25	2.8	0	250	13	0.5
Beets, raw, cooked	½ cup	31	0.75	0	0	6.75	0	2.5	0	49	11	0.6
Bok choy, chinese cabbage	½ cup	5	0.25	0	0	0.75	0	0.6	0	23	37	0.3
Broccoli, cooked	½ cup	24	1.75	0.11	0	4.25	0	2.5	0	15	68	0.8
Broccoli, raw	½ cup	12	0.75	0.11	0	2	0	1.5	0	12	21	0.4
Brussels sprouts	½ cup	32	1.5	0.33	0.11	5.75	0	2.4	0	18	24	0.8
Cabbage, raw or cooked	½ c rw, ¼ c ckd	9	0.25	0	0	1.75	0	1	0	7	13	0.2
Carrots, canned	½ cup	17	0.25	0.11	0	3.75	0	2.7	0	176	19	0.5
Carrots, raw or cooked	½ cup	26	0.5	0	0	5.75	0	2.2	0	43	21	0.4
Cauliflower, raw or cooked	½ cup	15	0.75	0.11	0	2.5	0	1.3	0	7	15	0.3
Celery, raw or cooked	½ cup	10	0.25	0	0	2.25	0	1.4	0	51	25	0.2
Coleslaw	½ cup	154	0.5	14.44	2.67	4.25	1	1.5	7	287	32	0.4
Corn	½ cup	80	1.75	0.33	0	17.5	0	4.6	0	4	2	0.5
Corn, canned	½ cup	83	1.5	0.44	0.11	13	5.5	4.7	0	324	5	0.4
Cucumber	½ cup	7	0.25	0	0	1.5	0	0.7	0	1	7	0.1
Eggplant	½ cup	13	0.25	0	0	3	0	1	0	2	3	0.2
French fries	½ cup	174	1.75	7.33	3.22	19	0	2.6	0	37	6	0.6
Fried vegetables/onions	½ cup, 6 rings	180	2	10.78	2.67	15.5	0	1	0	150	12	0.7
Green beans, canned	½ cup	13	0.75	0	0	2.5	0	1.5	0	170	18	0.6
Green beans, raw or cooked	½ cup	20	1	0	0	4	0	1.8	0	3	30	0.7

continued

Vegetables, continued

Name	Amount/Unit	Cal.	Pro. g	TFat g	SFat g	Carb. g	Sug. g	Fbr. g	Chol. mg	Sod. mg	Calc. mg	Iron mg
Greens, mustard, turnip, ckd	½ cup	15	1	0.11	0	2.5	0	1.4	0	16	87	0.7
Greens, mustard, turnip, raw	½ cup	7	0.5	0	0	1.5	0	0.9	0	9	41	0.4
Greens, turnip, canned	½ cup	17	1	0.22	0.11	2.5	0	2.2	0	325	138	1.8
Kale, raw or cooked	½ cup	20	0.75	0.11	0	3	0	1.7	0	15	47	0.6
Lettuce, endive	½ cup	4	0.25	0	0	0.75	0	0.7	0	6	13	0.2
Lettuce, iceberg	1 leaf	3	0	0	0	0.5	0	0.3	0	2	4	0.1
Miso	½ cup	284	14.25	7.33	1.11	39.25	0	7.4	0	5032	92	3.8
Mixed vegetables, canned	½ cup	39	1.25	0.11	0	8	0	3.5	0	122	22	0.9
Mixed vegetables, frozen	½ cup	22	0.75	0	0	4.5	0	2	0	22	27	0.6
Mushrooms, canned	½ cup	19	1	0.11	0	3.25	0	1.1	0	178	1	0.6
Mushrooms, fresh, cooked	½ cup	25	1.75	0.11	0	4.25	0	1.5	0	1	7	1.7
Mushrooms, raw	½ cup	9	0.5	0	0	1.5	0	0.6	0	1	2	0.4
Okra	½ cup	26	1	0.11	0	5.5	0	2.1	0	5	55	0.5
Onions	½ cup	29	0.5	0.11	0	6.25	0	1.4	0	8	20	0.3
Parsnips	½ cup	64	0.75	0.11	0	14.75	0	3.2	0	8	30	0.5
Peas, green	½ cup	63	3.75	0.11	0	11.5	0	3.5	0	70	19	1.2
Peas, green, canned	½ cup	59	3.25	0.11	0	8	2.75	5.3	0	186	17	0.8
Peas, snowpeas	½ cup	35	2.25	0.11	0	5.75	0	3.4	0	4	37	1.6
Peppers, hot	2 tablespoons	8	0.25	0	0	1.5	0	0.2	0	1	3	0.2
Peppers, sweet, green	½ cup	12	0.25	0.11	0	2.25	0	0.6	0	2	3	0.6
Peppers, sweet, red	½ cup	12	0.25	0.11	0	2.25	0	0.8	0	2	3	0.6
Potato, baked/boiled	½ bkd/1 bld	113	1.5	0	0	26.5	0	2.6	0	7	9	0.4
Potatoes, mashed	½ cup	118	1.5	4.56	1.44	17	0	1.8	4	340	40	0.3
Potato skins, cheese, bacon	2 halves	302	11	15.89	7.44	27.5	0	1.4	34	267	225	4.5
Rutabaga	½ cup	35	0.75	0.11	0	7.5	0	2.1	0	19	43	0.5
Salad, potato	½ cup	153	3	7.78	1.89	15	1.5	1.9	47	512	19	0.5
Salad, three bean	½ cup	80	2	0	0	16.25	1.75	5	0	540	20	3.6
Sauerkraut	½ cup	22	0.75	0.11	0	4.5	0	4.1	0	780	36	1.7
Soup, vegetable	1 cup	81	2	1.56	0.44	11.25	2.25	0.5	2	892	16	1
Spaghetti sauce	½ cup	118	2	5	0.89	12.75	1.5	3.3	0	589	20	1.1
Spaghetti sauce with meat	½ cup	80	2	3.11	0.67	12.5	2	3.3	2	630	20	1.1
Spinach, canned	½ cup	25	1.75	0.33	0.11	3.25	0	3.9	0	29	135	2.5
Spinach, fresh, cooked	½ cup	24	1.75	0.11	0	3.75	0	3	0	73	131	1.7
Spinach, raw	½ cup	6	0.5	0	0	0.75	0	1.1	0	22	28	0.8
Squash, summer	½ cup	18	0.5	0.11	0	3.75	0	1.5	0	3	22	0.4
Squash, winter	½ cup	41	0.75	0.11	0	9.5	0	3	0	4	23	0.6
Squash, zucchini, fresh, ckd	1 c rw, ½ c ckd	18	0.75	0	0	3.5	0	1.4	0	2	19	0.5
Sweet potato	½ cup	98	1.25	0	0	23	0	4	0	11	30	0.5
Sweet potato, candied	½ cup	190	1	0	0	26.5	20	4.4	0	60	20	0.7
Tomatoes, canned or stewed	½ cup	34	0.75	0.11	0	6.5	0.25	2.4	0	305	33	0.7
Tomatoes, raw	½ cup	17	0.5	0.11	0	3.5	0	1.3	0	8	6	0.5
Waterchestnuts, canned	½ cup	34	0.25	0	0	8.25	0	1.5	0	3	3	0.3
Waterchestnuts, raw	½ cup	66	0.75	0	0	15.75	0	1.4	0	9	7	0.4
Watercress, raw	½ cup	2	0.25	0	0	0.25	0	0.2	0	7	20	0

BEVERAGES

Name	Amount/Unit	Cal.	Pro. g	TFat g	SFat g	Carb. g	Sug. g	Fbr. g	Chol. mg	Sod. mg	Calc. mg	Iron mg
Beer, nonalcoholic	12 fluid ounces	55	0.75	0	0	11	0	0	0	19	25	0.1
Wine, nonalcoholic	5 fluid ounces	42	0.5	0	0	9.75	0	0	0	7	12	0.6
Cola	12 fluid ounces	150	0	0	0	0	37	0	0	70	0	0

continued

Beverages, continued

Name	Amount/Unit	Cal.	Pro. g	TFat g	SFat g	Carb. g	Sug. g	Fbr. g	Chol. mg	Sod. mg	Calc. mg	Iron mg
Cola, diet	12 fluid ounces	2	0.25	0	0	0.25	0	0	0	70	0	0
Cola, diet, no caffeine	12 fluid ounces	2	0	0	0	0	0	0	0	70	0	0
Cola, no caffeine	12 fluid ounces	155	0	0	0	0	38.75	0	0	73	0	0
Mellow Yellow, Mountain Dew	12 fluid ounces	177	0	0	0	0	44	0	0	30	0	0
Noncola, diet, no caffeine	12 fluid ounces	4	0	0	0	0.5	0	0	0	42	0	0
Noncola, no caffeine	12 fluid ounces	157	0	0	0	0	37.75	0	0	46	2	0.1
Juice drink	¾ cup/1 box	106	0	0	0	6.5	19.5	0	0	7	1	1
Coffee	1 cup	5	0.25	0	0	1	0	0	0	7	6	0.6
Coffee, decaffeinated	1 cup	3	0.25	0	0	0.75	0	0	0	8	8	0.1
Postum	1 teaspoon	12	0	0	0	3	0	1.3	0	0	0	0
Tea, herbal, no caffeine	1 cup	4	0	0	0	0.75	0	0	0	3	5	0.2
Tea, plain	1 cup	3	0	0	0	0.5	0	0	0	0	0	0

ALCOHOLIC BEVERAGES

Name	Amount/Unit	Cal.	Pro. g	TFat g	SFat g	Carb. g	Sug. g	Fbr. g	Chol. mg	Sod. mg	Calc. mg	Iron mg
Beer	12 fluid ounces	145	1	0	0	13.25	0	0	0	8	12	0
Beer, light	12 fluid ounces	110	1	0	0	7	0	0	0	8	15	0
Chianti	5 fluid ounces	106	0.25	0	0	2.5	0	0	0	8	12	0.6
Cocktail, mixed drink	1 cocktail	139	0	0	0	1	1.5	0	0	6	4	0.1
Liqueur	1 glass, 1½ oz	167	0	0.11	0	8.5	9.5	0	0	4	1	0
Liquor	1 jigger	110	0	0	0	0	0	0	0	0	0	0
Vermouth	5 fluid ounces	100	0.25	0	0	1	0	0	0	8	12	0.4
Wine	5 fluid ounces	104	0.25	0	0	2.5	0	0	0	12	12	0.4
Wine, light	5 fluid ounces	73	0.5	0	0	1	0	0	0	10	13	0.6
Wine cooler	12 fluid ounces	173	0.75	0	0	7.75	9.75	0	0	25	32	1.4

GRAINS

Name	Amount/Unit	Cal.	Pro. g	TFat g	SFat g	Carb. g	Sug. g	Fbr. g	Chol. mg	Sod. mg	Calc. mg	Iron mg
Cereal, bran, fiber	⅓ cup	62	2	0.78	0.22	7.75	2.75	3.8	0	113	13	3
Cereal, frosted	1 cup	147	1.75	0.11	0	18.75	14.75	0.5	0	93	4	2.4
Cereal, fruit-flavored	1 cup	110	1.75	0.22	0.11	12	13	0.5	0	168	5	4.5
Cereal, granola	¼ cup	130	3	4.89	0.89	13.5	4.5	1.7	0	55	19	0.9
Cereal, oat flakes	1 cup	182	5	1.78	0.44	24.75	4.5	3.2	0	115	32	5.8
Cereal, other, cold	1 cup	110	2	0.22	0.11	19.5	3	0.6	0	226	4	1.8
Cereal, other, hot	⅔ cup	100	3	0	0	22	0	0.7	0	54	18	1.1
Cereal, whole-grain	¾ cup	105	3	0.78	0.22	19	0	2.3	0	160	8	1.4
Granola, fat-free	¼ cup	90	2	0	0	21	0.25	2.5	0	20	0	0.4
Oatmeal, flavored	1 packet	140	4	2.22	0.44	18	8.25	2.4	0	181	100	4.5
Oatmeal, plain	⅔ cup cooked	109	4	1.78	0.33	18.25	0	3.3	0	1	15	1.9
Pancakes, waffles	2 pnck/2 wfl	173	4.75	4	1.11	26	3.5	1	44	503	100	1.5
Bagel	1 bagel	175	7	1.22	0.22	32.5	2.25	1.5	0	325	20	1.8
Biscuit	1 biscuit	100	2	3.78	1.22	13.5	0	0.5	2	262	47	0.7
Bread or roll, wheat	1 slice, 1 roll	65	2	0.89	0.22	10	2	1.4	0	106	20	0.7
Bread or roll, white	1 slice, 1 roll	70	2.75	1.11	0.33	11	2	0.5	0	132	20	0.7
Bread, mixed-grain	1 slice	65	2	0.89	0.22	9.75	2.25	1.4	0	106	27	0.8
Bread, oatmeal	1 slice	90	4	1.78	0.33	10.5	4	1.5	0	140	40	1.1
Bread, pita, wheat	1 pita (6" diam)	145	5.5	0.89	0.22	28.5	0.5	4.1	0	360	50	1.4

continued

Grains, continued

Name	Amount/Unit	Cal.	Pro. g	TFat g	SFat g	Carb. g	Sug. g	Fbr. g	Chol. mg	Sod. mg	Calc. mg	Iron mg
Bread, pita, white	1 pita (6″ diam)	160	6	1	0.22	30	1	1.1	0	300	80	0.7
Bread, raisin	1 slice	70	2	1	0.33	8.25	3	0.9	0	85	20	0.7
Bread, rye, pumpernickel	1 slice	80	2.75	0.89	0.11	13	1	1.1	0	185	22	1.1
Bread, wheat, diet	1 slice	40	2.5	0.56	0.11	4.25	2	2	0	120	40	0.7
Bread, white, diet	1 slice	40	3	0	0	6	1	2	0	110	40	0.7
Bread, whole wheat	1 slice, 1 roll	70	2.75	1.11	0.22	10	1.25	1.9	0	160	20	1
Breadsticks	⅓ lrg/2 sm	36	1.25	0.78	0.22	6	0.5	0.6	0	72	0	0.2
Cornbread, hushpuppies	2.5″ sq/3 hpup	166	3	5.33	1.78	25.75	0	1.6	42	421	87	0.8
Croissants	1 croissant	310	7	19	11.22	27	6	2	0	240	38	1.8
Danish, nonfat	1 piece	90	2	0	0	20	9.75	0.2	0	85	20	0
English muffin	1 muffin	130	5	0.89	0.33	25	1.5	1.6	0	280	96	1.7
Muffin	1 muffin	140	3	4.67	1.56	11.75	8	1.2	21	198	42	1.1
Muffins, fat free	1 muffin	155	3	0.11	0	35	11.5	0.9	0	140	50	0.5
Roll, hmbrgr, hot dog, wheat	1 roll	114	4	1.11	0.22	21.25	0.75	2.5	0	242	46	1
Roll, hmbrgr, hot dog, white	1 roll	138	3.25	2.44	0.67	22.5	2	1.4	0	271	67	1.3
Roll, hoagie, sub	½ roll	200	5.5	3.56	0.89	34.25	2	0.9	0	342	50	1.9
Stuffing	½ cup	210	4.5	12.67	3	17.5	2.5	0.5	22	578	40	1.1
Cake, nonfat	1 piece/slice	70	1.5	0	0	16	7.75	0.6	0	85	0	0
Cookies, nonfat	2 cookies	75	1	0	0	17.5	6.5	0.6	0	115	0	0.2
Cracker sandwiches	2 lrg, 5 sm	70	1.75	3.11	1.11	7.75	0.75	0.2	1	135	20	0.4
Crackers, butter type	5 lrg, 10 sm	70	1	3.56	1.11	8	0.25	0.2	1	193	4	0.4
Crackers, crispbread	1 lrg, 2 sm	40	1	0.89	0.33	8.5	0	1.6	0	112	0	0.5
Crackers, low-fat	2 lrg, 5 sm	60	2.25	2.33	0.33	10	0	0.6	0	100	0	0.4
Crackers, wheat	4 crackers	70	1	2.22	0.44	8	0.5	1.5	0	75	0	0.4
Matzo or melba toast	½ matzo, 5 melba	72	2.75	0.67	0.22	14	1.5	0.6	0	189	2	1
Barley, cooked	½ cup	84	2.25	0.11	0	18.5	0	2.5	0	3	11	0.5
Bulgur	½ cup	113	4.25	0.22	0	23.5	0	3	0	3	13	3.7
Couscous	⅔ cup	120	4	0	0	26	0	4.3	0	5	0	0.7
Grits	½ cup	73	1.5	0.11	0	16	0	0.3	0	136	0	0.8
Lasagna, meat	1 serving	350	27.5	23.11	6	31	1.5	2.6	73	1040	275	2.1
Lasagna, vegetable	1 serving	315	22	12	5.89	27	0.5	4.6	40	970	350	2.3
Macaroni and cheese	½ cup	191	6	8.56	2.67	22.75	0	1.4	18	434	71	1.2
Macaroni, whole-wheat	1 cup	202	8	1.11	0.22	39	0	7.4	0	10	20	4.5
Noodles, chow mein	½ cup	130	3	6.44	1.11	14.5	0	0.5	2	228	4	0.8
Noodles, egg, macaroni	1 cup	190	7	0.56	0.11	37	0	1.1	0	30	14	2.1
Pasta w/parmesan cheese	½ cup	252	6.5	14.67	6.33	22.5	0	1.1	38	479	78	1.5
Salad, pasta	½ cup	250	4	16	3.33	20.75	0	0.7	28	410	40	0.7
Spaghetti	1 cup	200	7.5	1	0.22	40.5	0	1.1	0	19	14	2
Spaghetti w/meatballs	1 cup	307	12	10.56	3.89	37	0	2.7	34	1220	53	3.3
Spaghetti, whole-wheat	1 cup	200	9	1.11	0.22	39.5	0	5.8	0	10	20	2.7
Rice cake	1 large cake	35	0.75	0	0	7.5	0	0.3	0	13	0	0
Rice, brown	½ cup	115	2.5	0.67	0.22	25	0	1.8	0	2	12	0.5
Rice, long-grain/wild, mix	½ cup	137	3	2	0.56	23	2	0.9	0	579	11	1.1
Rice, seasoned	½ cup	150	3.5	3.78	1.67	23	1	1	5	700	13	1.2
Rice, white	½ cup	92	2	0	0	20.5	0	0.5	0	225	10	0.7
Tabouli	½ cup	170	3	8.67	1.33	20	0	1.6	0	290	0	0.7
Taco shell	1 shell	50	0	2	1.11	8	0	0.2	0	5	0	0
Tortilla	1 tortilla	65	2	1	0.11	12	0	0.9	0	1	42	0.6

B

Name	Amount/Unit	Cal.	Pro. g	TFat g	SFat g	Carb. g	Sug. g	Fbr. g	Chol. mg	Sod. mg	Calc. mg	Iron mg
Buttermilk	1 cup	99	8.75	2	1.33	11.25	0	0	9	257	285	0.1
Hot cocoa prepared w/milk	1 cup	218	8	9	5.67	13.5	11.25	3	33	123	298	0.8
Meal replacement drinks	1 cup	200	14	1	0.44	36	17	4	5	230	500	6.3
Milk, chocolate	1 cup	179	8.5	4.67	3	10.5	14.5	1.1	17	150	284	0.6
Milk, low-fat	1 cup	112	8.75	3.56	2.22	11.25	0	0	14	123	299	0.1
Milk, skim	1 cup	86	9	0.44	0.33	11.5	0	0	4	126	302	0.1
Milk, whole	1 cup	150	8.5	7.67	5	11	0	0	33	120	291	0.1
Cheese spread	2 tablespoons	81	3.5	6.56	4.33	2	0	1	89	293	95	1
Cheese, American	1 ounce, 1 slice	106	6.75	8.22	5.44	0.5	0	0	27	406	174	0.1
Cheese, cheddar	1 ounce, 1 slice	113	7.5	8.67	5.89	0.5	0	0	30	177	203	0.2
Cheese, cottage	½ cup	113	14.5	4.78	3.11	3	0	0	17	440	65	0.2
Cheese, cottage, nonfat	½ cup	90	14	0	0	7	0	0	10	400	60	0
Cheese, cottage, low-fat	½ cup	96	15	1.22	0.78	4	0	0	5	440	74	0.2
Cheese, mozzarella	1 ounce, 1 slice	80	6	5.67	3.67	0.5	0	0	22	106	147	0.1
Cheese, mozzarella, light	1 ounce	72	7.25	4.11	2.78	0.75	0	0	16	150	183	0.1
Cheese, parmesan	1 tablespoon	23	2.25	1.44	0.89	0.25	0	0	4	93	69	0.1
Cheese, provolone	1 ounce, 1 slice	100	7.75	7	4.78	0.5	0	0	20	248	214	0.2
Cheese, reduced-fat	1 ounce	80	8	5	3	1	0	0	20	220	350	0
Cheese, ricotta	½ cup	216	15	14.89	10	3.75	0	0	63	104	257	0.5
Cheese, ricotta, part-skim	½ cup	166	14.5	8.67	5.67	6.25	0	0	37	143	369	0.3
Cheese, Swiss	1 ounce	101	8	6.89	4.67	0.75	0	0	25	231	246	0.1
Ice cream	½ cup	148	2.5	7.44	4.67	4.5	11.75	0.2	30	58	88	0.3
Ice milk	½ cup	110	3	2.78	1.89	10	8	0.3	8	75	100	1
Tofutti	½ cup	150	2.5	6.67	1.11	9	11	1.5	0	105	1	0.6
Yogurt, frozen	½ cup	100	3	1.78	1.11	8	10.25	0.1	7	59	100	1
Yogurt, low-fat w/fruit	1 container	240	9	3	2	27	16	0.3	10	120	330	1
Yogurt, nonfat w/fruit	1 container	95	3.5	0	0	8	12	0	0	70	150	1
Yogurt, plain, low-fat	1 container	142	11.25	3.67	2.44	15.75	0	0	15	160	422	0.6
Yogurt, plain, nonfat	1 container	110	11	0.22	0.22	16	0	0	4	160	430	1
Yogurt, plain, whole-milk	1 container	145	8.75	6.89	4.56	11.5	0	0	32	123	312	0.6
Yogurt, w/frt, art. swtner	1 container	90	7	0.67	0.44	14	0	0.5	5	110	250	1

Name	Amount/Unit	Cal.	Pro. g	TFat g	SFat g	Carb. g	Sug. g	Fbr. g	Chol. mg	Sod. mg	Calc. mg	Iron mg
Bacon	1 slice	36	5.25	1.78	0.67	0	0	0	12	360	2	0.2
Bacon bits	1 tablespoon	21	2.5	1.11	0.33	0	0	0	6	181	1	0.1
Butter	1 tablespoon	104	0	11.44	7.22	0	0	0	32	119	2	1
Gravy	¼ cup	30	1	1.44	0.56	2.25	0.5	0.1	1	260	3	0.4
Lard	1 tablespoon	115	0	12.22	5	0	0	0	12	0	0	0
Margarine, stick	1 tablespoon	101	0	10.56	2	0	0	0	0	133	4	0
Margarine, stick, light	1 tablespoon	60	0	6.67	1	0	0	0	0	110	1	1
Margarine, tub	1 tablespoon	101	0	8.89	2	0	0	0	0	152	4	0
Margarine, tub, light	1 tablespoon	50	0	5.89	1	0	0	0	0	110	1	1
Mayonnaise	1 tablespoon	100	0.25	11	1.89	0.25	0.25	0	8	74	1	1
Mayonnaise, light	1 tablespoon	48	0.25	4.56	1	0.75	1	0	5	95	1	1
Mayonnaise, nonfat	1 tablespoon	12	0	0	0	3	3	0	0	190	0	0
Miracle Whip	1 tablespoon	64	0	5.89	0.89	2.5	0.5	0	5	95	2	1
Miracle Whip, nonfat	1 tablespoon	20	0	0	0	5	5	0	0	210	0	0
Oil	1 tablespoon	120	0	12.78	1.89	0	0	0	0	0	0	0.1

continued

Name	Amount/Unit	Cal.	Pro. g	TFat g	SFat g	Carb. g	Sug. g	Fbr. g	Chol. mg	Sod. mg	Calc. mg	Iron mg
Salad dressing	1 tablespoon	80	0	8.22	1.33	0.25	0.25	1	0	146	2	1
Salad dressing, light	1 tablespoon	16	0.25	0.33	0.11	0.75	0.5	0.3	0	137	1	1
Salad dressing, no oil	1 tablespoon	12	0	0	0	2.5	0	0.7	0	0	1	1
Salad dressing, nonfat	1 tablespoon	16	0	0	0	3	3	0	0	143	0	0
Brownie	1¾" square	150	2	6.22	1.67	6.5	15	0.9	10	105	1	0.7
Cake	1 piece/slice	280	4	11.33	3	15.25	22.25	0.5	56	285	57	1
Candy, choc/peanut butter	1 pkg, 1½ oz	237	6	13.78	5.89	4	22	2.5	3	90	34	0.7
Candy, chocolate	1-ounce piece	150	2	8.22	4.78	2.25	15	0.8	6	24	50	0.3
Candy, chocolate-covered	1 ounce	132	1.25	5.56	2.11	3	13.25	1.5	3	43	33	0.4
Candy, fudge	1" cube	88	0.75	3	0.78	1.25	13.25	0.3	2	40	20	0.2
Candy, hard	5 pieces	110	0	0	0	0	27.5	0	0	7	1	0.1
Cookies, fig bars	2 fig bars	100	1	1.78	0.44	10.5	10.5	1.2	1	90	20	0.7
Cookies, oatmeal raisin	3 cookies	195	2.25	8.11	1.89	13.5	13.5	1.4	1	150	0	0.8
Cookies, other	3 cookies	180	1.5	8.11	2.89	10	15	0.3	3	131	1	0.7
Danish	1 roll	252	4.5	11.67	3.67	10.25	19	0.7	14	249	36	1.1
Diet bar	1 bar	120	2	4	1.44	19	9.5	3	1	30	150	2.7
Doughnut or sweet roll	1 serving	201	3	8.11	2.89	12.5	13.25	0.6	19	145	21	0.8
Frozen desserts, nonfat	½ cup	100	2	0.22	0.11	23.5	9.5	0.4	1	48	100	0
Frzn yogurt cone, low-fat	1 serving	105	4	1	0.56	22	13	0.1	3	80	112	0.2
Frzn yogurt sundae, low-fat	1 serving	240	6	3	2.33	50.5	43	0.8	6	170	190	0.1
Gelatin	½ cup	105	2	1	1	23	22	0	0	57	0	0
Gelatin, sugar-free	½ cup	8	1.5	0	0	0	0	0	0	31	0	0
Granola bars	1 bar	133	2	6	2	18.25	13	0.6	0	70	20	0.5
Pie, custard or cream	⅙ of 9" pie	346	6.75	13.11	6.22	20.75	25.75	1	125	375	122	0.8
Pie, fruit	⅙ of 9" pie	405	4	16.22	5.33	34.75	25.25	4	6	423	17	1.6
Pie, pecan	⅙ of 9" pie	575	7	29.67	5.67	33	37.25	2.2	100	305	65	4.6
Pudding	½ cup	150	4.5	2.22	1.44	10	18	0	9	443	152	0
Pudding, diet	½ cup	90	4	2.44	1.56	13	0	0.4	9	423	152	0.1
Cream, whipped	1 tablespoon	15	0.25	1.33	1.11	0.25	0.25	0	2	4	3	1
Dessert topping, no sugar	1 tablespoon	5	0	0.56	0.44	0	0	1	4	5	2	1
Jam or jelly	2 teaspoons	35	0	0	0	1	7.5	0.1	0	1	1	1
Cream, coffee, half & half	1 tablespoon	25	0.5	2.22	1.44	0.5	0	0	8	6	15	0
Nutrasweet, Equal	1 packet	4	0.5	0	0	0	0.5	0	0	0	0	0
Saccharin	1 packet	2	0	0	0	0	0	0	0	2	0	0
Salt	4 shakes	0	0	0	0	0	0	0	0	64	0	0
Sugar	1 teaspoon	15	0	0	0	0	3.75	0	0	0	0	0
Syrup, pancake, table	2 tablespoons	110	0	0	0	0	27.5	0	0	21	1	1
Coffee whitener	1 tablespoon	22	0	2.11	1.33	0	1	0	0	12	1	1
Cream cheese	2 tablespoons	106	2.5	10.22	6.67	1	0	0	34	90	24	0.4
Cream cheese, light	2 tablespoons	80	3	7	4	1	0	0	25	115	20	1
Sour cream	1 tablespoon	26	0.25	2.56	1.56	0.5	0	0	5	17	14	0
Sour cream, imitation	1 tablespoon	25	0.75	2.33	2	0.75	0	0	1	10	7	0
Sour cream, nonfat	1 tablespoon	8	1	0	0	1	0	0	0	10	20	0
Catsup	1 tablespoon	17	0	0	0	2.75	1.5	0.2	0	168	3	0.1
Cheese sauce	¼ cup	71	3.5	3.56	1.89	6.5	0	0	10	412	139	0.1
Chili sauce	1 tablespoon	17	0.25	0	0	2.75	1.25	0.9	0	196	2	0.1
Hollandaise sauce	¼ cup	230	2.25	23.22	8.44	2.5	0	0	140	316	50	1
Mustard	1 teaspoon	6	0.25	0.33	0	0.25	0	0	0	60	0	0
Olives	3 olives	15	0.25	1.56	0.22	0.25	0	0.3	0	234	8	0.2
Pickles, dill	2 spears	7	0	0.11	0	1	0.75	0.9	0	584	9	0.4
Pickles, sweet	1 pickle, 3 sl.	18	0	0	0	0.5	4	0.3	0	107	2	0.2
Soy sauce	1 tablespoon	10	1.25	0	0	1.25	0	0	0	1015	3	0.4

continued

Fats, Sweets, Other, continued

Name	Amount/Unit	Cal.	Pro. g	TFat g	SFat g	Carb. g	Sug. g	Fbr. g	Chol. mg	Sod. mg	Calc. mg	Iron mg
Steak, Worcestershire sauce	1 tablespoon	11	0	0	0	1	1.75	0	0	143	0	0
White sauce	¼ cup	99	2.5	5.67	2.22	6	0	0.1	8	222	73	0.2
Soup, beef or chicken	1 cup	74	4.25	2.22	0.67	8.5	0	1	7	910	17	0.9
Soup, bouillon, broth	1 cube/packet	9	0.75	0.22	0.11	0.25	1	0	1	965	1	0.1
Soup, broth-based, no-salt	1 cup	135	5.75	3.89	0.78	16.5	0	2.8	0	115	47	1.8
Soup, cream, chowder	1 cup	140	5.5	6.11	2.89	14	0	0.9	22	1010	150	0.6
Soup, low-salt	1 cup	110	4	3	1	12	0	0.5	2	100	17	1.3
Soup, miso	1 cup	152	4.5	6.44	0.89	19	0	3	0	490	20	1.3
Breakfast milk powder	1 packet	130	6	0	0	0	26.25	0.4	0	185	80	4.5
Hot chocolate mix	1 envelope	110	1.5	2.78	1.56	3.5	16	1.1	2	165	40	0.7
Meal replacement bar	1 serving	270	11	14	5	24	22.5	0	0	330	250	4.5
Milkshake	10 oz, 1¼ cup	368	10	12.78	8.22	26.5	19.25	0.5	54	243	375	0.5
Milkshake, low-fat	1 serving	320	10.75	1.33	0.56	66	44.75	0	10	170	327	0.1
Popcorn	1 cup	32	0.75	1.44	0.44	5.5	0	0.8	0	68	0	0.2
Potato chips, corn chips	1 cup	152	2	9.44	1.78	15	0	1.4	0	229	15	0.4
Pretzels	⅔ cup	110	2.75	0.89	0.22	21.75	1	0.9	0	610	9	1.4
Tortilla chips	1 cup	95	1.25	4.67	1.33	12	0	0.9	0	123	23	0.3

PROTEIN FOODS

Name	Amount/Unit	Cal.	Pro. g	TFat g	SFat g	Carb. g	Sug. g	Fbr. g	Chol. mg	Sod. mg	Calc. mg	Iron mg
Biscuit w/egg, meat, cheese	1 biscuit	489	18.75	31.22	9.67	29	4	0.8	347	1240	151	2.9
Egg salad	½ cup	267	11	22.89	5.78	1	3	0.3	418	513	43	1.8
Egg, boiled, poached	1 egg	79	6.5	5.56	2.11	0.5	0	0	274	69	28	1
Egg, fried, scrambled	1 egg	89	6.25	6.78	3	1	0	0	281	150	37	0.9
Egg, omelet	1 omelet	342	23.25	25.44	12.56	4	0	0	861	553	243	2.8
Egg, substitute	¼ cup	43	5.5	1.56	0.22	1.5	0	0	0	115	30	0.8
Chicken breast sandwich	1 sandwich	509	26	26.89	4.78	34.75	1.75	1.2	83	1082	80	2.7
Chicken salad	½ cup	179	14.75	12.22	2.89	0.75	0.75	0.3	118	329	21	0.9
Chicken wings	10 wings	1282	90	91.11	35.78	11.5	5	0.2	326	1750	62	4
Chicken, turkey, no skin	4 ounces	137	27.25	3.33	1.11	0	0	0	77	58	12	1.3
Chicken, turkey, w/skin	4 ounces	145	19.75	7.22	2.44	0	0	0	57	49	10	0.9
Chicken, fried, no skin	4 ounces	107	19.25	4.22	1.33	0.25	0	0	50	46	9	0.8
Chicken, fried, w/skin	4 ounces	206	21	11.22	3.22	6.25	0	0.2	69	199	14	1.1
Chicken, mixed dish	1 cup	365	15.25	17.78	5.56	13.5	0	1	103	600	30	2.2
Beef stew	1 cup	207	15.25	9	4.22	16.5	0.5	2.5	53	616	29	2.6
Beef, corned	4 ounces	242	24.25	16.11	7	0	0.25	0	87	1024	15	2
Beef, grnd, hmbrgr, not fried	4 ounces	200	21.25	13.67	6.11	0	0	0	70	60	8	1.9
Beef, grnd, hmbrgr, fried	4 ounces	207	21.25	13.56	5.89	0	0	0	68	62	8	1.9
Beef, mixed dish	1 cup	310	19.25	13.56	5.89	23.5	1.25	2.1	68	840	52	3.5
Beef, roast beef	4 ounces	198	21.25	11.11	4.89	0	0	0	59	47	6	2.1
Cheeseburger (large) w/roll	1 sandwich	711	32	43.33	16.78	33	4	1	113	1164	295	5
Cheeseburger (low-fat) w/roll	1 sandwich	370	24	14	5	35	3.5	1.6	75	890	200	3.6
Cheeseburger (small) w/roll	1 sandwich	461	29	27.56	13.67	25.25	3	0.8	95	906	245	3.3
Hamburger (large) w/roll	1 sandwich	594	27.5	33	12.67	33.25	2	0.9	101	688	87	4.8
Hamburger (low-fat) w/roll	1 sandwich	320	22	10	4	35	3.5	1.6	60	670	150	3.6
Hamburger (small) w/roll	1 sandwich	355	22	19.33	8.22	22.25	3	1.7	95	556	71	3.2
Liver	4 ounces	169	23.5	6	2.67	3.25	0	0	344	69	10	7.7
Pate	1 tablespoon	41	2	3.67	1.44	0	0	0	51	91	9	0.7
Roast beef sandwich	1 sandwich	353	27.25	14.89	7.33	30.25	2.25	0.7	49	766	87	4.1

continued

Protein Foods, continued

Name	Amount/Unit	Cal.	Pro. g	TFat g	SFat g	Carb. g	Sug. g	Fbr. g	Chol. mg	Sod. mg	Calc. mg	Iron mg
Tripe	4 ounces	61	12.5	1.11	0.67	0	0	0	58	44	77	0.3
Veal	4 ounces	177	21.75	9.78	4.78	0	0	0	78	52	9	2.7
Veal, mixed dish	1 serving	327	28.25	17.78	9.78	9.5	0.75	1.7	137	634	138	3.7
Bacon substitute	1 strip	52	3	4.11	1.56	0	0	0	13	207	1	0.2
Ham	4 ounces	165	21	8.67	3.11	0	0	0	54	1419	8	1
Hot dog	1 hot dog	144	5.75	12.89	5.22	0.25	1.25	0	30	547	20	0.7
Hot dog and roll	1 sandwich	298	9.25	17.56	6.67	20	2.5	0.7	29	880	60	2.2
Pork feet	8 ounces	138	14.5	8.78	3.22	0	0	0	71	597	32	1.1
Pork rinds	4 ounces	610	69	34.67	13.33	0	0	0	106	3033	25	0.7
Pork spareribs	4 ounces	176	13.75	13.11	5.22	0	0	0	54	41	21	0.8
Pork, fresh, fried	4 ounces	192	14.5	14.89	5.67	0	0	0	55	33	5	0.5
Pork, fresh, roasted	4 ounces	164	15.75	10.22	3.89	0	0	0	54	37	4	0.6
Sausage	1 ounce	88	4	7.44	2.89	0	0.5	0	14	258	4	0.4
Lamb	4 ounces	225	26.25	14.78	7.11	0	0	0	91	65	10	2
Caviar	1 tablespoon	40	4.25	2.11	0.78	0.5	0	0	94	240	44	1.8
Clams, oysters, shrimp, fried	4 pieces	103	5.25	6.11	1.11	6	0	0.1	23	183	20	0.6
Clams, oysters, shrimp	½ cup	71	12.25	1.22	0.33	2.5	0	0	62	108	41	6
Crabmeat	3 ounces	86	12.5	1	0.22	4.5	0	0	26	713	25	0.4
Fish casserole	1 cup	407	18.5	23.78	7.56	26.25	0.75	1.8	70	1314	182	2.3
Fish sandwich	1 sandwich	488	19	26.56	5.89	39.25	3.75	1.5	70	928	46	2
Fish, fried	4 ounces	279	11.5	15.33	3.56	21.5	1.5	0.9	52	467	0	0.7
Fish, not fried	4 ounces	108	22.75	1.33	0.44	10	0	0	60	76	17	0.5
Fish, smoked, pickled	1 ounce	56	6.25	2.33	0.67	0	0	0	14	235	5	0.3
Seafood or fish salad	½ cup	160	13.5	9.78	2.33	1.75	0.25	0.4	142	250	31	0.9
Tuna in oil	½ cup	142	22	5.44	1.11	0	0	0	18	275	7	0.8
Tuna in water	½ cup	90	19.25	1.44	0.44	0	0	0	28	400	0	0.7
Chili con carne	1 cup	286	15.75	12.44	5.78	28.5	0	6.5	43	964	86	3
Chili, vegetarian	1 cup	240	18	12	1.78	13	2	16.4	0	860	6	3.2
Luncheon meat, beef, pork	1 ounce slice	76	4.25	6.11	2.56	0	0.5	0	18	348	3	0.4
Luncheon meat, chkn, trky	1 ounce slice	32	5.75	0.67	0.22	0	0	0	12	358	3	0.3
Pepperoni	1 slice	27	1.25	2.33	0.89	0.25	0	0	5	112	1	0.1
Pizza, cheese topping	2 slices	352	21.75	13.44	7.33	36.25	0.75	3	33	890	474	2.3
Pizza, French bread	1 slice	410	17.5	19.22	8	39	2	2	35	1030	200	2.7
Pizza, meat topping	2 slices	445	25	17	8	50	0.5	4.3	31	906	263	3
Pizza, vegetable topping	2 slices	419	24.75	10.33	5.56	64.25	1	10	19	685	285	5
Chop suey	1 cup	300	26	16	4.33	13	0	1.5	68	1053	60	4.8
Chow mein, beef or chicken	¾ cup	65	6.5	1.44	0.56	5.25	0.75	1.4	26	845	80	1.3
Eggroll	1 eggroll	173	6.75	4.56	0.89	25	3	0.8	7	471	20	1.1
Sweet & sour chicken, pork	1 cup	426	17.5	13.89	3.33	23.5	31.75	1.3	83	1209	27	1.9
Burrito	2 burritos	426	16	14.33	7.11	57.75	0	6.4	65	1116	105	4.5
Chimichanga	1 chimichanga	425	18.5	17.11	8.33	41.25	0	5.2	30	933	145	4
Enchilada	1 enchilada	322	10.5	16.89	9.67	30	0	5.8	42	1052	276	2.2
Taco	1 small	370	21	18.44	11.11	26.5	0	3.4	57	802	221	2.4
Taco salad	1½ cups	279	13.5	13.33	6.67	24	0	4.3	44	763	192	2.3
Tostada	1 tostada	325	13.75	13.89	9.67	28	0	7.5	40	834	214	2.2
Beans, baked	½ cup	140	6	1.67	0.67	15	7.5	6	8	423	60	2.1
Beans, black	½ cup	113	6.5	0.33	0.11	20.75	0	4.4	0	1	24	1.8
Beans, kidney, pinto	½ cup	115	6.5	0.33	0.11	22.25	0	4.5	0	2	33	2.4
Beans, kidney, pinto, canned	½ cup	104	5.75	0.22	0	19.5	0	6.1	0	445	35	1.6
Beans, lima	½ cup	94	5.5	0.22	0.11	17.5	0	4.6	0	26	25	1.8
Beans, lima, canned	½ cup	93	4.75	0.22	0.11	17.5	0	5.8	0	309	35	2

continued

Protein Foods, continued

Name	Amount/Unit	Cal.	Pro. g	TFat g	SFat g	Carb. g	Sug. g	Fbr. g	Chol. mg	Sod. mg	Calc. mg	Iron mg
Beans, navy, chickpeas	½ cup	132	6.75	1	0.22	23.75	0	4.8	0	4	52	2.4
Beans, navy, chickpeas, cnd	½ cup	146	7	0.78	0.11	27.5	0	5	0	473	51	2
Beans, white, canned	½ cup	153	8.25	0.22	0.11	29.25	0	5	0	7	96	3.9
Beans, white, split peas	½ cup	125	7	0.22	0.11	23	0	5.3	0	2	66	2.6
Broadbeans, fava	½ cup	93	5.5	0.22	0	17	0	4.4	0	4	31	1.3
Broadbeans, fava, canned	½ cup	91	6	0.11	0	16.25	0	4.5	0	580	34	1.3
Chickpeas	½ cup	138	6.5	1.67	0.11	24.75	0	4.8	0	183	39	2
Lentils	½ cup	115	7.75	0.22	0	20.25	0	2.8	0	2	19	3.3
Peas, black-eyed	½ cup	100	5.75	0.33	0.11	18.25	0	8.3	0	3	21	2.2
Peas, black-eyed, canned	½ cup	92	5	0.33	0.11	16.5	0	8.2	0	359	24	1.2
Soybeans, roasted	¼ cup	205	14.25	10.22	1.56	13.5	0	1.9	0	1	89	2
Tahini	1 tablespoon	92	2.5	7.33	1.11	3.75	0	1.5	0	10	109	2.2
Nuts, mixed	3 tablespoons	170	4.25	13.56	2.22	6.25	0	1.6	0	170	20	1.1
Peanut butter	2 tablespoons	190	9	14.56	2.78	4.5	2	2.4	0	150	11	0.6
Peanuts	3 tablespoons	164	6.25	12.33	1.78	5.25	0	2.5	0	110	7	0.5

Nutritional Content of Popular Items from Fast-Food Restaurants

Arby's

	Serving size (g)	Calories	Protein (g)	Total fat (g)	Saturated fat (g)	Total carbohydrate (g)	Sugars (g)	Fiber (g)	Cholesterol (mg)	Sodium (mg)	Vitamin A	Vitamin C	Calcium	Iron	% calories from fat
											% Daily Value				
Regular roast beef	154	388	23	19	7	33	N/A	3	43	1009	N/A	N/A	N/A	N/A	44
Super roast beef	247	523	25	27	9	50	N/A	5	43	1189	N/A	N/A	N/A	N/A	46
Light roast beef deluxe	182	296	18	10	3	33	N/A	6	42	826	N/A	N/A	N/A	N/A	30
Roast chicken deluxe	216	433	24	22	5	36	N/A	2	34	763	N/A	N/A	N/A	N/A	46
French dip	195	475	30	22	8	40	N/A	3	55	1411	N/A	N/A	N/A	N/A	41
Turkey sub	277	550	31	27	7	47	N/A	2	65	2084	N/A	N/A	N/A	N/A	44
Light roast turkey deluxe	195	260	20	7	2	33	N/A	4	33	1262	N/A	N/A	N/A	N/A	21
Grilled chicken BBQ	201	388	23	13	3	47	N/A	2	43	1002	N/A	N/A	N/A	N/A	30
Cheddar curly fries	120	333	5	18	4	40	N/A	0	3	1016	N/A	N/A	N/A	N/A	49
Potato cakes	85	204	2	12	2	20	N/A	0	0	397	N/A	N/A	N/A	N/A	53
Red ranch dressing	14	75	0	6	1	5	N/A	0	0	115	N/A	N/A	N/A	N/A	72
French-toastix	124	430	10	21	5	52	N/A	3	0	550	N/A	N/A	N/A	N/A	44
Jamocha shake	340	384	15	10	3	62	N/A	0	36	262	N/A	N/A	N/A	N/A	23

N/A: not available.

Burger King

	Serving size (g)	Calories	Protein (g)	Total fat (g)	Saturated fat (g)	Total carbohydrate (g)	Sugars (g)	Fiber (g)	Cholesterol (mg)	Sodium (mg)	Vitamin A	Vitamin C	Calcium	Iron	% calories from fat
											% Daily Value				
Whopper®	270	640	27	39	11	45	8	3	90	870	N/A	N/A	N/A	N/A	55
Whopper Jr.®	164	420	21	24	8	29	5	2	60	530	N/A	N/A	N/A	N/A	51
Double Whopper® with cheese	375	960	52	63	24	46	8	3	195	1420	N/A	N/A	N/A	N/A	59
BK Big Fish™ sandwich	252	720	23	43	9	59	4	3	80	1180	N/A	N/A	N/A	N/A	54
BK Broiler® chicken sandwich	247	530	29	26	5	5	4	2	105	1060	N/A	N/A	N/A	N/A	44
Chicken Tenders® (8 pieces)	123	350	22	22	7	17	0	1	65	940	N/A	N/A	N/A	N/A	57
Ranch dipping sauce	28	170	0	17	3	2	1	0	0	200	N/A	N/A	N/A	N/A	90
Barbeque dipping sauce	28	35	0	0	0	9	7	0	0	400	N/A	N/A	N/A	N/A	0
Broiled chicken salad (no dressing)	302	190	20	8	4	9	5	3	75	500	N/A	N/A	N/A	N/A	38
Garden salad (no dressing)	215	100	6	5	3	8	4	4	15	115	N/A	N/A	N/A	N/A	45
Bleu cheese salad dressing	30	160	2	16	4	1	0	<1	30	260	N/A	N/A	N/A	N/A	90
French fries (medium, salted)	116	400	3	21	8	50	0	4	0	820	N/A	N/A	N/A	N/A	47
Onion rings	124	310	4	14	2	41	6	6	0	810	N/A	N/A	N/A	N/A	41
Chocolate shake (medium)	284	320	9	7	4	54	48	3	20	230	N/A	N/A	N/A	N/A	20
Croissan'wich® w/sausage, egg, and cheese	176	600	22	46	16	25	3	1	260	1140	N/A	N/A	N/A	N/A	69
French toast sticks	141	500	4	27	7	60	11	1	0	490	N/A	N/A	N/A	N/A	49
Dutch apple pie	113	300	3	15	3	39	22	2	0	230	N/A	N/A	N/A	N/A	45

N/A: not available.

Domino's Pizza

(1 serving = 2 of 12 slices or ⅙ of 14-inch pizza; 2 of 8 slices or ¼ of 12-inch pizza; 1 6-inch pizza)

	Serving size	Calories	Protein	Total fat	Saturated fat	Total carbohydrate	Sugars	Fiber	Cholesterol	Sodium	Vitamin A	Vitamin C	Calcium	Iron	% calories from fat
	g		g	g	g	g	g	g	mg	mg		% Daily Value			
14-inch lg. hand-tossed cheese	137	317	13	10	5	45	3	3	14	669	10	9	17	18	28
14-inch lg. thin crust cheese	99	253	11	11	5	29	2	2	14	757	9	4	20	5	39
14-inch lg. deep dish cheese	173	455	18	20	8	54	5	3	18	1029	11	5	22	21	39
12-inch med. hand-tossed cheese	149	347	14	11	5	50	3	3	15	723	11	8	18	20	29
12-inch med. thin crust cheese	106	271	12	12	5	31	3	2	15	509	10	4	22	5	40
12-inch med. deep dish cheese	180	477	18	22	8	55	5	3	19	1085	12	5	23	21	42
6-inch deep dish cheese	215	595	23	27	11	68	6	4	24	1300	13	5	28	26	41
Toppings: pepperoni	*	66	3	6	2	<1	<1	<1	14	212	†	†	†	†	82
ham	*	17	2	1	<1	<1	<1	0	7	156	†	†	†	†	53
Italian sausage	*	44	2	3	1	1	<1	<1	9	137	†	†	†	†	61
bacon	*	75	4	6	2	<1	<1	0	11	207	†	7	†	†	72
beef	*	44	2	4	2	<1	<1	<1	8	123	†	†	†	†	82
anchovies	*	23	3	1	<1	0	0	0	9	395	†	†	3	3	39
extra cheese	*	45	3	4	2	<1	<1	<1	7	140	3	†	12	†	80
cheddar cheese	*	48	3	4	2	<1	<1	0	12	73	3	†	9	†	75
Barbeque wings	25	50	6	2	1	2	1	<1	26	175	†	†	†	†	38
Hot wings	25	45	6	2	1	<1	<1	<1	26	354	3	†	†	†	40
Breadsticks (1 piece)	22	78	2	3	1	11	<1	<1	0	158	†	†	†	3	35
Cheesy bread (1 piece)	28	103	3	5	2	11	<1	<1	6	187	†	26	†	4	44

* Topping information is based on minimal portioning requirements for one serving of a 14-inch large pizza; add the values for toppings to the values for a cheese pizza. The following toppings supply fewer than 15 calories per serving: green and yellow peppers, onion, olives, mushrooms, pineapple.
† Contains less than 2% of the Daily Value of these nutrients.

Jack in the Box

	Serving size	Calories	Protein	Total fat	Saturated fat	Total carbohydrate	Sugars	Fiber	Cholesterol	Sodium	Vitamin A	Vitamin C	Calcium	Iron	% calories from fat
	g		g	g	g	g	g	g	mg	mg		% Daily Value			
Breakfast Jack®	126	280	17	12	5	30	3	1	195	920	8	4	15	20	39
Supreme croissant	163	520	21	32	13	39	6	2	245	1240	15	20	10	20	57
Hamburger	97	280	13	11	4	31	5	1	45	560	2	2	10	20	39
Jumbo Jack®	263	590	25	36	11	42	6	4	80	720	8	20	15	35	55
Sourdough Jack	229	690	31	46	15	38	3	3	110	1180	10	15	30	20	60
Chicken fajita pita	187	280	24	9	4	25	5	3	75	840	25	0	15	15	29
Grilled chicken fillet	231	520	27	26	6	42	9	4	140	1240	8	15	20	25	45
Chicken supreme	235	680	23	45	11	46	8	4	85	1500	10	15	20	15	60
Chicken Caesar sandwich	232	490	24	26	6	41	6	3	55	1050	15	15	20	20	48
Garden chicken salad	253	200	23	9	4	8	4	3	65	420	70	20	20	4	41
Blue cheese dressing	57	210	1	15	2.5	11	4	0	25	750	0	0	2	0	64
Chicken teriyaki bowl	502	670	26	4	1	128	27	3	15	1730	130	40	10	25	5
Monster taco	125	270	12	17	6	19	2	4	30	678	8	2	20	8	57
Egg rolls (3 pieces)	170	440	15	24	6	40	5	4	35	1020	15	20	8	25	49
Chicken breast pieces (5)	150	360	27	17	3	24	0	1	80	970	4	2	2	10	39
Stuffed jalapeños (10 pieces)	240	750	20	44	17	65	7	5	80	2470	30	50	45	10	53
Barbeque dipping sauce	28	45	1	0	0	11	7	0	0	310	0	0	0	0	0
Seasoned curly fries	125	410	6	23	5	45	0	4	0	1010	6	0	4	10	50
Onion rings	120	460	7	25	5	50	3	3	0	780	4	30	4	15	49
Cappuccino ice cream shake	16*	630	11	29	17	80	58	0	90	320	15	0	35	0	41

*Fluid ounces

KFC

	Serving size (g)	Calories	Protein (g)	Total fat (g)	Saturated fat (g)	Total carbohydrate (g)	Sugars (g)	Fiber (g)	Cholesterol (mg)	Sodium (mg)	Vitamin A (% DV)	Vitamin C (% DV)	Calcium (% DV)	Iron (% DV)	% calories from fat
Original Recipe®: breast	153	400	29	24	6	16	0	1	135	1116	*	*	4	6	54
thigh	91	250	16	18	4.5	6	0	1	95	747	*	*	2	4	65
Extra Tasty Crispy™: breast	168	470	31	28	7	25	0	1	80	930	*	*	4	6	54
thigh	118	370	19	25	6	18	0	2	70	540	*	*	2	4	61
Hot & Spicy: breast	180	530	32	35	8	23	0	2	110	1110	*	*	4	6	59
thigh	107	370	18	27	7	13	0	1	90	570	*	*	*	4	66
Tender Roast™: breast (as served)	139	251	37	11	3	1	<1	0	151	830	*	*	*	*	39
breast (skin removed)	118	169	31	4	1	1	0	0	112	797	*	*	*	*	21
thigh (as served)	90	207	18	12	4	<2	<1	0	120	504	*	*	*	*	52
thigh (skin removed)	59	106	13	6	2	<1	<1	0	84	312	*	*	*	*	51
Hot Wings™ Pieces	135	471	27	33	8	18	0	2	150	1230	*	*	4	8	63
Colonel's Crispy Strips™ (3)	92	261	20	16	4	10	0	3	40	658	*	*	*	3	55
Chunky chicken pot pie	368	770	29	42	13	69	8	5	70	2160	80	2	10	10	49
Corn on the cob	162	150	5	2	0	35	8	2	0	20	2	6	*	*	12
Mashed potatoes w/gravy	136	120	1	6	1	17	0	2	<1	440	*	*	*	2	45
Mean Greens™	152	70	4	3	1	11	1	5	10	650	60	10	20	10	39
BBQ baked beans	156	190	6	3	1	33	13	6	5	760	8	*	8	10	14
Potato salad	160	230	4	14	2	23	9	23	15	540	10	*	2	15	55
Cole slaw	142	180	2	9	1.5	21	20	3	5	280	*	60	4	4	45
Biscuit (1)	56	180	4	10	2.5	20	2	<1	0	560	*	*	2	6	50

*Contains less than 2% of the Daily Value of these nutrients.

McDonald's

	Serving size (g)	Calories	Protein (g)	Total fat (g)	Saturated fat (g)	Total carbohydrate (g)	Sugars (g)	Fiber (g)	Cholesterol (mg)	Sodium (mg)	Vitamin A (% DV)	Vitamin C (% DV)	Calcium (% DV)	Iron (% DV)	% calories from fat
Hamburger	107	260	13	9	3.5	34	7	2	30	580	*	4	15	15	31
Cheeseburger	121	320	15	13	6	35	7	2	40	820	6	4	20	15	37
Quarter-Pounder®	172	420	23	21	8	37	8	2	70	820	2	4	30	25	45
Quarter-Pounder® w/cheese	200	530	28	30	13	38	9	2	95	1290	10	4	15	25	51
Big Mac®	216	560	26	31	10	45	8	3	85	1070	6	4	25	25	50
Arch Deluxe™	239	550	29	31	11	39	8	4	90	1010	10	10	15	25	51
Fish Filet Deluxe™	228	560	23	28	6	54	5	4	60	1060	6	4	8	15	45
Grilled Chicken Deluxe™	223	440	27	20	3	38	6	4	60	1040	6	8	6	15	41
French fries (large)	147	450	6	22	4	57	0	5	0	290	*	30	2	6	44
Chicken McNuggets® (6 pieces)	106	290	18	17	3.5	15	0	0	60	510	*	*	2	6	53
Barbeque sauce	28	45	0	0	0	10	10	0	0	250	*	6	*	*	0
Garden salad (no dressing)	177	35	2	0	0	7	3	3	0	20	120	40	4	6	0
Grilled chicken salad (no dressing)	257	120	21	1.5	0	7	3	3	45	240	120	25	4	8	1
Ranch dressing (1 pkg.)	N/A	230	1	21	3	10	6	0	20	550	*	2	4	*	82
Fat-free herb vinaigrette (1 pkg.)	N/A	50	0	0	0	11	9	0	0	330	*	2	*	2	0
Egg McMuffin®	136	290	17	12	4.5	27	3	1	235	790	10	2	20	15	37
Hash browns	53	130	1	8	1.5	14	0	1	0	330	*	4	*	2	55
Hotcakes w/margarine & syrup	222	570	9	16	3	100	42	2	15	750	8	*	10	15	25
Chocolate shake, small	N/A	360	11	9	6	60	54	1	40	250	6	2	35	4	23
Baked apple pie	77	260	3	13	3.5	34	13	<1	0	200	*	40	2	6	45

*Contains less than 2% of the Daily Value of these nutrients.

Taco Bell

	Serving size	Calories	Protein	Total fat	Saturated fat	Total carbohydrate	Sugars	Fiber	Cholesterol	Sodium	Vitamin A	Vitamin C	Calcium	Iron	% calories from fat
	oz		g	g	g	g	g	g	mg	mg	% Daily Value				
Taco	2.75	180	9	10	4	12	1	3	25	330	10	0	8	6	50
Taco Supreme®	4	220	10	14	6	14	2	3	35	350	15	6	10	6	57
Double Decker Taco Supreme®	7	390	15	19	8	40	3	9	35	760	15	6	15	10	44
BLT soft taco	4.5	340	11	23	8	22	3	2	40	610	4	6	10	4	61
Burrito Supreme®	9	440	17	19	8	51	4	10	35	1230	50	8	15	15	39
Big Beef Burrito Supreme®	10.5	520	17	23	10	54	4	11	55	1520	60	8	15	15	40
Chili cheese burrito	5	330	10	13	6	37	2	5	35	870	60	0	20	8	35
Beef Gorditas Supreme®	5	300	21	13	6	31	3	3	35	390	10	4	8	15	39
Chicken Gorditas Supreme®	5	290	14	12	5	30	4	2	55	420	10	4	8	10	37
Big Beef MexiMelt®	4.75	290	21	15	7	23	0	4	45	850	25	6	20	6	47
Taco salad	19	850	9	52	15	65	1	16	60	1780	160	40	30	35	55
Taco salad w/o shell	16.5	420	5	21	11	32	1	15	60	1520	160	35	25	25	47
Chicken Fajita Wrap™	8	470	9	21	6	51		4	60	1290	35	6	15	8	42
Veggie Fajita Wrap™	8	420		19	5	53		3	20	980	35	6	15	8	41
Steak Fajita Wrap™ Supreme	9	510		25	8	52		3	50	1200	30	10	15	10	44
Big Beef Nachos Supreme	7	450		24	8	45		9	30	810	10	6	15	15	48
Nachos BellGrande®	11	720		39	11	84		17	35	1310	15	6	20	20	46
Pintos 'n cheese	4.5	190		9	4	18		10	15	650	50	0	15	10	43
Mexican rice	4.75	190		9	3.5	23		1	15	760	100	2	15	8	43
Fiesta breakfast burrito	3.5	280		16	6	25		2	25	580	15	0	8	4	51

Wendy's

	Serving size	Calories	Protein	Total fat	Saturated fat	Total carbohydrate	Sugars	Fiber	Cholesterol	Sodium	Vitamin A	Vitamin C	Calcium	Iron	% calories from fat
	g		g	g	g	g	g	g	mg	mg	% Daily Value				
Single w/everything	219	420	25	20	7	37	9	3	70	920	6	10	13	26	43
Big Bacon Classic	282	580	34	30	12	46	11	3	100	1460	15	25	25	30	47
Jr. hamburger	118	270	15	10	3.5	34	7	2	30	610	2	2	11	17	33
Jr. bacon cheeseburger	166	380	20	19	7	34	7	2	60	850	8	10	17	19	45
Grilled chicken sandwich	189	310	27	8	1.5	35	8	2	65	790	4	10	10	15	23
Caesar side salad (no dressing)	92	110	10	5	2.5	7	1	1	15	650	35	25	15	6	41
Grilled chicken salad (no dressing)	338	200	25	8	1.5	9	6	3	50	720	120	60	19	11	36
Taco salad (no dressing)	468	380	26	19	10	28	9	7	65	1040	45	45	37	23	45
Blue cheese dressing (2T)	28	180	1	19	3	0	0	0	15	180	2	0	2	0	95
Ranch dressing, reduced fat (2T)	28	60	1	5	1	2	1	0	10	240	0	0	1	0	75
Soft breadstick	44	130	4	3	0.5	23	N/A	1	5	250	0	0	4	9	21
French fries, medium	130	390	5	19	3	50	0	5	0	120	0	10	2	6	44
Baked potato w/broccoli & cheese	411	470	9	14	2.5	80	6	9	5	470	35	120	21	25	27
Baked potato w/chili & cheese	439	630	20	24	9	83	7	9	40	770	20	60	35	28	34
Chili, small, plain	227	210	15	7	2.5	21	5	5	30	800	8	6	8	16	30
Chili, large w/cheese & crackers	363	405	28	16.5	7	37	8	7	60	1380	14	10	25	26	37
Chicken nuggets (5)	75	230	11	16	3	11	0	0	30	470	0	2	2	2	63
Barbeque sauce	28	45	1	0	0	10	7	0	0	160	0	0	1	3	0
Frosty dairy dessert, medium	298	440	11	11	7	73	56	0	50	260	20	0	41	8	23
Chicken club sandwich	216	470	31	20	4	44	6	2	70	970	4	10	11	17	38

N/A: not available.

Monitoring Your Progress

Name _____ **Section** _____ **Date** _____

As you completed the 11 labs listed below, you entered the results in the Preprogram Assessment column of this lab. Now that you have been involved in a fitness and wellness program for some time, do the labs again and enter your new results in the Postprogram Assessment column. You will probably notice improvement in several areas. Congratulations! If you are not satisfied with your progress thus far, refer to the tips for successful behavior change in Chapter 1 and throughout this book. Remember—fitness and wellness are forever. The time you invest now in developing a comprehensive, individualized program will pay off in a richer, more vital life in the years to come.

	Preprogram Assessment	**Postprogram Assessment**
LAB 2-1 Activity Index	Activity index: ___60___ Classification: _active_	Activity index: _____ Classification: _____
LAB 3-1 Cardiorespiratory Endurance 1-mile walk test 3-minute step test 1.5-mile run-walk test Åstrand-Rhyming test	$\dot{V}O_{2max}$: _____ Rating: _____ $\dot{V}O_{2max}$: _____ Rating: _____ $\dot{V}O_{2max}$: _____ Rating: _____ $\dot{V}O_{2max}$: _____ Rating: _____	$\dot{V}O_{2max}$: _____ Rating: _____ $\dot{V}O_{2max}$: _____ Rating: _____ $\dot{V}O_{2max}$: _____ Rating: _____ $\dot{V}O_{2max}$: _____ Rating: _____
LAB 4-1 Muscular Strength Maximum bench press test Maximum leg press test Hand grip strength test	Weight: _____ lb Rating: _____ Weight: _____ lb Rating: _____ Weight: _____ kg Rating: _____	Weight: _____ lb Rating: _____ Weight: _____ lb Rating: _____ Weight: _____ kg Rating: _____
LAB 4-2 Muscular Endurance 60-second sit-up test Curl-up test Push-up test	Number: _____ Rating: _____ Number: _____ Rating: _____ Number: _____ Rating: _____	Number: _____ Rating: _____ Number: _____ Rating: _____ Number: _____ Rating: _____
LAB 5-1 Flexibility Sit-and-reach test	Score: _____ in. Rating: _____	Score: _____ in. Rating: _____

	Preprogram Assessment	Postprogram Assessment
LAB 6-1 Body Composition		
Body mass index	BMI: _____ kg/m^2 Rating: _____	BMI: _____ kg/m^2 Rating: _____
Skinfold measurements (or other method for determining percent body fat)	Sum of 3 skinfolds: _____ mm Percent body fat: _____% Rating: _____	Sum of 3 skinfolds: _____ mm Percent body fat: _____% Rating: _____
Waist circumference	Circumference: _____ Rating ($\sqrt{}$ high risk): _____	Circumference: _____ Rating ($\sqrt{}$ high risk): _____
Waist-to-hip-circumference ratio	Ratio: _____ Rating ($\sqrt{}$ high risk): _____	Ratio: _____ Rating ($\sqrt{}$ high risk): _____
LAB 8-1 Daily Diet		
Number of servings	Milk, cheese, etc.: ____	Milk, cheese, etc.: ____
Number of servings	Meat, poultry, fish, etc.: ____	Meat, poultry, fish, etc.: ____
Number of servings	Fruits: ____	Fruits: ____
Number of servings	Vegetables: ____	Vegetables: ____
Number of servings	Breads, cereals, rice, etc.: ____	Breads, cereals, rice, etc.: ____
LAB 8-2 Dietary Analysis		
Percentage of calories	From protein: _____%	From protein: _____%
Percentage of calories	From fat: _____%	From fat: _____%
Percentage of calories	From saturated fat: _____%	From saturated fat: _____%
Percentage of calories	From carbohydrate: _____%	From carbohydrate: _____%
LAB 9-1 Daily Energy Balance	Approximate daily energy expenditure: ____ cal/day	Approximate daily energy expenditure: ____ cal/day
LAB 10-1 Identifying Stressors	Average weekly stress score: ___	Average weekly stress score: ___
LAB 11-1 Cardiovascular Health		
CVD risk assessment	Score: ____ Estimated risk: ____	Score: ____ Estimated risk: ____
Hostility assessment	Score: _____ Rating: _____	Score: _____ Rating: _____

D

Behavior Change Workbook

This workbook is designed to take you step by step through the process of behavior change. The first eight activities in the workbook will help you develop a successful plan—beginning with choosing a target behavior and moving through the program planning steps described in Chapter 1, including the completion and signing of a behavior change contract. The final seven activities will help you work through common obstacles to behavior change and maximize your program's chances of success.

Part 1 Developing a Plan for Behavior Change and Completing a Contract

1. Choosing a Target Behavior
2. Gathering Information About Your Target Behavior
3. Monitoring Your Current Patterns of Behavior
4. Setting Goals
5. Examining Your Attitudes About Your Target Behavior
6. Choosing Rewards
7. Breaking Behavior Chains
8. Completing a Contract for Behavior Change

Part 2 Overcoming Obstacles to Behavior Change

9. Building Motivation and Commitment
10. Managing Your Time Successfully
11. Developing Realistic Self-Talk
12. Involving the People Around You
13. Dealing with Feelings
14. Overcoming Peer Pressure: Communicating Assertively
15. Maintaining Your Program over Time

ACTIVITY 1 CHOOSING A TARGET BEHAVIOR

Use your knowledge of yourself and the results of Lab 1-1 (Lifestyle Evaluation) to identify five behaviors that you could change to improve your level of wellness. Examples of target behaviors include smoking cigarettes, not exercising regularly, eating candy bars every night, not getting enough sleep, getting drunk frequently on weekends, and not wearing a safety belt when driving or riding in a car. List your five behaviors below.

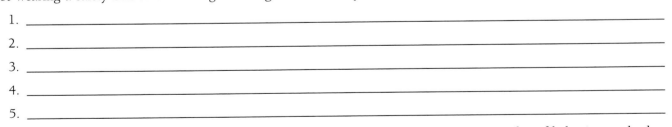

1. _____
2. _____
3. _____
4. _____
5. _____

   For successful behavior change, it's best to focus on one behavior at a time. Review your list of behaviors and select one to start with. Choose a behavior that is important to you and that you are strongly motivated to change. If this will be your first attempt at behavior change, start with a simple change, such as wearing your bicycle helmet regularly, before tackling a more difficult change, such as quitting smoking. Circle the behavior on your list that you've chosen to start with; this will be your target behavior throughout this workbook.

ACTIVITY 2 GATHERING INFORMATION ABOUT YOUR TARGET BEHAVIOR

Take a close look at what your target behavior means to your health, now and in the future. How is it affecting your level of wellness? What diseases or conditions does this behavior place you at risk for? What will changing this behavior mean to you? To evaluate your behavior, use information from this text, from the resources listed in the For More Information section at the end of each chapter, and from other reliable sources.

Health behaviors have short-term and long-term benefits and costs associated with them. For example, in the short term, an inactive lifestyle allows for more time to watch TV and hang out with friends but leaves a person less able to participate in recreational activities. In the long term, it increases risk for cardiovascular disease, cancer, and premature death. Fill in the blanks below with the benefits and costs of continuing your current behavior and of changing to a new, healthier behavior. Pay close attention to the short-term benefits of the new behavior—these are an important motivating force behind successful behavior change programs.

Target (current) behavior _____

Benefits   *Short-Term*   *Long-Term*

           _____   _____

           _____   _____

Costs   *Short-Term*   *Long-Term*

           _____   _____

           _____   _____

New behavior _____

Benefits   *Short-Term*   *Long-Term*

           _____   _____

           _____   _____

Costs   *Short-Term*   *Long-Term*

           _____   _____

           _____   _____

ACTIVITY 3 MONITORING YOUR CURRENT PATTERNS OF BEHAVIOR

To develop a successful behavior change program, you need detailed information about your own behavior patterns. You can obtain this information by developing a system of record keeping, geared toward your target behavior. Depending on your target behavior, you may want to monitor a single behavior, such as your diet, or you may want to keep daily activity records to determine how you could make time for exercise or another new behavior. Consider tracking factors such as the following:

- The behavior
- When and for how long it occurs
- Where it occurs
- What else you were doing at the time
- What other people you were with and how they influenced you
- Your thoughts and feelings
- How strong your urge for the behavior was (for example, how hungry you were or how much you wanted to watch TV)

continued

Figure 1-4 (p. 11) shows a sample log for tracking daily diet. Below, create a format for a sample daily log for monitoring the behavior patterns relating to your target behavior. Then use this sample log to monitor your behavior for a day. Evaluate the log you've created as you use it. Ask yourself if you are tracking all the key factors that influence your behavior; make any necessary adjustments to the format of your log. Once you've developed an appropriate format for your log, use a separate notebook (your health journal) to keep records of your behavior for a week or two. These records will provide solid information about your behavior that will help you develop a successful behavior change program. Later activities in this workbook will ask you to analyze your records.

ACTIVITY 4   SETTING GOALS

For your behavior change program to succeed, you must set meaningful, realistic goals. In addition to an ultimate goal, set some intermediate goals—milestones that you can strive for on the way to your final objective. For example, if your overall goal is to run a 5K road race, an intermediate goal might be to successfully complete 2 weeks of your fitness program. If you set a final goal of eating five servings of fruits and vegetables every day, an intermediate goal would be to increase your daily intake from two to three servings. List your intermediate and final goals below. Don't strive for immediate perfection. Allow an adequate amount of time to reach each of your goals.

Intermediate Goals   **Target Date**

_____   _____

_____   _____

_____   _____

_____   _____

_____   _____

Final Goal

_____   _____

ACTIVITY 5   EXAMINING YOUR ATTITUDES ABOUT YOUR TARGET BEHAVIOR

Your attitudes toward your target behavior can determine whether or not your behavior change program will be successful. Consider your attitudes carefully by completing the following statements about how you think and feel about your current behavior and your goal:

1. I like _____ because _____
               (current behavior)

_____

2. I don't like _____ because _____
                      (current behavior)

_____

3. I like _____ because _____
               (behavior goal)

_____

4. I don't like _____ because _____
                      (behavior goal)

_____

5. I don't _____ now because _____
                  (behavior goal)

_____

6. I would be more likely to _____ if _____
                                         (behavior goal)

_____

continued

If your statements indicate that you have major reservations about changing your behavior, work to build your motivation and commitment before you begin your program. Look carefully at your objections to changing your behavior. How valid and important are they? What can you do to overcome them? Can you adopt any of the strategies you listed under statement 6? Review the facts about your current behavior and your goals.

ACTIVITY 6 CHOOSING REWARDS

Make a list of objects, activities, and events you can use as rewards for achieving the goals of your behavior change program. Rewards should be special, relatively inexpensive, and preferably unrelated to food or alcohol: for example, tickets to a ball game, a CD, or a long-distance phone call to a family member or friend—whatever is meaningful for you. Write down a variety of rewards you can use when you reach milestones in your program and your final goal.

_____   _____

_____   _____

_____   _____

_____   _____

Many people also find it helpful to give themselves small rewards daily or weekly for sticking with their behavior change program. These could be things like a study break, a movie, or a Saturday morning bike ride. Make a list of rewards for maintaining your program in the short term.

_____   _____

_____   _____

_____   _____

And don't forget to congratulate yourself regularly during your behavior change program. Notice how much better you feel, and savor how far you've come and how you've gained control of your behavior.

ACTIVITY 7 BREAKING BEHAVIOR CHAINS

Use the records you collected about your target behavior in Activity 3 and in your health journal to identify what leads up to your target behavior and what follows it. By tracing these chains of events, you'll be able to identify points in the chain where you can make a change that will lead to your new behavior. The sample behavior chain on the next page shows a sequence of events for a person who wants to add exercise to her daily routine—but who winds up snacking and watching TV instead. By examining the chain carefully, one can identify ways to break it at every step. After you review the sample, go through the same process for a typical chain of events involving your target behavior. Use the blank behavior chain on the following page.

Some general strategies for breaking behavior chains include the following:

- _Control or eliminate environmental cues that provoke the behavior._ Stay out of the room where your television is located. Go out for an ice cream cone instead of buying a half gallon for your freezer.
- _Change behaviors or habits that are linked to your target behavior._ If you always smoke in your car when you drive to school, try taking public transportation instead.
- _Add new cues to your environment to trigger your new behavior._ Prepare easy-to-grab healthy snacks and carry them with you to class or work. Keep your exercise clothes and equipment in a visible location.

See also the suggestions in Chapter 1 and in the box "Maximizing Your Chances of Success" on p. 14.

continued

A Sample Behavior Chain and Strategies for Breaking It

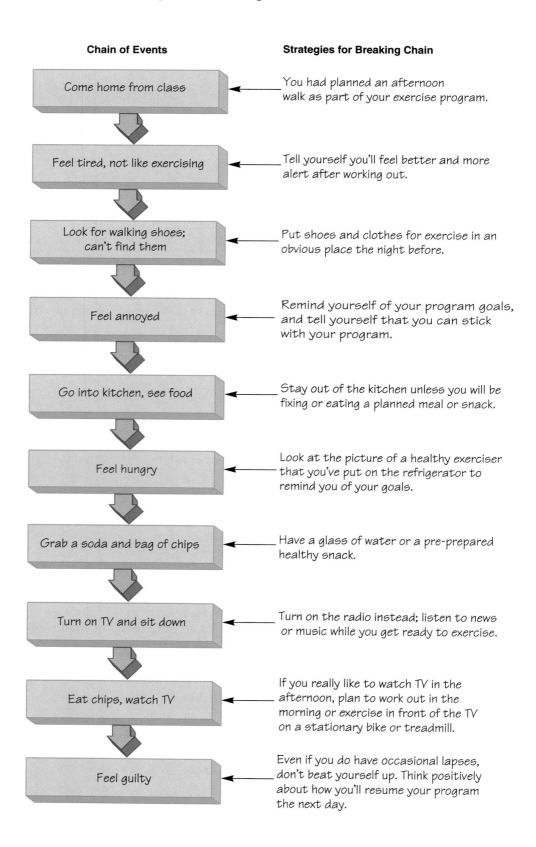

Chain of Events

Strategies for Breaking Chain

Come home from class → You had planned an afternoon walk as part of your exercise program.

Feel tired, not like exercising → Tell yourself you'll feel better and more alert after working out.

Look for walking shoes; can't find them → Put shoes and clothes for exercise in an obvious place the night before.

Feel annoyed → Remind yourself of your program goals, and tell yourself that you can stick with your program.

Go into kitchen, see food → Stay out of the kitchen unless you will be fixing or eating a planned meal or snack.

Feel hungry → Look at the picture of a healthy exerciser that you've put on the refrigerator to remind you of your goals.

Grab a soda and bag of chips → Have a glass of water or a pre-prepared healthy snack.

Turn on TV and sit down → Turn on the radio instead; listen to news or music while you get ready to exercise.

Eat chips, watch TV → If you really like to watch TV in the afternoon, plan to work out in the morning or exercise in front of the TV on a stationary bike or treadmill.

Feel guilty → Even if you do have occasional lapses, don't beat yourself up. Think positively about how you'll resume your program the next day.

continued

A Behavior Chain for Your Target Behavior

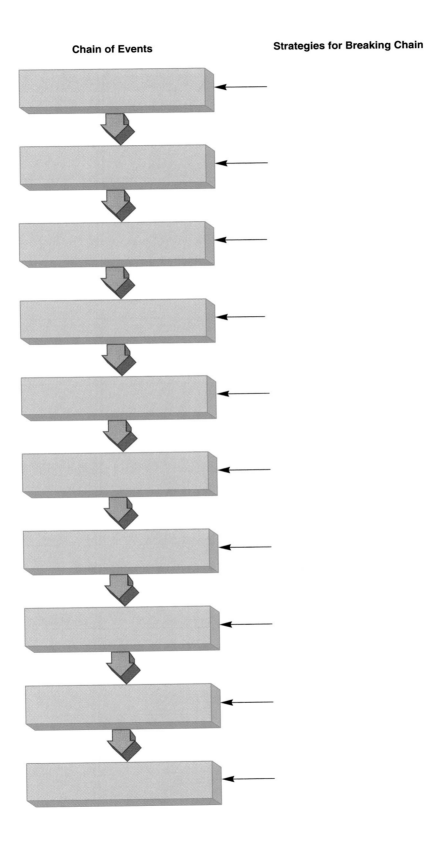

Chain of Events

Strategies for Breaking Chain

ACTIVITY 8   COMPLETING A CONTRACT FOR BEHAVIOR CHANGE

Your next step in creating a successful behavior change program is to complete and sign a behavior change contract. Your contract should include details of your program and indicate your commitment to changing your behavior. Use the information from previous activities in this workbook to complete the following contract. (If your target behavior relates to exercise, you may want to use the program plan and contract for a fitness program in Lab 7-1.)

1. I _____ agree to _____
                   (name)   (specify behavior you want to change)

   _____

2. I will begin on _____ and plan to reach my goal of _____
                           (start date)   (specify final goal)

   _____ by_____
                                                                  (final target date)

3. In order to reach my final goal, I have devised the following schedule of mini-goals. For each step in my program, I will give myself the reward listed.

   _____   _____   _____
   (mini-goal 1)   (target date)   (reward)

   _____   _____   _____
   (mini-goal 2)   (target date)   (reward)

   _____   _____   _____
   (mini-goal 3)   (target date)   (reward)

   _____   _____   _____
   (mini-goal 4)   (target date)   (reward)

   _____   _____   _____
   (mini-goal 5)   (target date)   (reward)

   My overall reward for reaching my final goal will be _____

4. I have gathered and analyzed data on my target behavior and have identified the following strategies for changing my behavior: _____

   _____

   _____

5. I will use the following tools to monitor my progress toward reaching my final goal:

   _____
                                         (list any charts, graphs, or journals you plan to use)

   _____

   I sign this contract as an indication of my personal commitment to reach my goal.

   _____   _____
   (your signature)   (date)

   I have recruited a helper who will witness my contract and _____

   _____
                    (list any way in which your helper will participate in your program)

   _____   _____
   (witness's signature)   (date)

continued

Describe in detail any special strategies you will use to help change your behavior (refer to Activity 7).

Create a plan below for any charts, graphs, or journals you will use to monitor your progress. The log format you developed in Activity 3 may be appropriate, or you may need to develop a more detailed or specific record-keeping system. Examples of journal formats are included in Labs 3-2, 4-3, 5-2, 7-2, 8-1, and 10-1. You might also want to develop a graph to show your progress; posting such a graph in a prominent location can help keep your motivation strong and your program on track. Depending on your target behavior, you could graph the number of push-ups you can do, the number of servings of vegetables you eat each day, or your average daily stress level.

BEHAVIOR CHANGE WORKBOOK

Complete the following checklist to determine whether you are motivated and committed to changing your behavior. Check the statements that are true for you.

_____ I feel responsible for my own behavior and capable of managing it.

_____ I am not easily discouraged.

_____ I enjoy setting goals and then working to achieve them.

_____ I am good at keeping promises to myself.

_____ I like having a structure and schedule for my activities.

_____ I view my new behavior as a necessity, not an optional activity.

_____ Compared with previous attempts to change my behavior, I am more motivated now.

_____ My goals are realistic.

_____ I have a positive mental picture of the new behavior.

_____ Considering the stresses in my life, I feel confident that I can stick to my program.

_____ I feel prepared for lapses and ups-and-downs in my behavior change program.

_____ I feel that my plan for behavior change is enjoyable.

_____ I feel comfortable telling other people about the change I am making in my behavior.

Did you check most of these statements? If not, you need to boost your motivation and commitment. Consider these strategies:

• Review the potential benefits of changing your behavior and the costs of not changing it (see Activity 2). Pay special attention to the short-term benefits of changing your behavior, including feelings of accomplishment and self-confidence. Post a list of these benefits in a prominent location.

• Visualize yourself achieving your goal and enjoying its benefits. For example, if you want to manage time more effectively, picture yourself as a confident, organized person who systematically tackles important tasks and sets aside time each day for relaxation, exercise, and friends. Practice this type of visualization regularly.

• Put aside obstacles and objections to change. Counter thoughts such as "I'll never have time to exercise" with thoughts like "Lots of other people do it and so can I."

• Bombard yourself with propaganda. Take a class dealing with the change you want to make. Read books and watch television shows on the subject. Post motivational phrases or pictures on your refrigerator or over your desk. Talk to people who have already made the change.

• Build up your confidence. Remind yourself of other goals you've achieved. At the end of each day, mentally review your good decisions and actions. See yourself as a capable person, one who is in charge of her or his behavior.

List two strategies for boosting your motivation and commitment; choose from the list above or develop your own. Try each strategy, and then describe how well it worked for you.

Strategy 1: _____

How well it worked: _____

_____

Strategy 2: _____

How well it worked: _____

_____

"Too little time" is a common excuse for not exercising or engaging in other healthy behaviors. Learning to manage your time successfully is crucial if you are to maintain a wellness lifestyle. The first step is to examine how you are currently spending your time; use the following grid broken into blocks to track your activities.

Time	Activity	Time	Activity
6:00 A.M.		6:00 P.M.	
6:30 A.M.		6:30 P.M.	
7:00 A.M.		7:00 P.M.	
8:00 A.M.		8:00 P.M.	
9:00 A.M.		9:00 P.M.	
10:00 A.M.		10:00 P.M.	
11:00 A.M.		11:00 P.M.	
12:00 P.M.		12:00 A.M.	
1:00 P.M.		1:00 A.M.	
2:00 P.M.		2:00 A.M.	
3:00 P.M.		3:00 A.M.	
4:00 P.M.		4:00 A.M.	
5:00 P.M.		5:00 A.M.	

continued

Next, list each type of activity and the total time you engaged in it on a given day in the chart below (for example, sleeping, 7 hours; eating, 1.5 hours; studying, 3 hours; working, 3 hours; and so on). Take a close look at your list of activities. Successful time management is based on prioritization. Assign a priority to each of your activities according to how important it is to you: essential (A), somewhat important (B), or not important (C). Based on these priority rankings, make changes in your schedule by adding and subtracting hours from different categories of activities; enter a duration goal for each activity. Add your new activities to the list, and assign a priority and duration goal to each.

Activity	Current Total Duration	Priority (A, B, or C)	Goal Total Duration

Prioritizing in this manner will involve tradeoffs. For example, you may choose to reduce the amount of time you spend watching television, listening to music, and chatting on the telephone while you increase the amount of time spent sleeping, studying, and exercising. Don't feel that you have to miss out on anything you enjoy. You can get more from less time by focusing on what you are doing. Strategies for managing time more productively and creatively are described in Chapter 10.

ACTIVITY 11   DEVELOPING REALISTIC SELF-TALK

Self-talk is the ongoing internal dialogue we have with ourselves throughout much of the day. Our thoughts can be accurate, positive, and supportive, or they can be exaggerated and negative. Self-talk is closely related to self-esteem and self-concept. Realistic self-talk can help maintain positive self-esteem, the belief that one is a good and competent person, worthy of friendship and love. A negative internal dialogue can reinforce negative self-esteem and can make behavior change very difficult. Substituting realistic self-talk for negative self-talk can help you build and maintain self-esteem and cope better with the challenges in your life.

First, take a closer look at your current pattern of self-talk. Use your health journal to track self-talk, especially as it relates to your target behavior. Does any of your self-talk fall into the common patterns of distorted negative self-talk shown in Chapter 10 (p. 263)? If so, use the examples of realistic self-talk from Chapter 10 to develop more accurate and rational responses. Write your current negative thoughts in the left-hand column, and then record more realistic responses in the right-hand column.

Current Self-Talk About Target Behavior

More Realistic Self-Talk

Your behavior change program will be more successful if the people around you are supportive and involved—or at least are not sabotaging your efforts. Use your health journal to track how other people influence your target behavior and your efforts to change it. For example, do you always skip exercising when you're with certain people? Do you always drink or eat too much when you socialize with certain friends? Are friends and family members offering you enthusiastic support for your efforts to change your behavior, or do they make jokes about your program? Have they even noticed your efforts? Summarize the reactions of those around you in the chart below.

Target behavior: _____

Person	Typical Effect on Target Behavior	Involvement in/Reaction to Program

It may be difficult to change the actions and reactions of the people who are close to you. For them to be involved in your program, you may need to develop new ways of interacting with them (for example, taking a walk rather than going out to dinner as a means of socializing). Most of your friends and family members will want to help you—if they know how. Ask for exactly the type of help or involvement you want. Do you want feedback, praise, or just cooperation? Would you like someone to witness your contract or to be involved more directly in your program? Do you want someone to stop sabotaging your efforts by inviting you to watch TV, eat rich desserts, and so on? Look for ways that the people who are close to you can share in your behavior change program. They can help to motivate you and to maintain your commitment to your program. Develop a way that each individual you listed above can become involved in your program in a positive way.

Person	Target Involvement in Behavior Change Program

Choose one person on your list to tackle first. Talk to that person about her or his current behavior and how you would like her or him to be involved in your behavior change program. Below, describe this person's reaction to your talk and her or his subsequent behavior. Did this individual become a positive participant in your behavior change program?

_____

_____

_____

_____

BEHAVIOR CHANGE WORKBOOK

Longstanding habits are difficult to change in part because many represent ways people have developed to cope with certain feelings. For example, people may overeat when bored, skip their exercise sessions when frustrated, or drink alcoholic beverages when anxious. Developing new ways to deal with feelings can help improve the chance that a behavior change program will succeed.

Review the records on your target behavior that you kept in your health journal. Identify the feelings that are interfering with the success of your program, and develop new strategies for coping with them. Some common problematic feelings are listed below, along with one possible coping strategy for each. Put a check mark next to those that are influencing your target behavior, and fill in additional strategies. Add the other feelings that are significant roadblocks in your program to the bottom of the chart, along with coping strategies for each.

✔	Feeling	Coping Strategies
	Stressed out	Go for a 10-minute walk.
	Anxious	Do one of the relaxation exercises described in Chapter 10.
	Bored	Call a friend for a chat.
	Tired	Take a 20-minute nap.
	Frustrated	Identify the source of the feeling, and deal with it constructively.

- Julia is trying to give up smoking; her friend Marie continues to offer her cigarettes whenever they are together.
- Emilio is planning to exercise in the morning; his roommates tell him he's being antisocial by not having brunch with them.
- Tracy's boyfriend told her that in high school he once experimented with drugs and shared needles; she wants him to have an HIV test, but he says he's sure the people he shared needles with were not infected.

Peer pressure is the common ingredient in these situations. To successfully maintain your behavior change program, you must develop effective strategies for resisting peer pressure. Assertive communication is one such strategy. By communicating assertively—firmly, but not aggressively—you can stick with your program even in the face of pressure from others. Review your health journal to determine how other people affect your target behavior. If you find that you often do give in to peer pressure, try the following strategies for communicating more assertively.

- Collect your thoughts, and plan in advance what you will say. You might try out your response on a friend to get some feedback.
- State your case—how you feel and what you want—as clearly as you can.
- Use "I" messages—statements about how you feel—rather than statements beginning with "You."
- Focus on the behavior rather than the person. Suggest a solution, such as asking the other person to change his or her behavior toward you. Avoid generalizations. Be specific about what you want.
- Make clear, constructive requests. Focus on your needs ("I would like . . .") rather than the mistakes of others ("You always . . .").
- Avoid blaming, accusing, and belittling. Treat others with the same respect you'd like to receive yourself.
- Ask for action ahead of time. Tell others what you would like to happen; don't wait for them to do the wrong thing and then get angry at them.
- Ask for a response to what you have proposed. Wait for an answer, and listen carefully to it. Try to understand other people's points of view, just as you would hope that others would understand yours.

With these strategies in mind, review your health journal and identify three instances in which peer pressure interfered with your behavior change program. For each of these instances, write out what you might have said to deal with the situation more assertively. (If you can't find three situations from your own experiences, choose one or more of the three scenarios described at the beginning of this activity.)

1. _____
_____
_____
_____

2. _____
_____
_____
_____

3. _____
_____
_____

Assertive communication can help you achieve your behavior change goals in a direct way by helping you keep your program on track. It can also provide a boost for your self-image and increase your confidence in your ability to successfully manage your own behavior.

BEHAVIOR CHANGE WORKBOOK

If you maintain your new behavior for at least 6 months, your chances of lifetime success are greatly increased. However, you may find yourself sliding back into old habits at some point. If this happens, there are some things you can do to help maintain your new behavior.

• Remind yourself of the goals of your program (list them here).

_____

_____

_____

_____

_____

• Pay attention to how your new pattern of behavior has improved your wellness status. List the major benefits of changing your behavior, both now and in the future.

_____

_____

_____

_____

_____

• Consider the things you enjoy most about your new pattern of behavior. List your favorite aspects.

_____

_____

_____

_____

_____

• Think of yourself as a problem solver. If something begins to interfere with your program, devise strategies for dealing with it. Take time out now to list things that have the potential to derail your program, and develop possible coping mechanisms.

Problem	Solution
_____	_____
	_____
_____	_____
	_____
_____	_____
	_____
_____	_____

• Remember the basics of behavior change. If your program runs into trouble, go back to keeping records of your behavior to pinpoint problem areas. Make adjustments in your program to deal with new disruptions. And don't feel defeated if you lapse. The best thing you can do is to renew your commitment and continue with your program.

Index

Boldface numbers indicate pages on which glossary definitions appear. "*t*" indicates that the information is in a table.

for flexibility, 29t, 114, 163
   in weight training, 29t, 76–77, 163
dynamic flexibility, 110

eating disorders, 230, 237, **238–240**
   assessment of, 251–252
   helping someone with, 240
   treatment of, 239
   types of, 238–239
   See also body image
eating habits
   for college students, 210
   weight management and, 232, 233, 241
   See also diet; nutrition
eccentric loading, **74**
eccentric muscle contractions, **72,** 73, 74
educational attainment, 7, 20t, 277
elastin, **110,** 111
emergency care, A-8–A-9
emotional wellness, 2, 3
   cardiorespiratory endurance exercise and, 47
   See also mind-body connection; stress
emotions
   behavior change and, 12–13, W-14
   stress and, 256
   weight management and, 234–235
endocrine system, **254–255**
endorphins, **46,** 47, **254,** 255
endurance. *See* cardiorespiratory endurance; muscular endurance
energy balance, 229–230
   assessment of, 245–248
   exercise and, 145
   to gain weight, 230, 242
   to lose weight, 230, 240
energy expenditures. *See* calorie costs
energy systems, 42, 43–44, 43t
environment
   for changing behavior, 10–11, W-5–W-7
   stressors in, 260
   wellness and, 7
environmental tobacco smoke (ETS), **274,** 289
environmental wellness, 2–3
ephedrine, 96t, 236
epinephrine, **46,** 47, **254,** 255
equipment. *See* exercise equipment
essential fat, 138, **139**
essential nutrients. *See* nutrients, essential
Estimated Minimum Requirements, 198, 199t
Estimated Safe and Adequate Daily Dietary Intakes (ESADDIs), 198,199t
estrogen, 196, 278, 285
ethnic groups
   cardiovascular disease (CVD) among, 278, 279
   diabetes among, 7, 140
   diet of, 211
   eating disorders among, 238
   exercise among, 20t
   overweight/obesity among, 228t
   wellness and, 7
   See also specific groups
eustress, **256,** 257
exercise
   advice on, 32
   benefits of, 21
   body composition and, 145, 146
   body image and, 141
   cancer and, 46
   cardiovascular disease (CVD) and, 46, 276, 284, 289
   clothing for, 57, 164–165, 169
   cool down after, 30, 53, 77, 166
   defined, 20–**21**

designing program for, 27–31
   diabetes and, 46, 140, 167–168
   duration of, 26, 28, 29t, 30, 35, 53, 162–163, 164–165
   energy systems and, 43–44
   fluids and, 57, 58, 209
   frequency of, 25, 28, 29t, 30, 35, 51, 77, 114, 162–163, 165, 168
   frequently asked questions about, 32, 57–58, 95, 126, 146, 168–169
   intensity of, 26, 28, 29t, 30, 35, 51–53, 76, 114, 162–163, 164–165
   isokinetic, **74**
   isometric, **72,** 73, 75, 88
   isotonic, **72,** 73–74, 75
   metabolism and, 45, 70, 145, 230
   osteoporosis and, 46, 168, 196
   for physical fitness, 22, 27
   recommended amount of, 27, 29t
   safety of, 32, 37, 57–58, 78–80, 168–169
   scheduling, 32
   with special health concerns, 32, 57–58, 167–168
   stress management and, 260–261, 262, 271
   warm up before, 30, 53, 77, 166
   weather and, 58, 166
   weight management and, 45, 70, 95, 138–139, 233–234
   See also cardiorespiratory endurance exercise; personal fitness programs; physical training; stretching; weight training
exercise equipment
   bicycling, 169, 173
   consumer guidelines on, 57, 59
   in-line skating, 169, 177
   safety and, 169, A-5
   swimming, 175
   weight training, 74, 75, 81–83, 82t, 84–94, 99–101
exercise injuries. *See* injuries
exercise machines
   Nautilus weight machines, 74, 81, 82t, 83, 89–94
   safety with, 79–80
   Universal weight machines, 82t, 83, 99–101
   in weight training, 74, 75, 79–80, 81–83, 82t, 99–101
exercise stress test, **32,** 281

fast food, 212, 225–226
   guidelines for choosing, 210
   nutritional content of, C-1–C-10
fast-twitch fibers, **72**
fat-free foods. *See* reduced-fat foods
fat-free mass, 24, **25**
   See also body composition
fats, 42, 186–189
   in butter vs. margarine, 212
   calories from, 184, 188, 189, 231–232
   cancer and, 189
   cardiovascular disease and, 188–189, 276, 283–284
   as essential nutrient, 185t, 186–190
   goals for intake of, 189
   in meat, 213, 214
   reducing intake of, 203–204, 205, 206, 231, 242, 283–284
   types of, 186–188
   See also body fat; cholesterol
fats, oils, and sweets food group, 203–204
fatty acids
   monounsaturated, 186, **187,** 283, 302
   omega-3, **188**–189, 285
   polyunsaturated, 186, **187,** 188–189, 283

saturated, 186, **187,** 188, 212, 276, 283
   trans, **187,** 188, 212, 276, 284
feelings. *See* emotions
females. *See* women
fenfluramine, 236–237
fen-phen, herbal, 236
fiber, dietary, **190,** 191–192, 192t
   cancer and, 191
   cardiovascular disease and, 190, 191, 284
   diabetes and, 140, 191
   in diet aids, 236
   in foods, 192t, B-1–B-10, C-1–C-4
   increased intake of, 191–192, 284
   insoluble vs. soluble, **190,** 191
fibers, muscle, 72
fight-or-flight reaction, **254,** 255, 256
fitness. *See* cardiorespiratory fitness; physical fitness
fitness centers, 32, 33
fitness programs. *See* personal fitness programs
flexibility, 24, **25,** 110–136
   activities for developing, 28, 29, 160–161t
   aging and, 24, 110
   assessment of, 112, 129–134
   benefits of, 110–111
   creating program for, 112–119, 135–136, 163
   duration of exercise for, 29t, 114, 163
   dynamic, 110
   exercises for, 115–127
   frequency of exercise for, 25, 28, 29t, 114
   frequently asked questions about, 126
   injuries and, 110–111
   intensity of exercise for, 114, 163
   jogging and, 126
   joint structure and, 111
   low-back pain and, 110–111, 119–126
   physiological determinants of, 111–112
   safe stretching for, 114, 126, 127
   sample programs for, 115–127, 173, 174, 177, 178
   static, 110
   stretching techniques for, 112–113
   types of, 110
   weight training and, 126
   See also stretching
fluids, exercise and, 57, 58, 209
folate, 192, 193t, 194, 198, 201t
food
   fast, 210, 212, 225–226, C-1–C-4
   nutritional content of, B-1–B10, C-1–C-4
   reduced-fat, 204, 242
   reducing calorie intake from, 231
   serving sizes of, 203, 212, 213, 231
   See also diet; nutrition
Food Guide Pyramid, **197,** 201–205, 208
   vs. actual diet, 204t, 217–220
   food groups in, 202–204
   food labels and, 206
   servings in, 202, 212–213
food journals, 11, 217–224, 241
food labels, 206, 207, 225
food poisoning, 213
footwear, 164–165
fractures, 55t
free radicals, **44,** 45, **197**
free weights, in weight training, 74, 75, 79, 81, 82, 83, 84–88
frequency of exercise, 25, 28, 29t, 30, 35, 51, 77, 114, 162–163, 165, 168
   for cardiorespiratory endurance, 25, 28, 51, 163, 168, 170
   for flexibility, 25, 28, 29t, 114
   in stretching, 114, 163
   in weight training, 28, 77, 95, 163, 168

frequently asked questions
about body composition, 145–146
about cardiorespiratory endurance exercise, 57–58
about cardiovascular disease (CVD), 285–286
about nutrition, 212–213
about personal fitness programs, 168–169
about physical fitness, 32
about stress, 267
about stretching and flexibility, 126
about weight management, 242
about weight training, 95
fruits
fiber in, 192t
food group, 202–203, 204t
nutritional content of, B-1–B-2

GAS (general adaptation syndrome), **256**, 257
gender differences
in body composition, 138, 153
in cardiorespiratory endurance, 51
in cardiovascular disease (CVD), 277, 278, 285
in muscular strength, 71
in rates of exercise, 20t
weight training and, 70, 71, 95
wellness and, 7
See also men; women
general adaptation syndrome (GAS), **256**, 257
genetics
body composition and, 144, 145–146
cardiovascular disease (CVD) and, 277, 279, 289
obesity/overweight and, 228–229, 232
physical training and, 26–27
wellness and, 7
glucose, **42**, 43t, **190**
glycogen, **42**, 43t, **190**
goals
for behavior change, 10, 11–12, W-4
for cardiorespiratory endurance programs, 50
for fat, protein, and carbohydrate intake, 189
of Healthy People initiative, 8t
for personal fitness programs, 27, 158, 163
time management and, 261–262
for weight loss, 238, 249–250
in weight management, 144–145, 240
grains
fiber in, 192t
nutritional content of, B-4–B-5
whole, 191, 192
See also bread, cereals, rice, and pasta food group; carbohydrates

hatha yoga, 265
HDLs (high-density lipoproteins), 46, **188**, 189, **274**, 275, 276, 285, 289
health
body composition and, 139–141
obesity and, 139, 141
See also wellness
health care, 7
health clubs, 32, 33
health information, evaluating, 286, 287
health journals, 10, 12, W-2–W-3
food journals, 11, 217–224, 241
Healthy People initiative, 8, 8t
heart
blood supply to, 282
cardiorespiratory endurance exercise and, 44–45
circulation in, 40–41
See also cardiorespiratory system
heart attacks, 274, 278, **280**, 281–282, 283, 285
heart disease. See coronary heart disease (CHD)

heart rate
monitoring, 49, 50
physical fitness and, 45
target heart rate zone, **51**–52
heat disorders, 58
herbal fen-phen, 236
heredity. See genetics
high blood pressure. See hypertension (high blood pressure)
high-density lipoproteins (HDLs), 46, **188**, 189, **274**, 275, 276, 285, 289
Hispanic Americans
cardiovascular disease (CVD) among, 278
diabetes among, 7, 140
diet of, 211
exercise among, 20t
obesity among, 228t
HIV infection, 4t
homeostasis, **254**, 255–256
homocysteine, 278–279, 286
hormone replacement therapy (HRT), 196
hormones
androgens, 71
estrogen, 196, 278, 285
stress and, **254**, 255
testosterone, **70**
hostility, 277, 285, 290
hot weather, and exercise, 58, 166
hydrogenation, 186–**187**
See also trans fatty acids
hydrostatic (underwater) weighing, 143–144, 145, 153
hypertension (high blood pressure), 46, **274**, 279–280
body composition and, 139, 143
diet and, 210, 284
among ethnic groups, 7, 278, 279
exercise and, 168
weight training and, 81
hypertrophy, **72**

illness, exercise and, 32
imagery, 264
immediate energy system, **42**, 43, 43t, 44
immune system
cardiorespiratory endurance exercise and, 47
stress and, 258, 261
inactivity. See physical inactivity
income. See socioeconomic status
Indian food, guidelines for choosing, 211
Indians. See Native Americans
infectious diseases, **2**, 3
See also sexually transmitted diseases (STDs)
injuries, 4t, 53–56, 70, A-1–A-10
alcohol and, 4t, A-1, A-2, A-5, A-8
exercise and, 53–56, 70, 81, A-5
flexibility and, 110–111
intentional, A-6–A-10
medical attention for, 54
motor vehicle–related, 4t, A-1, A-2
preventing, 54, 56, 70, A-1–A-10
rehabilitation after, 55
R-I-C-E treatment for, 55, 81
sports and, A-5
treatment for minor, 54, 55, 55t
unintentional, 4t, **5**, 7, A-1–A-6
violence and, A-6–A-10
in weight training, 81
See also low-back pain
in-line skating
calorie costs for, 178
equipment for, 177
injury prevention for, 177, A-5
sample program for, 177–178

insoluble fiber, **190**, 191, 294
insomnia, 259
intellectual wellness, 2, 3
intensity of exercise, 26, 28, 29t, 30, 35, 51–53, 76, 114, 162–163, 164–165
for cardiorespiratory endurance, 51–52, 54, 162–163, 170
for flexibility, 114, 163
in weight training, 76, 163
interpersonal wellness, 2, 3
interval training, **167**, 170
intervertebral disks, **119**–121
Ionamin, 236
iron, 194, 195t, 199t, 205, 208
isokinetic exercise, **74**
isometric exercise, **72**, 73, 75, 88
isotonic exercise, **72**, 73–74, 75
Italian food, guidelines for choosing, 211

Japanese food, guidelines for choosing, 211
jobs, stress related to, 259–260
jogging
calorie costs for, 171t
flexibility and, 126
progression in, 25, 172t
safety when, 168–169
sample program for, 168–173
shoes for, 164–165
See also running
joint capsules, **110**, 111
joints, 110, 111
journals. See health journals

kilocalories (kcalories), **184**

lactic acid, **42**, 43
lacto-ovo-vegetarians, **208**
lacto-vegetarians, **208**
Latinos. See Hispanic Americans
LDLs (low-density lipoproteins), 46, **188**, 275, **276**, 279, 285
legumes, **190**, 191, 192t, 202, B-9–B-10
life events
changing behavior and, 9
stressful, 258–259, 269
life expectancy, 3, 5
lifestyle
assessment of, 17–18
for cardiovascular disease (CVD) prevention, 283–285
daily physical activity in, 21–22, 163
inactive, 4, 6, 20, 276, 284
stress management and, 258–260, 271
weight management and, 230–235
for wellness, 4–7
lifestyle management, 8–15, W-1–W-16
behavior change plan for, 10–13
locus of control and, 9–10
motivation for, 9, 13
persistence with, 13–14
physical training and, 30–31
stress and, 13–14
support for, 13, 14
target behavior in, 10
workbook for, W-1–W-16
ligaments, **70**
lipids. See cholesterol; fats
lipoproteins, **46**, **274**, 275–276
high-density (HDLs), 46, **188**, 189, **274**, 275, 276, 285, 289
lipoprotein(a) [Lp(a)], 279
low-density (LDLs), 46, **188**, 275, **276**, 279, 285
liposuction, 146
liver, cirrhosis of, 4t